CANCER THERAPY

PRESCRIBING AND ADMINISTRATION BASICS

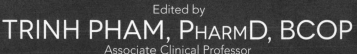

Edited by

TRINH PHAM, PharmD, BCOP
Associate Clinical Professor
University of Connecticut School of Pharmacy
Storrs, Connecticut

LISA HOLLE, PharmD, BCOP
Assistant Clinical Professor
University of Connecticut School of Pharmacy
Storrs, Connecticut

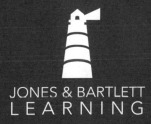

JONES & BARTLETT
LEARNING

World Headquarters
Jones & Bartlett Learning
5 Wall Street
Burlington, MA 01803
978-443-5000
info@jblearning.com
www.jblearning.com

Jones & Bartlett Learning books and products are available through most bookstores and online booksellers. To contact Jones & Bartlett Learning directly, call 800-832-0034, fax 978-443-8000, or visit our website, www.jblearning.com.

Substantial discounts on bulk quantities of Jones & Bartlett Learning publications are available to corporations, professional associations, and other qualified organizations. For details and specific discount information, contact the special sales department at Jones & Bartlett Learning via the above contact information or send an email to specialsales@jblearning.com.

Production Credits
Executive Publisher: William Brottmiller
Executive Editor: Rhonda Dearborn
Associate Editor: Teresa Reilly
Editorial Assistant: Sean Fabery
Production Editor: Cindie Bryan
Marketing Manager: Grace Richards
VP, Manufacturing and Inventory Control:
  Therese Connell
Composition: Laserwords Private Limited, Chennai,
  India

Cover Design: Kristin E. Parker
Photo Research and Permissions Coordinator:
  Amy Rathburn
Cover and Title Page Images: Background: © _Lonely_/
  ShutterStock, Inc., Left: © Li Wa/ShutterStock, Inc.,
  Middle: © Wavebreakmedia ltd/ShutterStock, Inc.,
  Right: © jordache/ShutterStock, Inc.
Printing and Binding: Edwards Brothers Malloy
Cover Printing: Edwards Brothers Malloy

Library of Congress Cataloging-in-Publication Data
Pham, Trinh, author.
  Cancer therapy : prescribing and administration basics / Trinh Pham, Lisa Holle.
    p. ; cm.
  Includes bibliographical references and index.
  ISBN 978-1-4496-3397-4 (pbk.) – ISBN 1-4496-3397-8 (pbk.)
  I. Holle, Lisa, author. II. Title.
  [DNLM: 1. Neoplasms–drug therapy. 2. Antineoplastic Agents–administration & dosage. 3. Antineoplastic Agents–therapeutic use. QZ 267]
  RC271.C5
  616.99'4061–dc23
                                                                          2013028713
6048

Printed in the United States of America
17 16 15 14 13   10 9 8 7 6 5 4 3 2 1

Dedication

This book is dedicated to all of our patients who have undergone the journey of cancer and from whom we've learned so much about cancer therapy and so much more.

Contents

Preface   xiii

About the Editors   xv

Contributors   xvii

Reviewers   xxi

CHAPTER 1   **Overview of Cancer Therapy**   1
Lisa Holle, Jane Pruemer, Hyejin Kim
   Introduction   1
      What Is Cancer?   1
      Modalities of Cancer Treatment   4
      Cancer Therapy Medications   5
   Classes of Chemotherapy Agents   5
      Microtubule-Targeting Drugs   5
         Vinca Alkaloids   6
         Taxanes   6
         Epothilones   7
         Eribulin   14
         Estramustine   15
      Alkylating Agents   15
         Nitrogen Mustard and Its Derivatives   15
         Nitrosoureas   16
         Nonclassical Alkylating Agents   16
      Heavy Metal Compounds   17
      Antimetabolites   17
         Pyrimidines   18
         Cytidine Analogs   18
         Purine Antimetabolites   19
         Antifolates   19

Topoisomerase Inhibitors 20
    Camptothecin Derivatives 20
    Podophyllotoxin Derivatives 21
    Anthracene Derivatives 21
Miscellaneous Agents 22
Targeted Therapy 24
  Monoclonal Antibodies 24
  Angiogenesis Inhibitors 26
  Immunomodulators 26
  Tyrosine Kinase Inhibitors 26
  Miscellaneous Targeted Agents 29
  Interferon and Interleukin-2 30
Hormonal Agents 30
  Antiestrogens 30
  Aromatase Inhibitors 30
  *Luteinizing Hormone Releasing Hormone Analogs
    and Antagonists* 31
  Antiandrogens 31
Response to Treatment 32
  Performance Status 32
Summary 35
References 35
Suggested Reading 38

CHAPTER 2   **Basics of Systemic Anticancer Therapy Prescribing
and Verification 39**
Trinh Pham, Joan Rivington
Introduction 40
Oncology Training 40
Education 43
Cancer Therapy Prescribing 44
  *Computerized Provider-Order-Entry for Anticancer
    Agents* 45
  *Strategies to Prevent Errors in Cancer Therapy
    Prescribing* 46
  *The Prescribing Vocabulary–Anticancer Therapy
    Regimen Cycle* 51
  Dose Calculation 52
  References 54
  *Investigational Anticancer Regimens or
    Medications* 54
Cancer Therapy Verification 55

Oral Anticancer Therapy   58
Intrathecal Anticancer Therapy   60
  *Anticancer Agents for Intrathecal Administration
    and Dosing Considerations*   60
  Avoid Intrathecal Vincristine Injection   61
Supportive Care and Ancillary Medications   62
  Infusion-Related Reactions   63
  Tumor Lysis Syndrome   64
  Chemotherapy-Induced Nausea and Vomiting   64
  *Febrile Neutropenia and Colony-Stimulating Growth
    Factors*   68
Nononcology Indications for Anticancer Therapy   68
Resources   69
Summary   69
References   70
Suggested Reading   71

CHAPTER 3   **Dosing Calculations   73**
Trinh Pham, Man Yee Merl, Jia Li
Introduction   73
Methods for Dose Calculation   74
BSA-Based Dosing   75
  *Dose Calculation in Obese and Underweight
    Patients*   78
  Dose Calculation in Adult Amputees   81
Pharmacokinetic-Based Dosing—Area Under the
    Curve   82
  Carboplatin Dosing   82
Flat Fixed-Dose Dosing System   85
Genotype-Guided Dosing   85
Dose Rounding   88
Organ Function Assessment and Anticancer Therapy
    Dosing   88
  *Renal Function Assessment and Anticancer Therapy
    Dosing*   89
  *Dose and Administration Modification in Hemodialysis
    Setting*   102
  *Hepatic Function Assessment and Anticancer Therapy
    Dosing*   105
Summary   106
References   107
Suggested Websites and Readings   110

CHAPTER 4   **Cancer Therapy Preparation   111**
Michele Rice, Jeanne Adams, James G. Stevenson
Introduction   112
Cancer Therapy Preparation Area: The Cleanroom   113
Environmental Controls   113
Cancer Therapy Production: Cleanroom
Processes   120
Personal Protective Equipment   120
Cleaning Regimens   123
Chemotherapy Spills   124
Storage and Dispensing   124
Refrigeration   128
Safe Disposal of Hazardous Drug Waste   131
Cancer Therapy Preparation Personnel: The
Multidisciplinary Team   133
The Pharmacist   134
The Nurse   135
The Pharmacy Technician   136
Ideal Staffing   137
Summary   137
References   137

CHAPTER 5   **Oral Cancer Therapy   139**
Beth Chen, Lisa Holle
Introduction   139
Dosing and Administration   141
Side Effects   145
Skin Toxicity   147
Cardiovascular Toxicity   148
Gastrointestinal Toxicity   149
Fatigue   150
Toxicities of Hormonal Agents   151
Drug and Food Interactions   152
Counseling and Monitoring   156
Adherence   158
Safe Prescribing and Dispensing Practices   160
*Risk Evaluation Mitigation Strategy (REMS)
Requirements*   162
Safe Handling   164
Financial Considerations   165
Summary   168
References   169

CHAPTER 6   **Drug Safety and Risk Management   171**
Karen R. Smethers
Introduction   172
Types of Chemotherapy Errors in the Medication Use
    Process   174
    Procurement   174
    Prescribing   177
    Transcribing/Documenting   178
    Compounding/Dispensing   179
    Administering   183
    Monitoring   186
Preventing Chemotherapy Medication Errors   186
    Ready Access to Pertinent Patient Information   186
    Ready Access to Medication Information   187
    Standardized Chemotherapy Order Forms and Checking
        Process   188
    Preventing Look-Alike and Sound-Alike Medication
        Errors   189
    Preventing Wrong-Route Errors Associated With
        Intrathecal Therapy   192
    Employ Technology   193
    Provide a Safe Work Environment   193
Medication Error Reporting   194
Sentinel Event Reporting   194
Adverse Event Reporting   195
Risk Evaluation and Mitigation Strategies   196
Summary   198
References   199

CHAPTER 7   **Inventory and Reimbursement   203**
Timothy Tyler, Lisa Holle
Introduction   203
Inventory   204
    Accounting   204
    Purchasing   206
    340B Pricing   212
Reimbursement   212
    Payers   212
        Medicare   213
        Medicaid   216
        Private Insurance   216

Coverage   217
   Patient Assistance Programs   218
Summary   220
References   221

CHAPTER 8   **High-Dose Cancer Therapy   223**
Laura E. Wiggins, Ashley Richards
Overview of Hematopoietic Stem Cell
   Transplantation   223
   Types of HSCT   226
   Collection of Hematopoietic Stem Cells   229
   Infusion of HSCs   231
Supportive Care and Transplant-Related
   Complications   233
   Chemotherapy-Induced Nausea and Vomiting   233
   Cytopenias   235
   Graft-Versus-Host Disease   236
      Prevention of Acute GVHD   238
      Pharmacologic Prophylaxis of Acute GVHD   238
      GVHD Treatment   239
   Steroid Refractory GVHD   245
      Supportive Care for Acute GVHD   246
      Chronic GVHD   246
      Treatment of Chronic GVHD   247
Sinusoidal Obstruction Syndrome   252
   Treatment of SOS   253
   Infection in HSCT Patients   254
Summary   262
References   262

CHAPTER 9   **Pediatric Oncology   267**
Brooke Bernhardt, Susannah E. Koontz
Introduction   267
Role of Cooperative Research Groups   268
Initial Presentation and Oncologic Emergencies   269
   Initial Presentation   269
   Oncologic Emergencies   270
      Hyperleukocytosis   270
      Tumor Lysis Syndrome   270
      Superior Vena Cava Syndrome   271

Acute Leukemias   271
   Acute Lymphoblastic Leukemia   271
      Down Syndrome and ALL   274
   Acute Myeloid Leukemia   274
      Down Syndrome and AML   275
   Acute Promyelocytic Leukemia   276
Lymphomas   276
   Hodgkin's Lymphoma   276
   Non-Hodgkin's Lymphoma   277
Central Nervous System Tumors   278
Common Solid Tumors of Childhood   280
   Neuroblastoma   280
   Wilms' Tumor   281
   Rhabdomyosarcoma   281
   Osteosarcoma   282
   Ewing's Sarcoma   282
   Retinoblastoma   283
Supportive Care   284
Chemotherapy-Induced Nausea and Vomiting   284
Bone Marrow Support   285
Survivorship and Long-Term Toxicities   285
Special Dosing Considerations   286
Fluid Management   289
Chemotherapy Dosing in Infants   290
Obese Children   293
Outpatient Pediatric Oncology   294
   Medication Errors in the Outpatient Setting   294
   Oral Chemotherapy Formulations   294
   Outpatient Pediatric Oncology   297
Summary   298
References   299

CHAPTER 10   **Investigational Drugs**   **303**
Theresa A. Mays, Leslie Smetzer
Introduction   303
Documentation   304
Standard Operating Procedures   305
Issues Affecting the Patient's Enrollment in the Clinical
   Trial   310

Common Terminology Criteria for Adverse Events   313
Clinical Trial Medication Issues   316
    Drug Accountability Records   316
    Drug Preparation and Administration Issues   319
    Dispensing Oral Agents   320
    Bioequivalence and Bioavailability Studies   320
    Hazardous Versus Biohazardous Drugs   321
Code of Federal Regulations Title 21(1) and the
    International Conference on Harmonization Guideline
    for Good Clinical Practice   322
Summary   323
References   323

CHAPTER 11   Pharmacogenetics and Pharmacogenomics in Cancer
               Therapy   325
               Trinh Pham, Man Yee Merl, Jia Li
Introduction   325
Terminology   326
Biomarkers That Predict Treatment Toxicity   327
    Thiopurine S-Methyltransferase   327
    Dihydropyrimidine Dehydrogenase   329
    Uridine Diphosphoglucuronosyltransferase 1A1   329
Biomarkers That Predict Treatment Response and/or
    Prognosis   330
    Estrogen Receptor/Progesterone Receptor   330
    Human Epidermal Growth Factor Receptor 2   333
    Epidermal Growth Factor Receptor   334
    K-RAS   335
    EML4-ALK Fusion Gene   337
    BRAF   338
    BCR/ABL Chromosomal Translocation (Philadelphia
        Chromosome)   339
    Promyelocytic Leukemia/Retinoic Acid Receptor-
        Alpha   339
    Deletion of Chromosome 5q   340
    O^6-Methyl Guanine Methyl Transferase   340
Summary   341
References   341
Suggested Reading   345

Index   347

Preface

As practicing oncology pharmacists, we are often asked about the practical, day-to-day aspects of cancer therapy prescribing, verification, admixing, administration, and cost/reimbursement. As teachers, we find that there is not one comprehensive reference source that addresses all of these issues in the available pharmacy, nursing, or medicine textbooks. For these reasons, we decided to publish *Cancer Therapy: Prescribing and Administration Basics* to fulfill this unmet need for practicing or in-training nurses, nurse practitioners, physician assistants, pharmacists, and hematology/oncology physician fellows who work with cancer patients. Healthcare professionals whose primary area of practice is not hematology/oncology but who may be responsible for verifying, preparing, dispensing, or administering cancer therapy agents will also find this textbook useful. The goal of this book is to optimize safe and effective care of cancer patients in a variety of healthcare settings, including hospitals, ambulatory care clinics, and private oncology practices.

The purpose is to provide a multidisciplinary, comprehensive, hands-on, practical guide of cancer therapy basics for oncology clinicians. Each chapter focuses on the various clinical and practice-related aspects of the delivery of cancer therapies, from prescribing through reimbursement, and chapters on special populations such as pediatrics and stem cell transplantation are included. The information is presented in a simple and direct way and includes the following:

- Checklists to ensure safe and consistent reviews of cancer therapy orders
- Common equations used in oncology
- Tables with key information for an easy-to-read and refer-to format
- Clinical pearls that are often learned on the job rather than in textbooks

- Comprehensive patient case examples with answers to emphasize key concepts and provide the reader an opportunity to apply the knowledge
- Listings of additional practical resources and recommended readings to enhance depth of knowledge for those who desire it

We thank each contributing author for offering his or her expertise and insightful clinical pearls to make this textbook complete. Your contributions are truly appreciated. We are also grateful to the peer reviewers for offering their time and outstanding critiques of each of the chapters. Finally, we thank our colleagues and mentors for their support and inspiration, our students and trainees for continually challenging us, and our patients for reminding us why we do what we do.

Trinh and Lisa

About the Editors

Trinh Pham, PharmD, BCOP, is an Associate Clinical Professor at the University of Connecticut's School of Pharmacy. Her practice site is at the Smilow Cancer Center at the Yale-New Haven Hospital, where she provides education to the oncology pharmacists, pharmacy residents, and pharmacy students along with the medical oncology team in the areas of pain management and supportive care. Dr. Pham completed her bachelor of science in pharmacy degree at the University of Texas in Austin. She also completed a post-baccalaureate doctor of pharmacy degree and a specialized oncology residency and fellowship at the University of Oklahoma. Dr. Pham is a board-certified oncology pharmacist. Her clinical and research interests include pain management and supportive care. Dr. Pham is a member of the Hematology/Oncology Pharmacy Association and the American Society of Clinical Oncology.

Lisa Holle, PharmD, BCOP, is an Assistant Clinical Professor at the University of Connecticut's School of Pharmacy. Her practice site is at the University of Connecticut Health Center's Carole and Ray Neag Comprehensive Cancer Center, where she works with the medical oncology team to provide management of oral cancer therapy, supportive care, and pain management. Dr. Holle completed her bachelor of science degree in pharmacy and a post-baccalaureate doctor of pharmacy degree from the University of Wisconsin at Madison. She completed a specialized oncology residency at The University of Texas M.D. Anderson Cancer Center and is a board-certified oncology pharmacist. Dr. Holle is a past president of the Hematology/Oncology Pharmacy Association and is a member of many professional pharmacy and oncology organizations. Her clinical research program focuses on oncology quality improvement initiatives, drug shortages, oral cancer therapy management, and supportive care reimbursement for clinical pharmacy services.

Contributors

Jeanne Adams, CPhT
IV Prep Supervisor
Illinois CancerCare
Peoria, Illinois

Brooke Bernhardt, PharmD, MS, BCOP
Group Pharmacist, Children's Oncology Group
Clinical Pharmacy Specialist, Oncology
Texas Children's Hospital
Houston, Texas

Beth Chen, PharmD, BCOP
Oncology Clinical Specialist
Biologics, Inc
Cary, North Carolina

Hyejin Kim, PharmD
Pharmacist
Department of Pharmacy Services
The William W. Backus Hospital
Norwich, Connecticut

Susannah E. Koontz, PharmD, BCOP
Principal and Consultant—Pediatric Hematology/Oncology/HSCT
Koontz Oncology Consulting, LLC
Houston, Texas

Jia Li, MD, PhD
Assistant Professor
VA Connecticut Healthcare System
Yale Cancer Center
Yale School of Medicine
New Haven, Connecticut

Theresa A. Mays, BS, PharmD, BCOP, FASHP
Director, Investigational Drug Section
South Texas Accelerated Research Therapeutics
San Antonio, Texas

Man Yee Merl, BS, PharmD, BCOP
Senior Clinical Specialist, Oncology Pharmacy Services
Department of Oncology Pharmacy Services
Smilow Cancer Hospital at Yale–New Haven
New Haven, Connecticut

Jane Pruemer, PharmD, BS Pharm, BCOP, FASHP
Clinical Professor of Pharmacy Practice
Department of Pharmacy Practice and Administrative Sciences
University of Cincinnati James L. Winkle College of Pharmacy
Cincinnati, Ohio

Michele Rice, PharmD, BCOP
Director of Pharmacy and Research
Illinois CancerCare
Peoria, Illinois

Ashley Richards, PharmD, BCOP
Clinical Pharmacy Specialist, BMT/Leukemia
Department of Pharmacy
UF Health Shands Hospital
Clinical Assistant Professor
Department of Pharmacotherapy and Translational Research
University of Florida College of Pharmacy
Gainesville, Florida

Joan Rivington, MPharm, BCOP
Clinical Oncology Pharmacist
Lawrence and Memorial Cancer Center
Waterford, Connecticut

Karen R. Smethers, BS, PharmD, BCOP
National Clinical Pharmacy Integration Leader
Ascension Health
St. Louis, Missouri

Leslie Smetzer, BSN, RN, OCN
Director, Phase I Nursing
South Texas Accelerated Research Therapeutics (START)
San Antonio, Texas

James G. Stevenson, PharmD, FASHP
Chief Pharmacy Officer
University of Michigan Health System
Professor and Associate Dean for Clinical Sciences
University of Michigan College of Pharmacy
Ann Arbor, Michigan

Timothy Tyler, PharmD, FCSHP
Director of Pharmacy Services
Comprehensive Cancer Center
Desert Regional Medical Center
Associate Adjunct Professor
University of Southern California School of Pharmacy
Palm Springs, California

Laura E. Wiggins, PharmD, BCOP
Clinical Chief, Oncology Pharmacy Services
UF Health Shands Hospital
Clinical Assistant Professor
Department of Pharmacotherapy and Translational Research
University of Florida College of Pharmacy
Gainesville, Florida

Reviewers

Sandra Cuellar, PharmD, BCOP
Director, PGY-2 Oncology Pharmacy Residency
Clinical Assistant Professor
Department of Pharmacy Practice
University of Illinois Medical Center
Chicago, Illinois

Ryan A. Forrey, PharmD, MS
Associate Director, Pharmacy and Infusion Services
The Ohio State University Comprehensive Cancer Center: Arthur G. James
    Cancer Hospital and Richard J. Solove Research Institute
Clinical Assistant Professor
College of Pharmacy
The Ohio State University
Columbus, Ohio

Rebecca E. Greene, PharmD, BCOP
Orlando VA Medical Center
Orlando, Florida

Suzanne Jones, PharmD
Scientific Director
Sarah Cannon Research Institute
Nashville, Tennessee

James J. Natale, PharmD, BCOP
Clinical Pharmacy Specialist
UPMC Cancer Center
Pittsburgh, Pennsylvania

Lisa A. Thompson, PharmD, BCOP
Assistant Professor
Department of Clinical Pharmacy
University of Colorado Skaggs School of Pharmacy and
    Pharmaceutical Sciences
Aurora, Colorado

Scott Wirth, PharmD, BCOP
Clinical Assistant Professor
Department of Pharmacy Practice
Clinical Pharmacist, Oncology
University of Illinois at Chicago
Chicago, Illinois

CHAPTER 1

Overview of Cancer Therapy

Lisa Holle
Jane Pruemer
Hyejin Kim

LEARNING OBJECTIVES

Upon completion of the chapter, the reader will be able to:
1. Identify differences between normal cells and malignant cells.
2. Classify cancer drugs based on their mechanism of action.
3. Describe toxicities that are common to a given class of cancer drugs.
4. Identify the different definitions used to evaluate the response of the tumor to therapy.

INTRODUCTION

What Is Cancer?

Cancer is a group of diseases, not one single entity. An understanding of the characteristics of cancer is important to understanding the principles and practices of cancer management. This chapter will outline the basic characteristics of cancer, its potential causes, the basic pharmacology and pharmacotherapy of medications used in the treatment of cancer, and the terms used to determine response to anticancer therapy. This chapter is meant to be an introduction to cancer therapy rather than a comprehensive review. For a more thorough review of cancer therapy, please see the *References* and the *Suggested Reading* list.

Normal cells grow, divide, and die in an orderly, predictable fashion. Cancer cells are different than normal cells in that they continue to grow, divide, and form new, abnormal cells. Although there are many different types of cancer, they have several characteristics in common. Both normal and cancer cells progress through 4 distinct phases of cell division known as the cell cycle: G_1 phase (growth), S phase (synthesis), G_2 phase (2nd growth phase), and M phase (mitosis). Following cell division, the cell will enter a resting phase (G_0 phase). Cancer cells, however, exhibit excessive growth, possess an extended life span, and have metastatic potential. They have the means to invade tissues surrounding them and to spread throughout the body, destroying distant tissues and organs. If allowed to continue to grow, the cancer will ultimately cause death.

One of the first steps in cancer cell development is DNA damage. Damaged DNA is inheritable and accounts for 5%–10% of all cancers.[1,2] More often, mutations in the DNA may occur by exposure to environmental factors or random cellular events. Substances that may act as carcinogens or initiators of cancer include chemical, physical, and biologic agents.[3] Exposure to chemicals (eg, aniline dye, benzene) may occur through occupational and environmental contact, as well as lifestyle habits. Physical agents that act as carcinogens include ultraviolet light and ionizing radiation. These types of radiation induce mutations by forming free radicals that damage DNA and other cellular components. Viruses are biologic agents that may be associated with certain cancers.[4] The Epstein-Barr virus is believed to be an important factor in the initiation of Burkitt's lymphoma. Likewise, infection with the human papillomavirus is known to be a major cause of head and neck cancer and cervical cancer (**Table 1-1**).[4–13]

Recently, because of advances in genomic information, there is significant progress in the understanding of genetic changes that lead to the development of cancer. Two major classes of genes have been identified in the course of cancer development: oncogenes and tumor suppressor genes. Oncogenes develop from normal genes (proto-oncogenes) and can have effects in all phases of cancer development. Changes of proto-oncogenes can occur through point mutation, chromosomal rearrangement, or gene amplification by exposure to carcinogenic agents (**Table 1-2**).[14–17] The result is dysregulation of normal cell growth and proliferation.

In contrast, tumor suppressor genes regulate and inhibit inappropriate cellular growth and proliferation. The p53 gene is an example of a tumor suppressor gene. Mutation of p53 is one of the most common genetic changes associated with cancer, and it is estimated to occur in half of all malignancies.[18] Inactivation of p53 is linked to a variety of malignancies including astrocytomas, breast, colon, lung, cervix, and bone cancers.

Table 1-1 Potential Causes of Cancer[4-13]

Risk Factor	Associated Cancer
Environmental	
Radiation	Leukemia, breast, thyroid
UV radiation	Melanoma, skin
Radon	Lung
Viruses	Leukemia, lymphoma, anal, nasopharyngeal, cervical, oropharyngeal, liver
Lifestyle	
Alcohol	Esophageal, larynx, liver, gastric, oropharynx
Tobacco	Bladder, esophageal, lung, larynx, lip, mouth, pharynx
Dietary	
Low fiber, high fat	Colorectal, breast, endometrial, gallbladder
Reproductive history	
Late first pregnancy, 0 or low parity	Breast, ovarian
Medications	
Alkylating agents	Leukemia, bladder
Azathioprine	Lymphoma
Chloramphenicol	Leukemia
Diethylstilbestrol	Vaginal in daughters of users
Estrogens	Breast, endometrial
Tamoxifen	Endometrial
Occupational exposure	
Aniline dye	Bladder
Asbestos	Lung, mesothelioma
Benzene	Leukemia
Cadmium	Lung
Chromium	Lung
Nickel	Lung, nasal sinus
Vinyl chloride	Leukemia, liver

The current theory for the development of cancer supports the concept that carcinogenesis is a multistep process. The first step is *initiation*, which requires a cell to be exposed to carcinogenic substances (Table 1-1) that produce genetic damage (Table 1-2). If not repaired, the damage results in irreversible cellular mutations and selective growth advantage, allowing the mutated cells the potential to develop into a clonal population of cancer cells. The second step, *promotion*, occurs as the environment is altered to favor the growth of the mutated cell population over normal cells. The promotion phase may be a reversible process. The third step is the *transformation* phase, when the mutated cells become cancerous.

Table 1-2 Types of Genetic Mutations[14–17]

Mutation	Description	Example
Point mutations	Change in 1 base pair in the genetic material may lead to a single amino acid substitution in a critical portion of the protein.	K-Ras gene in non–small cell lung cancer
Deletions	Removal of 1 or more base pairs may result in loss of expression of a protein.	13q in multiple myeloma
Insertions	Addition of 1 or more base pairs may result in altered expression of a protein.	Epidermal growth factor receptor (EGFR) exon 20 in lung adenocarcinoma
Translocations	All or part of a gene recombines with other genes, which may result in altered expression of a protein.	Philadelphia chromosome (also known as bcr-abl or translocation [9;22]) in chronic myeloid leukemia
Amplifications	Increase in the amount of DNA from a specific region of a chromosome, which may result in altered expression of a protein.	Overexpression of HER-2 in breast cancer

Progression is the final stage of neoplastic growth, which involves further genetic changes, increased cell proliferation, tumor invasion into local tissues, and metastases to distant sites.[19]

Modalities of Cancer Treatment

The following 3 major modalities exist for the treatment of cancer: surgery, radiation, and drug therapy. This chapter will focus on the use of pharmacotherapy to treat cancer. Drug therapy may have systemic effects (eg, intravenous cisplatin) or local effects (eg, carmustine wafers) and can treat the primary cancer as well as metastatic sites. Chemotherapy is a group of drugs that interfere with DNA (genes) of fast-growing cells. Biologic therapies are made from a living organism or its products and include cytokines, antibodies, vaccines, and growth factors. Targeted therapies are drugs that are designed to target specific tumor antigens or molecules critical to the survival and growth of cancer cells.

Cancer Therapy Medications

While surgery and radiation specifically target the tumor, cancer therapy medications affect the whole body through various mechanisms of action. New cancer therapy drugs have greater efficacy and less toxicity than first-generation cancer therapy drugs developed 50 years ago. Additionally, due to greater knowledge of cancer therapy delivery, including optimal dose and frequency of dosing, they are more efficacious and less toxic in the treatment of cancer.[20]

Cancer therapy medications can be given as the primary treatment for some cancers, such as lymphoma and leukemia. It can also be given as adjuvant therapy, after the cancer has been surgically removed, to improve survival and delay or prevent disease recurrence. Neoadjuvant therapy is given before surgery to shrink tumors to permit less extensive surgery. Maintenance therapy is the continued use of cancer medications to help lower the risk of recurrence after the first cancer therapy treatment or to prevent the spread of disease in patients with advanced cancer. When cancer is not curable, cancer therapy may be administered palliatively to reduce symptoms caused by tumors.

CLASSES OF CHEMOTHERAPY AGENTS

Chemotherapy agents (also referred to as antineoplastics) are commonly classified by their mechanism of action or by their source of origin.[19] Traditional antineoplastics target rapidly dividing cells and have activity in 1 or more sites of the cell cycle. Those drugs with major activity at 1 site of the cell cycle are known as cell-cycle specific drugs, whereas those with activity at multiple sites are known as cell-cycle nonspecific drugs. However, not all cytotoxicity is a result of disruption of the cell cycle. Intracellular activity may also result in cytotoxicity, such as direct lymphocyte toxicity or inhibition of signal transduction pathways involved in proliferation, survival, and metastases of cancer cells. The following sections describe the various classes of antineoplastics used in the treatment of cancer. The clinical uses, mechanism of action, side effects, and practical patient management for these agents are reviewed. For more thorough information about each of these drugs, please see the *Suggested Reading* list at the end of this chapter.

Microtubule-Targeting Drugs

Mitotic inhibitors disrupt mitosis, a phase of cell division in which a cell duplicates and separates the chromosomes in its cell nucleus. These agents are considered to be cell-cycle specific (mostly in the M phase of the cell cycle) chemotherapy drugs and include the vinca alkaloids, taxanes, epothilones, eribulin, and estramustine.

Vinca Alkaloids

The vinca alkaloids include vinblastine, vincristine, and vinorelbine, which are used to treat some solid tumors, as well as lymphomas and leukemias. Vinca alkaloids are derived from the periwinkle plant and bind to tubulin, the structural protein that polymerizes to form the microtubules that make up the mitotic spindle. The vinca alkaloids inhibit the assembly of microtubules; thus, they inhibit microtubule polymerization. The microtubules are also important in nerve conduction and neurotransmission, and loss of this function results in some of the toxicities seen with these agents. Although structurally similar with the same mechanism of action, the vinca alkaloids possess different activities and toxicity profiles. Vinblastine and vinorelbine are more often associated with dose-limiting myelosuppression, whereas vincristine causes less bone marrow suppression but more neurotoxicity.[19] In regimens such as CHOP (cyclophosphamide, doxorubicin, vincristine, prednisone) and CVP (cyclophosphamide, vincristine, prednisone) used to treat lymphomas, the maximum single dose limit for vincristine is generally 2 mg because of the high risk of neurotoxicity.[21] The neurotoxicity is a neuropathy that affects sensation and motor function with paresthesias of the fingers and toes as the most common clinical manifestations. Hoarseness, facial palsies, or jaw pain occur due to damage of cranial nerves and constipation or colicky abdominal pain occur due to autonomic neuropathy. These side effects are often reversible, however, in some cases, the neuropathy may persist. Therapy should be discontinued when the effects are disabling. Recently, a liposomal formulation of vincristine was approved for use in Philadelphia chromosome-negative (t [9;22] chromosomal translocation) acute lymphoblastic leukemia patients. The formulation was developed to allow higher doses of the drug to be administered with fewer side effects. The liposomal vincristine dose is 2.25 mg/m^2, nearly double the usual dose of vincristine; however, the toxicity profile is comparable to standard vincristine.[22]

Taxanes

The taxanes are plant alkaloids and include paclitaxel, docetaxel, and cabazitaxel. Paclitaxel was isolated from the bark of the North American Pacific yew tree, *Taxus brevifolia*, in the early 1970s.[19] Docetaxel is a semisynthetic

compound produced from 10-deacetylbaccatin-III, which is found in the needles of the European yew tree, *Taxus baccata*. Cabazitaxel is a semisynthetic taxane from a diastereoisomer of 10-deacetylbaccatin-III, derived from the needles
of various *Taxus* species. These agents possess antimitotic activity by binding
to tubulin and promoting its assembly into microtubules while simultaneously
inhibiting disassembly. In contrast to vinca alkaloids, these agents promote
microtubule polymerization. This leads to the stabilization of microtubules and
results in the inhibition of mitotic and interphase cellular functions. Taxanes
also have other actions that can cause cancer cell death, such as antiangiogen-
esis. Cross-resistance between the taxanes is incomplete.[23] Myelosuppression
is a dose-limiting toxicity of the taxanes.[24] Fluid retention is more common
with docetaxel, whereas paclitaxel has increased neurotoxicity and hypersensitivity reactions.[25] The diluent (eg, Cremophor EL [polyoxyethylated castor
oil] with paclitaxel) and the emulsifier (eg, polysorbate 80 with docetaxel and
cabazitaxel) used to formulate these drugs are associated with hypersensitivity
reactions; thus, patients require premedications to prevent this side effect. See
Table 1-3 for premedication recommendations and precautions associated with
the taxanes.[26–33]

Recently, a nanoparticle albumin-bound paclitaxel product, which is not
associated with hypersensitivity reactions, became available for the treatment of
breast cancer. No premedications are thus needed for this product. It is important to note that the dosing for nanoparticle albumin-bound paclitaxel is different than paclitaxel. Other side effects are similar between the different taxanes,
including myelosuppression, neuropathy, and myalgias.

Epothilones

The epothilones work in the mitotic phase of the cell cycle by promoting microtubule polymerization.[19] The only currently available epothilone derivative in
the United States is ixabepilone, approved as monotherapy to treat metastatic
or locally advanced breast cancer following failure with anthracyclines, taxanes,
and capecitabine. It can also be used in combination with capecitabine following failure of an anthracycline and a taxane. Mitotic inhibitors are known for
their potential to cause peripheral nerve injury, which can be a dose-limiting side
effect for this class of chemotherapy agents. The other toxicities associated with
ixabepilone are similar to those of the taxanes, with the exception of fluid retention, which does not occur with ixabepilone.

Table 1-3 Anticancer Agents Requiring Special Premedications/ Precautions[26-33]

Agent (Brand Name)	Premedications	Precautions
Alemtuzumab (Campath)	Diphenhydramine 50 mg and acetaminophen 500-1000 mg PO 30 minutes prior to first infusion and each dose escalation	Monitor and premedicate for infusion-related reactions. Prophylaxis against *Pneumocystis jiroveci* pneumonia and herpes simplex virus recommended upon initiation of treatment and continuing 2 months after or until CD4+ count is ≥ 200 cells/microliter, whichever occurs later.
Bevacizumab (Avastin)		Monitor for infusion-related reactions (uncommon); no premedications required. Do not administer to patients with recent hemoptysis, GI perforation, serious bleeding, or nephrotic syndrome. Monitor blood pressure every 2–3 weeks during treatment; treat with appropriate antihypertensive therapy as necessary. Check urine for protein; hold for proteinuria > 2 grams/24 hours. Do not initiate bevacizumab for at least 28 days after surgery and until the surgical wound is fully healed.
Bleomycin (Blenoxane)		Hypersensitivity reactions can occur with any dose of bleomycin, regardless of test dosing; more common in lymphoma patients. Test dosing and premedication vs close clinical monitoring is controversial. Pulmonary fibrosis can occur; risk higher in elderly patients, lifetime cumulative dose > 400 units, smoking, patients receiving concurrent oxygen therapy, and possibly with concurrent granulocyte colony-stimulating factor use.

Agent (Brand Name)	Premedications	Precautions
Busulfan (Busulfex, Myleran)	Prevent seizures with high doses (transplant regimens) by using phenytoin or high dose clonazepam or lorazepam, during and for at least 48 hours following completion of therapy	
Cabazitaxel (Jevtana)	Premedicate with an antihistamine (eg, diphenhydramine 25 mg IV), a corticosteroid (dexamethasone 8 mg IV), and an H_2 antagonist (eg, ranitidine 50 mg IV) 30 minutes prior to administration	Avoid in patients with sensitivity to polysorbate 80. Severe hypersensitivity reactions require discontinuation.
Carboplatin (Paraplatin)		Hypersensitivity reactions can occur with any cycle, but most common after 6-8 cycles. Discontinuation or desensitization is recommended for future doses after a hypersensitivity reaction occurs.
Cetuximab (Erbitux)	Diphenhydramine 50 mg IV 30-60 minutes prior to first dose	Premedication prior to subsequent treatments based on clinical judgment and presence/severity of prior infusion reactions. Observe patient for 1 hour after infusion. Interrupt infusion if infusion-related reaction occurs, and rechallenge with 50% reduction in infusion rate if reaction was not severe.
Cisplatin (Platinol)	Prehydrate with 1-2 liters of fluid over 1 to 12 hours prior to administration; maximum rate of 500 mL/hour	Consider mannitol (50-gram to 100-gram dose) or furosemide for diuresis if patient cannot tolerate fluid load
Cytarabine (Cytosar)	For doses > 1.5 g/m^2: initiate corticosteroid ophthalmic drops (eg, prednisolone 1%, 1 drop to each eye every 8 hours during treatment and until 24-72 hours after therapy)	For doses > 1.5 g/m^2, monitor for neurotoxicity with neurology checks (have patient sign name) before each dose, or every 8 hours.

(continues)

Table 1-3 Anticancer Agents Requiring Special Premedications/
Precautions[26-33] (*continued*)

Agent (Brand Name)	Premedications	Precautions
Docetaxel (Taxotere)	Dexamethasone 8 mg PO BID × 3 days, starting the day prior to treatment. Weekly docetaxel: Dexamethasone 8 mg PO every 12 hours × 3 doses (24 mg/week) beginning the evening before docetaxel dosing. **Note**: Dose may be omitted in patients who have developed tolerance to the drug Hormone-refractory metastatic prostate cancer: given the concurrent use of prednisone, the recommended premedication regimen is oral dexamethasone 8 mg, at 12 hours, 3 hours, and 1 hour before docetaxel	Avoid in patients with severe hypersensitivity to polysorbate 80. Severe hypersensitivity reactions require discontinuation.
Ibritumomab tiuxetan (Zevalin)	Diphenhydramine 50 mg PO and acetaminophen 650 mg PO 30 minutes prior to treatment	
Interferon-alfa (Roferon-A, Intron A)	Acetaminophen 650 mg PO 30 minutes prior to treatment, repeat q 4 h prn for flu-like symptoms, including fever and chills	Roferon-A no longer manufactured. Intron A still available
Interleukin-2 (Aldesleukin)	Acetaminophen 650 mg PO prior to each dose q 4 h plus nonsteroidal anti-inflammatory drug (NSAID) (indomethacin 25 mg PO prior to each dose q 6 h or naproxen 500 mg PO BID during therapy). High dose, bolus (> 600,000 units/kg): H_2 receptor antagonist (cimetidine, famotidine, or ranitidine)	**Note**: Do *not* use corticosteroids with high-dose IL-2.

Agent (Brand Name)	Premedications	Precautions
Irinotecan (Camptosar)	**Acute diarrhea** (1st 24 hours after administration): 0.25 mg to 1 mg atropine as needed. **Delayed diarrhea**: (> 24 hours): 4 mg loperamide load, then 2 mg q 2 h or alternatively, 4 mg q 4 h around the clock until diarrhea free for 12 hours. **Note**: Will exceed package insert recommended dose of 16 mg/day.	
Ixabepilone (Ixempra)	Oral H₁ (diphenhydramine) and H₂ (cimetidine, famotidine, or ranitidine) antagonists 1 hour prior to infusion. If history of hypersensitivity, premedication with corticosteroid is recommended	Contains 39.8% dehydrated alcohol Formulated with Cremophor EL (polyoxyethylated castor oil; (hypersensitivity possible)
Methotrexate (Trexall)	High dose (> 100 mg/m²) requires: • Administration of leucovorin at 24 hours, or no later than 42 hours, after methotrexate administration and continue until methotrexate level is less than 0.05 μmol • Hydrate with IV fluids containing sodium bicarbonate to maintain urine pH above 7 to enhance solubility of methotrexate in urine and precipitation in kidneys	Avoid all NSAIDS prior to and during therapy. Consider interactions with drugs known to alter plasma protein binding or renal elimination of methotrexate (eg, salicylates, sulfisoxazole, NSAIDs, penicillin, probenecid). Avoid high-dose vitamin C supplementation including excessive consumption of juice containing vitamin C (eg, orange juice).
Ofatumumab (Arzerra)	Acetaminophen (1000 mg), oral or IV antihistamine (eg, cetirizine 10 mg orally or equivalent), and corticosteroid 30–120 min prior to administration. Full-dose corticosteroid recommended	Monitor and premedicate for infusion-related reactions. Interrupt infusion and institute treatment if reaction occurs; may require subsequent rate modification. Avoid live vaccine administration during treatment.

(continues)

Table 1-3 Anticancer Agents Requiring Special Premedications/ Precautions[26-33] (*continued*)

Agent (Brand Name)	Premedications	Precautions
Ofatumumab (Arzerra) (*continued*)	for doses 1, 2, and 9; in absence of grade 3 infusion-related reaction, gradually reduce corticosteroid dose for doses 3 through 8; administer full or half-dose corticosteroid with doses 10 through 12 if grade 3 infusion-related reaction did not occur with dose 9	
Oxaliplatin (Eloxatin)		Hypersensitivity reactions can occur with any cycle, but most commonly after 6-8 cycles. Discontinuation or desensitization is recommended for future doses after a hypersensitivity reaction occurs.
Paclitaxel (Taxol)	Dexamethasone 20 mg PO at 12 hours and 6 hours prior to therapy, or 10 mg to 20 mg, once, IV at 30 minutes prior to paclitaxel infusion with diphenhydramine 50 mg IV/PO and H_2-receptor antagonist (famotidine or ranitidine). **Note**: Weekly paclitaxel, 8-10 mg IV dexamethasone with diphenhydramine and H_2 receptor antagonist as above prior to paclitaxel; dexamethasone can be decreased to 4 mg with subsequent cycles if tolerated	Avoid in patients with severe hypersensitivity to Cremophor EL (polyoxyethylated castor oil). Severe hypersensitivity reactions require discontinuation. **Note**: Cimetidine usually not given due to potential drug–drug interactions.
Panitumumab (Vectibix)	While there are no premedications recommended, monitor for infusion-related reactions	

Agent (Brand Name)	Premedications	Precautions
Pemetrexed (Alimta)	Dexamethasone 4 mg PO BID day before, day of, and day after treatment. Folic acid 350-1000 mcg PO daily starting 5-7 days prior to treatment, continued throughout treatment and for 21 days after last treatment. Vitamin B_{12} 1000 mcg IM, once, 7 days prior to treatment and every 3 cycles (or every 9 weeks) thereafter	
Pralatrexate (Folotyn)	Folic acid 1 to 1.25 mg orally once daily beginning 10 days before the first dose of pralatrexate; continue during the full course of therapy and for 30 days after the last dose. Vitamin B_{12} 1 mg IM within 10 weeks prior to the first dose and every 8-10 weeks thereafter (may be given the same day as treatment with pralatrexate) Diphenhydramine 50 mg PO and acetaminophen 650 mg PO 30 minutes prior to treatment	
Rituximab (Rituxan)		Interrupt infusion if infusion-related reaction occurs, and rechallenge with 50% reduction in infusion rate unless reaction is severe. Screen patients at high risk of hepatitis B virus (HBV) infection before initiation of rituximab and closely monitor carriers of hepatitis B for clinical and laboratory signs of active HBV infection for several months following rituximab therapy.
Temsirolimus (Torisel)	Diphenhydramine 25 mg to 50 mg IV 30 minutes before the start of each dose	Significant drug–drug interactions. Use caution with inhibitors and inducers of CYP3A4.

(continues)

Table 1-3 Anticancer Agents Requiring Special Premedications/ Precautions[26-33] (*continued*)

Agent (Brand Name)	Premedications	Precautions
Tositumomab (Bexxar)	Diphenhydramine 50 mg PO and acetaminophen 650 mg PO 30 minutes prior to or during treatment	Thyroid-protective premedication: Initiate thyroid-protective drugs 24 hours prior to the dosimetric dose and continue daily dosing for a minimum of 14 days following the therapeutic dose. The following regimens are recommended: • Saturated solution of potassium iodide (SSKI) 4 drops orally 3 times daily or • Lugol's solution 20 drops orally 3 times daily or • Potassium iodide tablets 130 mg orally once daily Do not administer tositumomab dose unless the patient has received at least 3 doses of SSKI, 3 doses of Lugol's solution, or 1 dose of 130-mg potassium iodide tablet.
Trastuzumab (Herceptin)	Diphenhydramine 50 mg PO and acetaminophen 650 mg PO 30 minutes prior to treatment	Infusion-related symptoms most commonly occur during infusion or within 24 hours.

Eribulin

Eribulin is the newest mitotic inhibitor that is a synthetic analog of halichondrin B, a compound found in a marine sponge.[34] It was approved by the Food and Drug Administration (FDA) in 2010 for the treatment of metastatic breast cancer in patients who have previously received at least 2 chemotherapeutic regimens that should have included an anthracycline and a taxane in either the adjuvant or metastatic setting.[26] Eribulin inhibits microtubule growth by depolymerization without affecting the shortening phase and sequesters tubulin into nonproductive aggregates.[34] This leads to disruption of mitotic spindles, arrest of the cell cycle at the G_2/M phase, and subsequent apoptotic cell death. The most common side effects associated with eribulin are neutropenia, anemia, fatigue, peripheral neuropathy, and constipation.[34]

Estramustine

A combination of an alkylating agent (*nor*-nitrogen mustard) that is linked by a carbamate bridge with estradiol, estramustine is a unique drug.[19] It was developed with the intent that the estrogenic portion of the molecule would facilitate the uptake of the alkylating agent into hormone-sensitive prostate cancer cells. However, the compound was found to be devoid of alkylating activity due to unanticipated stability of the carbamate bridge and lack of alkylating activity of the intact molecule. Furthermore, the intact estramustine molecule did not show any significant binding to estrogen receptors. Although the drug did not exert the expected hormonal or alkylating effects for which it was developed, estramustine exerts cytotoxic effects by microtubule depolymerization and inhibits mitosis.[35] Common side effects include gynecomastia, edema, and elevated hepatic enzymes.[26]

Alkylating Agents

Alkylating agents are active against blood-related cancers, such as non-Hodgkin's lymphoma, Hodgkin's lymphoma, chronic leukemias, and multiple myeloma, and are also effective in breast, ovarian, lung, and some gastrointestinal cancers.[19] Alkylating agents work by damaging the DNA of cancer cells to prevent them from dividing. Their specific mechanism of action is covalent bonding of highly reactive alkyl groups or substituted alkyl groups with nucleophilic groups of proteins and nucleic acids. These covalent interactions result in cross-linking between 2 DNA strands or between 2 bases in the same strand of DNA. Reactions between DNA and RNA and between the alkylators and proteins may also occur, but the main damage that results in cell death is inhibition of DNA replication. These agents are considered non–cell-cycle specific chemotherapy drugs.

Nitrogen Mustard and Its Derivatives

Classical alkylators include the original nitrogen mustard drug, mechlorethamine; cyclophosphamide; ifosfamide; bendamustine; and thiotepa. Mechlorethamine is a common component of one of the regimens used to treat Hodgkin's lymphoma and is highly emetogenic, with nausea and vomiting occurring in over 90% of patients within the first 3 hours of administration.[36] Cyclophosphamide and ifosfamide are nitrogen mustard derivatives and are not active as parent compounds. They must be activated by metabolism via the cytochrome

P450 enzyme CYP3A4.[19] Acrolein, a metabolite of both of these agents, has little antitumor effect but is responsible for the hemorrhagic cystitis adverse effect associated with these drugs. Mesna is a chemoprotectant agent, which is given prior to, during, and after ifosfamide and sometimes cyclophosphamide in order to prevent hemorrhagic cystitis.[37] Bendamustine has a benzimidazole ring that makes it only partially cross-resistant with the other alkylating agents.[38] Thiotepa and busulfan are polyfunctional alkylating agents, which are mostly used in hematopoietic stem cell transplantation conditioning regimens. All of the nitrogen mustard agents cause myelosuppression as one of their primary side effects.

Nitrosoureas

A unique feature of the nitrosoureas is their lipophilicity and ability to cross the blood–brain barrier.[19] These agents play a very important role in the management of primary brain cancers. Carmustine (BCNU) and lomustine (CCNU) are metabolized to reactive alkylating compounds and isocyanate moieties that exert cytotoxic effects. In addition to being available as an intravenous medication, carmustine is also available in a biodegradable wafer for direct implantation into the surgical cavity after resection of brain tumors.[19] The most common side effects of carmustine and lomustine are nausea and vomiting, nephrotoxicity, and myelosuppression. Streptozocin is another nitrosourea that possesses a glucose moiety rather than the chlorethyl side chain that most nitrosoureas have. The glucose moiety is responsible for streptozocin's specificity for pancreatic islet cells and reduced myelotoxicity.[36]

Nonclassical Alkylating Agents

Although they do not have the structures of classical alkylating agents, dacarbazine, procarbazine, and temozolomide are capable of binding covalently to DNA, causing cellular damage. Both dacarbazine and temozolomide are metabolized to the same intermediary, MTIC (5–[3–methyltriazen–1–yl] imidazole–4–carboxamide).[39] Dacarbazine requires the liver for activation; temozolomide does not. Dacarbazine has poor absorption and is available only in an intravenous form. Temozolomide is nearly 100% bioavailable when taken on an empty stomach and is an orally available medication. Dacarbazine penetrates the central nervous system poorly, but temozolomide readily crosses the blood–brain barrier, achieving therapeutically active concentrations in the central nervous system.

Heavy Metal Compounds

Cisplatin, carboplatin, and oxaliplatin are platinum derivatives with cytotoxicity due to platinum binding to DNA and the formation of intrastrand cross-links between neighboring guanines.[19] These are non–cell-cycle specific agents. Cisplatin is a platinum-chloride complex, carboplatin is a structural analog of cisplatin with the chloride groups replaced by a carboxycyclobutane ring, and oxaliplatin is a platinum compound complexed with an oxalate ligand and diaminocyclohexane. Cross-resistance between cisplatin and carboplatin is common, whereas oxaliplatin's spectrum of activity is different from the other platinums and includes significant activity against colorectal cancer.[19,40] The side effects profile for the platinums vary significantly for individual agents. Cisplatin causes significant nephrotoxicity, ototoxicity, peripheral neuropathy, emesis, and anemia.[19] Supportive care measures, including hyperhydration and antiemetic therapy, are vital to the effective use of cisplatin. Carboplatin has less nephrotoxic, neurotoxic, ototoxic, and emetogenic potential than cisplatin, but causes more myelosuppression.[19] Carboplatin is most often dosed via pharmacokinetic parameters using the Calvert formula [Dose in mg = AUC × (CrCl + 25)].[41] For more information on pharmacokinetic dosing and the factors involved in calculating the creatinine clearance see the chapter titled, *Dosing Calculations*, elsewhere in this text. Oxaliplatin is only rarely associated with clinically significant nephrotoxicity and does not appear to cause ototoxicity.[42] It has less emetogenic potential than cisplatin, but it can cause unusual peripheral neuropathies, including cold-induced neuropathies and pharyngolaryngeal dysesthesias.[42] All platinum agents have the potential to cause hypersensitivity reactions.[19]

Antimetabolites

Antimetabolites are in a class of drugs that interfere with DNA and RNA production. They are often analogs of the nucleotides that make up DNA and RNA.[19] In general, the antimetabolites are effective in a specific cycle of cell growth (S phase). The most common adverse effects associated with the antimetabolites are those seen on the rapidly dividing cells of the body, such as the bone marrow, gastrointestinal tract, hair follicles, and reproductive system. The subclasses of antimetabolites include the pyrimidines, cytidine analogs, purine antimetabolites, and folate antagonists.

Pyrimidines

Fluorinated analogs of the pyrimidine uracil include fluorouracil and its oral prodrug, capecitabine. The metabolites of these drugs (fluorodeoxyuridine monophosphate [FdUMP], fluorodeoxyuridine triphosphate [FdUTP], and fluorouridine triphosphate [FUTP]) are incorporated into RNA and DNA and inhibit the enzyme thymidylate synthase (TS) to interfere with cancer cell growth.[19,43] The administration of leucovorin forms a stable ternary complex between fluorouracil, TS, and leucovorin that enhances inhibition of TS and blocks the synthesis of thymidylate. The mechanism of cytotoxicity is influenced by the method of administration; continuous infusion of fluorouracil is associated with thymidylate synthase inhibition, whereas the incorporation into RNA and DNA is associated with the bolus administration of fluorouracil. Pyrimidines are effective in colorectal, breast, gastric, and head and neck cancers. The most common side effects of pyrimidines include myelosuppression, stomatitis, diarrhea, and hand-foot syndrome. Myelosuppression is more common with the bolus administration of fluorouracil, whereas diarrhea and hand-foot syndrome are more common with capecitabine and the continuous infusion of fluorouracil.

Cytidine Analogs

Cytidine analogs include cytarabine, gemcitabine, azacitidine, decitabine, and nelarabine. Cytarabine is an analog of cytosine and is phosphorylated within tumor cells to inhibit DNA polymerase, ultimately preventing DNA elongation.[19,43] Cytarabine is effective in leukemias and lymphomas and may be administered as a low-dose continuous infusion, high-dose intermittent infusion, or intrathecally. A liposomal formulation is also available for intrathecal use. The toxicity of cytarabine is dose dependent but includes myelosuppression and, at high doses, cerebellar toxicity and ophthalmic irritation. Gemcitabine is a deoxycytidine analog, similar in structure to cytarabine. It also inhibits DNA polymerase as well as ribonucleotide reductase, resulting in prevention of DNA elongation. It is used in pancreatic, breast, lung, and ovarian cancers, non–small cell lung cancer, and in some lymphomas. Myelosuppression, flu-like symptoms within the first 24 hours after administration, and rash are the most common side effects associated with gemcitabine. Azacitidine and decitabine are directly incorporated into DNA, inhibiting DNA methyltransferase and causing hypomethylation of DNA, which ultimately causes cellular differentiation and apoptosis. These drugs are used to treat myelodysplastic syndrome and acute myeloid leukemia. Myelosuppression is the most common side effect. Additionally, renal dysfunction and injection-site reactions can occur with azacitidine, and decitabine is associated with constipation, edema, headache, and nausea. Nelarabine, a treatment for T-cell acute lymphoblastic leukemia, is a prodrug that accumulates in leukemic blasts to prevent DNA synthesis and cell death.[26,43] Myelosuppression and fatigue are the most common side effects associated with nelarabine.

Purine Antimetabolites

Purine antimetabolites are represented by mercaptopurine, thioguanine, fludarabine, cladribine, clofarabine, and pentostatin. Mercaptopurine and thioguanine are oral purine analogs that are converted to ribonucleotide to inhibit purine synthesis.[19,26,43] These drugs are metabolized by thiopurine S-methyltransferase (TPMT). Genetic polymorphisms of TMPT may result in reduced activity and decreased tolerance. In addition to myelosuppression that occurs with all purine antimetabolites, rash, mild nausea, and cholestasis often occur with mercaptopurine and thioguanine. Fludarabine, a purine adenine analog, interferes with DNA polymerase to cause chain termination and inhibits transcription by RNA incorporation. It is used in the treatment of chronic lymphocytic leukemia, some lymphomas, and refractory acute myelogenous leukemia. Significant myelosuppression and immunosuppression can occur, resulting in an increased risk of opportunistic infections. Prophylactic antibiotics and antivirals are recommended until CD4 counts normalize. Cladribine, once phosphorylated into an active form, is incorporated into DNA, resulting in DNA synthesis inhibition and chain termination. It is used to treat hairy cell leukemia, chronic lymphocytic leukemia, and some forms of lymphoma. In addition to myelosuppression and immunosuppression, fever is common. Clofarabine is a deoxyadenosine analog that is active in myeloid leukemia and myelodysplastic syndrome. Side effects include myelosuppression, liver dysfunction (severe but transient), skin rashes, and hand-foot syndrome. Pentostatin is an inhibitor of adenosine deaminase, which ultimately blocks DNA synthesis through RNA ribonucleotide reductase inhibition. Pentostatin is used in hairy cell leukemia. Side effects for pentostatin include myelosuppression, immunosuppression, rash, conjunctivitis, and myalgias.

Antifolates

The antifolates include methotrexate, pemetrexed, and pralatrexate. Methotrexate, a folic acid analog, inhibits dihydrofolate reductase in both malignant and nonmalignant cells, ultimately reducing purine and thymidylic acid synthesis, which are needed for DNA formation and cell division.[19,43] When methotrexate is administered in high doses, leucovorin, a reduced folate, is administered 24 hours after methotrexate to bypass the dihydrofolate reductase block in normal cells. Similarly to the other antimetabolites, myelosuppression, nausea/vomiting, and stomatitis can occur with methotrexate. Renal tubular necrosis can occur with high-dose methotrexate; thus, vigorous hydration with sodium bicarbonate to maintain an alkaline pH is recommended to increase the solubility of methotrexate and prevent precipitation in the renal tubules. Methotrexate is used in lymphoma, acute lymphocytic leukemia, and gastric, esophageal, bladder, and breast cancers. It can also be administered via the intrathecal route. Pemetrexed is an antifolate that inhibits the following 3 enzymes involved in thymidine and purine synthesis: dihydrofolate reductase, thymidylate synthase, and glycinamide ribonucleotide formyltransferase. This drug is used in mesothelioma and non–small cell lung cancer. Common side effects include myelosuppression, rash, diarrhea, and nausea/vomiting. Patients should receive both folic acid and cyanocobalamin (vitamin B_{12}) to reduce bone marrow suppression and diarrhea. To prevent rash, a corticosteroid, such as dexamethasone, should be administered the day before, the day of, and the day after pemetrexed administration. Pralatrexate inhibits DNA, RNA, and protein synthesis by selectively entering cells expressing reduced folate carrier and competing for the dihydrofolate reductase-binding site to inhibit dihydrofolate reductase. It is used in T-cell lymphomas. Side effects include myelosuppression, mucositis, fatigue, and edema. As with pemetrexed, folic acid and cyanocobalamin should be administered to patients receiving pralatrexate (see Table 1-3 for specific premedication dosing information).

Topoisomerase Inhibitors

The enzymes responsible for maintaining DNA structure during replication and transcription are the topoisomerases I and II.[19] These enzymes relieve the torsional strain during the unwinding of DNA by producing strand breaks. Topoisomerase I produces single-strand breaks; topoisomerase II causes double-strand breaks. There are 3 major groups of antineoplastic agents that affect topoisomerase enzymes. They include camptothecin, podophyllotoxin, and the anthracene derivatives.

Camptothecin Derivatives

Topoisomerase inhibitors, such as irinotecan and topotecan, interfere with enzymes that are important for accurate DNA replication and arrest cells in the S phase.[19] Both of these agents inhibit topoisomerase I. Irinotecan must undergo metabolism to SN–38 by uridine diphosphate glucosyltransferase (UGT), an enzyme, which may be variably inherited with a mutation. Inheritance of this genetic mutation may result in an increased risk of diarrhea and neutropenia associated with irinotecan use. These agents are used to treat colorectal, lung, ovarian, gastrointestinal, and other cancers.

Podophyllotoxin Derivatives

Etoposide and teniposide are semisynthetic podophyllotoxins that arrest cells in the S or early G_2 phase and are considered cell-cycle, phase specific.[19] In addition to binding to tubulin and interfering with microtubule formation, they also damage cells by causing strand breakage by inhibiting topoisomerase II. Etoposide is used for a variety of both hematologic and solid tumors; whereas, teniposide is primarily used for hematologic malignancies. Etoposide is available as solution for intravenous injection, oral formulation, and as etoposide phosphate (the prodrug formulation of etoposide) for intravenous injection; teniposide is available as an intravenous injection. The intravenous formulation of etoposide is formulated in polyethylene glycol (PEG) and polysorbate 80. Teniposide is solubilized in polyoxyethylated castor oil (Cremophor EL). These formulations contribute to hypersensitivity reactions and hypotension associated with rapid infusions. These effects may be minimized by slowly infusing the drug over 30 minutes to 1 hour and if necessary, premedicating with diphenhydramine and hydrocortisone. Other toxicities associated with these agents include myelosuppression and peripheral neuropathies.

Anthracene Derivatives

The anthracyclines of the anthracene group include doxorubicin, daunorubicin, idarubicin, and epirubicin.[19] Mitoxantrone is an anthracenedione. Anthracyclines are classified as antitumor antibiotics that interfere with enzymes involved in DNA replication. They are intercalating agents that insert between base pairs of DNA resulting in structural changes that interfere with DNA and RNA synthesis. They are also topoisomerase II inhibitors causing double-strand DNA breaks. The anthracyclines also undergo electron reduction to form oxygen free-radicals that are responsible for anthracycline's cardiotoxicity and extravasation ulceration profile. Because they can damage the heart, anthracyclines have a lifetime dose limit.[44] Refer to **Clinical Pearl 1-1** for calculating total anthracycline cumulative dose when multiple, different anthracycline drugs have been administered. Mitoxantrone is also an intercalating topoisomerase II inhibitor but it has less potential to form oxygen free radicals, thus, less cardiotoxicity. Anthracyclines treat a variety of tumors and work in all phases of the cell cycle.

CLINICAL PEARL 1-1

A 5% risk of cardiotoxicity occurs with anthracyclines when the maximum cumulative dose is reached. The following table shows the cumulative dose at which a 5% cardiotoxicity risk occurs and the conversion factor between anthracyclines. This allows the clinician to calculate a total anthracycline cumulative dose if a patient has received multiple, different anthracyclines.[44]

Anthracycline	Conversion Factor	% Cardiotoxicity at Cumulative Dose
Doxorubicin	1	5% at 450 mg/m^2
Daunorubicin	0.5	5% at 900 mg/m^2
Epirubicin	0.5	5% at 935 mg/m^2
Idarubicin	2	5% at 225 mg/m^2
Mitoxantrone	2.2	5% at 200 mg/m^2

Examples:

A patient received a total of 120 mg/m^2 of daunorubicin. What is the equivalent in doxorubicin dosing?

Take 120 mg/m^2 × 0.5 = 60 mg/m^2 of doxorubicin.

A patient received a total of 36 mg/m^2 of idarubicin. What is the equivalent doxorubicin dose?

Take 36 mg/m^2 × 2 = 72 mg/m^2 of doxorubicin.

Note: It is common in clinical practice to calculate the risk of cardiotoxicity in terms of the total cumulative doxorubicin dose.

Miscellaneous Agents

Arsenic trioxide is an organic element that acts as a differentiating agent in the treatment of acute promyelocytic leukemia (APL). It induces the maturation of cancer cells into normal cells. It also can cause programmed cell death or apoptosis.[19] The most common toxicities of this agent include the APL differentiation syndrome, which is characterized by fever, dyspnea, weight gain, pulmonary infiltrates, and pleural or pericardial effusions, with or without leukocytosis.[45]

Asparaginase is an enzyme derived from *Escherichia coli* or *Erwinia chrysanthemi*. L-asparagine is a nonessential amino acid that can be made by most mammalian cells, except for some lymphoid malignancies.[19] Asparaginase causes degradation of any available asparagine in these tumor cells, resulting in inhibition of protein synthesis and ultimate cell death. The primary side effects seen with asparaginase include glucose intolerance and bleeding disorders, due to a decreased production of insulin and clotting factors. Hypersensitivity may also occur with asparaginase; however, pegaspargase is a pegylated formulation of asparaginase that allows for less frequent administration and less hypersensitivity than the native formulation.[46] In 2012, production of *E coli* derived asparaginase was discontinued.

Bleomycin, an antitumor antibiotic, is derived from a fungal species and is a mixture of several proteins. It is cell-cycle specific (G_2 phase).[19] Bleomycin causes DNA strand breakage via free radical formation. It is inactivated by an enzyme called aminohydrolase, which is in low concentrations in the skin and lungs, thus accounting for the pulmonary toxicity of the drug. Baseline pulmonary tests and monitoring for pulmonary toxicity is a must during bleomycin treatment. Other side effects include fever, nausea, and vomiting. Bleomycin is used in the treatment of testicular cancer and Hodgkin's lymphoma. The agent is dosed in either units or milligrams, and 1 unit = 1 mg.

Histone deacetylase (HDAC) inhibitors cause an accumulation of acetylated histones and induce cell cycle arrest or apoptosis of transformed cancer cells.[19,26] Two HDAC inhibitors, romidepsin and vorinostat, are currently marketed. Both of these drugs are used in the treatment of T-cell lymphoma. Romidepsin is an intravenous agent, whereas vorinostat is an oral agent. The most common side effects of these drugs include fatigue, myelosuppression, and gastrointestinal disturbances, such as nausea and diarrhea. Vorinostat is also associated with an increase in serum glucose, creatinine, and urine protein.[47] A high risk of infection and electrocardiogram changes have been seen with romidepsin.[26]

Hydroxyurea inhibits ribonucleotide reductase, causing the production of short strands of DNA.[19] Its primary role in the management of cancer lies in its ability to rapidly reduce white blood cell counts in patients with acute or chronic leukemias. It has a greater role today in the management of patients with sickle cell disease by increasing the production of hemoglobin F. The most common side effect is myelosuppression.

Retinoids (vitamin A and its metabolites) regulate the expression of genes that control cell growth and differentiation by binding to retinoid receptors.[19,43] Tretinoin (all-trans retinoic acid) is a naturally occurring derivative of vitamin A, which is not cytotoxic but promotes the maturation of promyelocytic cells with the t(15;17) cytogenetic marker. It is used in the treatment of APL. Headache, fatigue, weakness, and fever are the most common side effects. Retinoic acid syndrome is a life-threatening syndrome characterized by fever, respiratory distress, and hypotension, which can occur at any time during therapy. Prompt recognition and treatment with corticosteroids is required. Bexarotene is a synthetic retinoid that activates retinoid X receptors, affecting cellular differentiation and proliferation. It is used in cutaneous T-cell lymphoma in patients who are refractory to other therapy. Common side effects include hypercholesterolemia, pancreatitis, hypothyroidism, leukopenia, and triglyceride elevations.

TARGETED THERAPY

Researchers have learned more about specific molecular changes responsible for cancer growth, resulting in a new class of drugs called targeted therapies.[19] These targeted agents are designed to interfere with biochemical processes and signaling pathways that control cancerous cell growth, ultimately resulting in suppression of cell cycle progression, proliferation, and survival.

Targeted therapies include monoclonal antibodies that target cell surface glycoproteins, growth factor receptors, and ligands; agents that inhibit epidermal growth factors or vascular endothelial growth factors; agents that inhibit enzymes responsible for degrading proteins that control cell cycles; agents that inhibit the activity of intracellular signaling pathways involved in cancer cell growth and proliferation; immunomodulating agents that have anticancer activity; and cytokines that have antitumor and immune stimulation activity.

Monoclonal Antibodies

Monoclonal antibodies (MoABs) were among the first targeted agents. The original MoABs were made entirely from mouse cells; today, the MoABs are chimeric, humanized, or fully human where they differ in the amount of foreign component.[19] MoABs are classified into those that target cell-surface antigens and those that target growth factor receptors or ligands. MoABs may also be conjugated to a toxin, chemotherapy agent (eg, ado-trastuzumab, brentuximab vedotin), or radioactive particle (eg, ibritumomab tiuxetan, tositumomab). **Table 1-4** describes the nomenclature of MoAB names, which can provide insight into the target/disease class and the source of the MoAB.[48] The suffix -*mab* is used for all MoABs and is always preceded by identification of the animal source of the product and the target or general disease state the MoAB is treating.

Table 1-4 Nomenclature of Monoclonal Antibodies[48]

Monoclonal antibody name = <u>prefix</u> + **target/disease class infix** + *source infix* + stem (mab)[a]

Prefix (Identifies the Distinctive Product)	Target/Disease Infix	Source Infix	Example
ibri	**-t(u)(m)** tumor	-o- mouse	<u>ibri**tu**m*o*</u>mab tiuxetan
beva	**-c(i)(m)** Cardiovascular	-zu- humanized	<u>beva**ci**z*u*</u>mab
ipi	**-l(i)(m)** Immunomodulating	-u- fully human	<u>ipi**li**m*u*</u>mab
deno	**-s(o)** Bone	-u- fully human	<u>deno**s***u*</u>mab
ofa	**-t(u)(m)** tumor	-u- fully human	<u>ofa**tu**m*u*</u>mab
tras	**-t(u)(m)** tumor	-zu- humanized	<u>tras**tu**z*u*</u>mab
ri	**-t(u)(m)** tumor	-xi- chimeric	<u>ri**tu**x*i*</u>mab

Hypersensitivity and infusion-related reactions may occur with MoABs administration along with development of human antimouse antibodies (HAMA); risks are generally greatest with murine MoAB, least with humanized MoAB, and are not expected with fully human MoAB.[19] These symptoms can be mild with fever, chills, nausea, and rash, to severe with manifestations of life-threatening anaphylaxis with cardiopulmonary collapse. Chest or back pain may also occur with MoAB administration. The reactions are generally more severe with initial infusion and should subside with subsequent treatments. Patients must be closely monitored while receiving MoAB and premedication with antihistamines and acetaminophen is recommended for most MoABs. Starting with slower infusion rates with incremental increases as the patient tolerates also minimizes infusion-related reactions.[19] Table 1-3 lists drugs, including MoABs, that require premedications to prevent infusion-related reactions.

Alemtuzumab, brentuximab vedotin, ibritumomab tiuxetan, ofatumumab, rituximab, and tositumomab are used for the treatment of hematologic malignancies; ado-trastuzumab emtansine, bevacizumab, cetuximab, ipilimumab, panitumumab, and trastuzumab are used in the treatment of solid tumors.

Angiogenesis Inhibitors

Angiogenesis is the development of new blood vessels, and when this process is unregulated in cancer, it can lead to tumor growth, invasion, and metastasis. Angiogenesis inhibitors prevent the formation of new blood vessels in the tumor, thus decreasing the delivery of nutrients and oxygen, resulting in growth delay of the tumor. Most antiangiogenic drugs target vascular endothelial growth factors (VEGFs), the VEGF receptors, platelet-derived growth factor receptors (PDG-FRs), or the production of endothelial cells that are involved in the formation of blood vessels. Bevacizumab was the first successful MoAB to inhibit angiogenesis. Antiangiogenic drugs that are not MoABs include the immunomodulators thalidomide, lenalidomide, and pomalidomide; the tyrosine kinase inhibitors axitinib, cabozantinib, pazopanib, sorafenib, sunitinib, and vandetanib; and the recombinant fusion-protein ziv-aflibercept.

Immunomodulators

Thalidomide, lenalidomide, and pomalidomide are immunomodulators thought to act primarily as antiangiogenic agents in the treatment of malignancies.[19,26] They may, however, have additional mechanisms of action. They are primarily used in the treatment of multiple myeloma. The most common side effects of these agents are peripheral neuropathies, somnolence, constipation, rash, dizziness, and orthostatic hypotension. Lenalidomide and pomalidomide cause less somnolence and peripheral neuropathies than thalidomide, but are associated with myelosuppression. All of these immunomodulators are associated with thrombotic issues, especially when given in combination with steroids for the treatment of multiple of myeloma, and prophylactic thrombotic therapy should be considered. Because of the teratogenic potential of these drugs, all pharmacies and prescribers must be enrolled in the respective risk evaluation and mitigation strategy programs, THALOMID REMS (risk evaluation and mitigation strategy) (formerly known as the System for Thalidomide Education and Prescribing Safety [S.T.E.P.S.] program) for thalidomide, the REVLIMID REMS (formerly known as the RevAssist program) for lenalidomide, and the POMALYST REMS for pomalidomide. For more information on the REMS program, see the chapter titled, *Drug Safety and Risk Management,* elsewhere in this text.

Tyrosine Kinase Inhibitors

Tyrosine kinases are mediators of the signaling cascade that is important in cell proliferation, differentiation, migration, metabolism, and apoptosis.

These enzymes are tightly regulated in normal cells, but mutations, overexpression, and stimulation can result in malignant cell transformation.[49] Tyrosine kinase inhibitors (TKIs) block enzymes with a variety of functions, including angiogenesis and inhibition of cancer cell growth.

Erlotinib is an oral agent that is a selective epidermal growth factor receptor– (EGFR-) tyrosine kinase inhibitor that blocks signal transduction pathways involved in proliferation, survival, and metastases of cancer cells.[19] Rash and diarrhea are the most common side effects. Clinical studies suggest that the development of a rash is predictive of its antitumor effect and response to therapy. There are drug interactions with CYP3A4 inducers and inhibitors. Erlotinib is indicated for non–small cell lung cancer and pancreatic cancer.

Sunitinib and sorafenib inhibit multiple tyrosine kinases, including VEGFR-2 and PDGFR, which are involved in angiogenesis; c-KIT, which is involved with gastrointestinal tumors; and FLT3, which is involved in leukemia.[19] Diarrhea, rash, fatigue, and hypertension occur with both agents. Sunitinib can cause congestive heart failure, and sorafenib has been reported to cause hand-foot syndrome. These agents have activity against renal cell cancers, gastrointestinal stromal tumors, and are being evaluated for other cancers. Similar to erlotinib, drug interactions occur with CYP3A4 inducers and inhibitors.[49,50]

Lapatinib inhibits EGFR and HER-2 (also known as human epidermal growth factor receptor 2, ErbB-2).[19] It is effective in combination with capecitabine in breast cancer patients overexpressing HER-2 who have previously received trastuzumab and chemotherapy. Diarrhea, rash, hepatotoxicity, and QT interval prolongation are most common side effects. Significant CYP450-mediated drug interactions exist.

Imatinib, often considered the first designer targeted agent, is an inhibitor of the tyrosine kinase activity of the BCR-ABL fusion gene of patients with chronic myelogenous leukemia (CML).[19] Prevention of tyrosine-kinase phosphorylation of the fusion gene inhibits downstream activation of cellular proliferation. Bosutinib, dasatinib, and nilotinib are second-generation TKIs that also bind to the BCR-ABL tyrosine kinase domain.[19,51] The advantage of these agents is that they have activity in CML patients with BCR-ABL fusion gene mutations that confer resistance to imatinib. Patients with the T315I gene mutation are resistant to all of the 3 TKI inhibitors. Ponatinib is also a TKI but was designed to be effective in patients with T315I mutation.[26] Adverse effects of imatinib include rash, fluid retention, myelosuppression, nausea, muscle cramps, elevation of liver enzymes, and headaches. Dasatinib and nilotinib have toxicities similar to that of imatinib, although dasatinib also has been reported to cause hypocalcemia and more significant pleural effusions. Bosutinib is associated with diarrhea, nausea, and thrombocytopenia, and ponatinib is associated with rashes, dry skin, abdominal pain, headache, and constipation.[51] All of these agents have extensive drug–drug interactions with substrates, inducers, and inhibitors of CYP3A4 and other CYP450 enzymes.

Other newly approved tyrosine kinase inhibitors target a variety of tyrosine kinases and are used in several different types of malignancies (**Clinical Pearl 1-2**). Afatinib is a tyrosine kinase inhibitor of EGFR, HER2, and HER4. It is FDA approved for the first-line treatment of patients with metastatic non–small cell lung cancer whose tumors have EGFR exon 19 deletions or exon 21 substitution mutations detected by an FDA-approved test.[51] Common side effects include diarrhea, rash, acneiform, stomatitis, paronychia, dry skin, decreased appetite, and pruritis. Axitinib is an inhibitor of VEGFR–1, –2, and –3, approved for the treatment of advanced renal cell carcinoma. Common side effects include diarrhea, hypertension, fatigue, decreased appetite, and hand-foot syndrome. Cabozantinib is a pan-tyrosine kinase inhibitor. It is used in medullary thyroid cancer. Common side effects include diarrhea, stomatitis, hand-foot syndrome, and decreased weight. Crizotinib is an ALK and ROs1 inhibitor that is approved for ALK-positive non–small cell lung cancer. Common side effects include vision disorders, nausea, diarrhea, constipation, and edema. Dabrafenib selectively inhibits mutated forms of BRAF kinases that result from mutations in the BRAF gene, including BRAFV600E, which is found in 70% of melanomas. It is approved for patients with unresectable or metastatic melanoma with the BRAFV600E mutation. Side effects include hyperkeratosis, headache, pyrexia, arthralgia, papilloma, alopecia, and hand-foot syndrome. Regorafenib is a multikinase inhibitor, which targets angiogenic, stromal, and oncogenic tyrosine kinase receptors. It is approved for metastatic colorectal cancer and is associated with fatigue, decreased appetite, hand-foot syndrome, and diarrhea. Trametinib is mitogen-activated protein kinase (MEK) inhibitor, which specifically binds and inhibits MEK 1 and 2, resulting in inhibition of cell signaling and cellular proliferation of various cancers. It is specifically indicated in patients with unresectable or metastatic melanoma with BRAFV600E or BRAFV600K mutations as detected by an FDA approved test. Common side effects include rash, diarrhea, and lymphedema. Vemurafenib also selectively inhibits the BRAFV600E gene and is indicated for metastatic melanoma with BRAFV600E mutation. Side effects include arthralgia, rash, alopecia, fatigue, and photosensitivity reactions. Vandetanib blocks VEGF and EGF. It is indicated for medullary thyroid cancer. Side effects include diarrhea, rash, acne, nausea, and hypertension. Most of these drugs are metabolized by CYP450 enzymes; therefore, drug interactions should be reviewed before administration.

CLINICAL PEARL 1-2

FDA Approved Drugs on the CenterWatch website (http://www
.centerwatch.com/drug-information/fda-approvals/) is a good
source to keep updated with newly approved oncology drugs.
For more in-depth information for verifying/prescribing the regimens
and reported side effects, primary literature should be reviewed.

Miscellaneous Targeted Agents

Bortezomib is a proteasome inhibitor with significant activity in the treatment of multiple myeloma and mantle cell lymphoma.[19] Carfilzomib is a second-generation proteasome inhibitor.[51] The proteasome is an enzyme complex that breaks down proteins that regulate the cell cycle. Inhibition of the proteasome ultimately results in inactivation of NFκB, which prevents the transcription of genes that promote cancer growth.[19] The most common side effects of bortezomib and carfilzomib include fatigue, malaise, weakness, nausea, and diarrhea. Serious side effects that have been reported include myelosuppression and peripheral neuropathies (bortezomib greater than carfilzomib).

Temsirolimus and everolimus are known as mTOR (mammalian target of rapamycin) inhibitors. An mTOR is a part of the signaling pathway important in the growth and replication of various cell pathways.[19] Temsirolimus and everolimus are indicated for the treatment of renal cell cancer; everolimus is also indicated in advanced breast cancer and primary neuroendocrine tumors.[26] Adverse reactions include rash, fatigue, mucositis, nausea, hyperglycemia, hyperlipidemia, myelosuppression, and abnormal liver function tests. Drug interactions with CYP3A4 inducers or inhibitors can occur with both of these agents.

Vismodegib is a hedgehog signaling pathway inhibitor.[51] The hedgehog pathway promotes cellular development and cell division. It is indicated for metastatic basal cell carcinoma, in which this pathway is overactivated. Side effects include muscle spasms, alopecia, dysgeusia, weight loss, and nausea.

Ziv-aflibercept is a recombinant fusion protein designed to bind to VEGF and placental growth factor, with angiogenic properties.[51] This drug is indicated for colorectal cancer when combined with 5-flouroruacil, leucovorin, and irinotecan. Common side effects include myelosuppression, diarrhea, proteinuria, and stomatitis.

Interferon and Interleukin-2

Interferon-alfa and interleukin-2 are immunologic agents that have demonstrated anticancer effects. Interferon-alfa has cell growth inhibiting and apoptosis inducing characteristics, and exerts direct cytotoxic effects via caspase activation.[52] Adverse effects include flu-like symptoms, fever, extreme fatigue, psychiatric symptoms (depression, anxiety), sleep disturbances, and dose-related myelosuppression.[26] Interleukin-2 enhances lymphocyte mitogenesis and induces lymphocyte killing of cancer cells. Interleukin-2 may cause capillary leak syndrome, as well as associated hypotension, pulmonary edema, total body edema, cardiac arrhythmias, and renal abnormalities.[26]

HORMONAL AGENTS

Hormonal agents are typically used in the treatment of breast, uterine, and prostate cancers. These agents do not work directly on cancer cells. Rather, they inhibit the hormonal activation of cancer cell growth, either by competing for hormone receptors or by limiting the endogenous production of hormones.

Antiestrogens

Antiestrogens bind to estrogen receptors, inhibiting receptor-mediated gene transcription. This in turns prevents the effect of estrogen.[53] Selective estrogen receptor modulators (SERMs), such as tamoxifen, toremifene, and raloxifene, act as estrogen antagonists in breast tissue, but mimic estrogen in other tissues, such as uterine (eg, tamoxifen and toremifene), bone (eg, tamoxifen and raloxifene), and lipid tissue (eg, tamoxifen, toremifene, and raloxifene). Tamoxifen and toremifene can be used for treatment of breast cancer and risk reduction of breast cancer in high-risk patients. For cancer therapy, raloxifene is only indicated for risk reduction of invasive breast cancer in postmenopausal women at high risk of developing invasive breast cancer with or without osteoporosis. Adverse effects of SERMs include hot flashes, vaginal dryness, and thrombosis. Due to the estrogen-like effects on the uterus with tamoxifen and toremifene, endometrial hyperplasia is another potential adverse effect of these agents. Unlike SERMs, fulvestrant is a pure antiestrogen that down-regulates estrogen receptors and only has antagonist effects.

Aromatase Inhibitors

Aromatase inhibitors block estrogen production by inhibiting the enzyme aromatase, which is involved in the synthesis of estrogens from androstenedione.[53]

These agents are used mainly in postmenopausal women because the main source of estrogen in these women is from peripheral conversion of androstenedione into estrone and estradiol by aromatases. Anastrozole and letrozole are nonsteroidal agents that reversibly inactivate aromatase, while exemestane is a steroidal agent that permanently inactivates the enzyme. Common adverse effects of this class include bone loss/osteoporosis, hot flashes, arthralgias/myalgias, mild fatigue, and nausea.

Luteinizing Hormone Releasing Hormone Analogs and Antagonists

Chemical or surgical estrogen/androgen ablation is the common hormonal therapy in premenopausal women with breast cancer and men with prostate cancer, respectively.[19] Chemical castration is accomplished with the administration of luteinizing hormone releasing hormone (LHRH) analogs (leuprolide, goserelin, triptorelin). These drugs work by down-regulating LHRH receptors in the pituitary gland, subsequently leading to castrate levels of estrogens or testosterone. However, the initial administration of LHRH analogs can cause a flare response that stimulates cancer growth in the first few weeks due to the temporary rise in luteinizing hormone (LH) and follicle-stimulating hormone (FSH) levels.[19,54] Other side effects include hot flashes and bone loss, as well as amenorrhea in women and decreased libido (more commonly reported in men). Degarelix is an LHRH antagonist that reversibly binds to LHRH receptors in the pituitary gland, decreasing testosterone to castrate levels. It causes a rapid decrease in testosterone levels without a flare response. Liver enzyme increases and bone loss are common side effects.

Antiandrogens

Bicalutamide, flutamide, and nilutamide are nonsteroidal antiandrogens that competitively inhibit dihydrotestosterone and testosterone at their binding sites. These agents can be used as monotherapy or in addition to LHRH agonists in prostate cancer patients.[19] The combination of antiandrogens with LHRH analogs often reduce the flare symptoms associated with the administration of LHRH agonists. Adverse effects of the antiandrogens agents include hot flashes, gynecomastia, diarrhea, and liver function abnormalities. Enzalutamide, a second-generation antiandrogen, has a higher affinity for the androgen receptor and no agonist effects.[51] It is used in metastatic castration-resistant prostate cancer patients who have previously received docetaxel. Enzalutamide is associated with fatigue, diarrhea, flushing, and musculoskeletal pain. Abiraterone acetate is a prodrug that is hydrolyzed to abiraterone, a steroidal progesterone derivative that selectively and irreversibly inhibits CYP17A1 enzyme that is involved with testosterone production.[55-57] It is used in combination with prednisone for metastatic castration-resistant prostate cancer. Common side effects include joint swelling/discomfort, hypokalemia, edema, hot flushes, and diarrhea.

RESPONSE TO TREATMENT

Various terms are used to describe a patient's response to cancer therapies. Clinicians often describe these responses as a cure, complete response, partial response, stable disease, or progressive disease. **Table 1-5** includes some common definitions related to treatment response for solid tumors.[58,59] These response definition guidelines for solid tumors were developed to provide a more uniform reporting of tumor responses. The RECIST (response evaluation criteria in solid tumors) criteria were first developed in 2000 and then revised in 2009.

The response criteria for hematological tumors are different because they are not defined by measurable masses. Leukemias, lymphomas, and multiple myeloma responses are defined by the elimination of abnormal cells, return of tumor markers to normal levels, or improved function of affected organs (eg, normal peripheral blood counts). Additionally, measuring the cytogenetic response is often performed in patients with known cytogenetic abnormalities and is often correlated with disease relapse. The National Comprehensive Cancer Network Guidelines for Treatment of Cancer include response criteria and the corresponding supporting references in each of their cancer site guidelines.[60]

In addition, various survival end points are used to describe treatment responses. Overall survival, disease-free survival, progression-free survival, and clinical benefit response (Table 1-5) are all used to describe cancer treatment responses. The challenge to the clinical researcher is to correlate the patient's quality of life to these various responses.

Performance Status

One of the most likely factors to help predict response to chemotherapy is a patient-specific factor referred to as performance status. The presence or absence of other disease states affects the overall functional status of a patient, which has a great impact on patient response to cancer treatment. The overall functional status of a patient may be described using performances scales such as the Karnofsky score or the Eastern Cooperative Oncology Group (ECOG) scale (**Table 1-6**).[61-63] For many cancers, the patient's performance status at the time of diagnosis is the most important predictor of response.

Table 1-5 Common Definitions of Responses to Cancer Treatments[58,59]

Term	Definition
Cure	The patient is entirely free of disease and has the same life expectancy as a cancer-free individual.
Stable disease (SD)[a]	Solid tumor mass that is neither decreasing nor increasing in extent or severity.
Complete response (CR)[a]	Complete disappearance of all solid tumor masses without evidence of new disease for a least 1 month after treatment.
Partial response (PR)[a]	A 30% or greater decrease in the solid tumor size and no evidence of any new disease for at least 1 month.
Overall response (OR)[a]	CR + PR
Clinical benefit response	Subjective improvement in the symptoms caused by cancer without a defined response.
Progression free survival (PFS)	The length of time during and after treatment in which a patient is living with disease that does not get worse.
Overall survival (OS)	The percentage of people in a study or treatment group who are alive for a certain period of time after they were diagnosed with or treated for a disease.
Time to progression (TTP)	A measure of time after a disease is diagnosed (or treated) until it starts to get worse.

[a] Generally for solid tumors based on the RECIST criteria. For hematologic malignancies, see National Comprehensive Cancer Network guidelines for specific response criteria definitions.

Table 1-6 Performance Status Scales[61–63]

ECOG		Karnofsky		
Grade	**Description**	**Status**	**Score**	**Description**
			100%	Normal activity; no complaints; no evidence of disease.
0	Fully active, able to carry on all predisease performance without restriction.	Able to carry on normal activity and work; no special care needed.	90%	Able to carry on normal activity; minor signs or symptoms of disease.
1	Restricted in physically strenuous activity but ambulatory and able to carry out work of a light or sedentary nature (eg, light housework, office work).		80%	Normal activity with effort; some signs or symptoms of disease.
2	Ambulatory and capable of all self-care but unable to carry out any work activities. Up and about more than 50% of waking hours.		70%	Cares for self; unable to carry on normal activity or do active work.
3	Capable of only limited self-care, confined to bed or chair more than 50% of waking hours.	Unable to work; able to live at home and care for most personal needs; varying amount of assistance needed.	60%	Requires occasional assistance, but is able to care for most personal needs.
4	Completely disabled. Cannot carry on any self-care. Totally confined to bed or chair.		50%	Requires considerable assistance and frequent medical care.
5	Dead		40%	Disabled; requires special care and assistance.
			30%	Severely disabled; hospital admission is indicated; death not imminent.
		Unable to care for self; requires equivalent of institutional or hospital care; disease may be progressing rapidly.	20%	Very sick; hospital admission necessary; active supportive treatment necessary.
			10%	Moribund; fatal processes progressing rapidly.
			0%	Dead

SUMMARY

Carcinogenesis is a multistep process that includes initiation, promotion, transformation, and progression. Cancer therapy medications are the cornerstone of systemic treatment and include chemotherapy, hormonal therapy, biologic therapy, and targeted therapies. Typically, common toxicities are associated with a class of therapies that are often classified based on the mechanism of action. A thorough understanding of the mechanism of action and toxicity of cancer therapies as well as assessing the response to therapy is important for safe preparation and administration of the first and subsequent cycles of cancer therapy. Additional chapters in this text provide more details.

REFERENCES

1. American Cancer Society. Heredity and cancer. http://www.cancer.org/Cancer /CancerCauses/GeneticsandCancer/heredity-and-cancer. Revised March 28, 2013. Accessed June 13, 2013.
2. American Cancer Society. *Cancer Facts & Figures 2013*. Atlanta, GA: American Cancer Society; 2013.
3. US Department of Health and Human Services. Public Health Service, National Toxicology Program. *Report on Carcinogens*. 12th ed; 2011. http://ntp.niehs.nih.gov /ntp/roc/twelfth/roc12.pdf. Accessed June 13, 2013.
4. Liao JB. Viruses and human cancer. *Yale J Biol Med*. 2006; 79:115–122.
5. Initiative for Vaccine Research. Viral cancers. World Health Organization website. http://www.who.int/vaccine_research/diseases/viral_cancers/en/index1.html. Accessed June 13, 2013.
6. Schiffman M, Castle PE, Jeronimo J, Rodriguez AC, Wacholder S. Human papillomavirus and cervical cancer. *Lancet*. 2007; 370:890–907.
7. D'souza G, Dempscy A. The role of HPV in head and neck cancer and review of the HPV vaccine. *Prev Med*. 2011; 53(suppl 1):S5-S11.
8. American Cancer Society. Known and probable human carcinogens. http://www.cancer .org/cancer/cancercauses/othercarcinogens/generalinformationaboutcarcinogens /known-and-probable-human-carcinogens. Revised May 10, 2013. Accessed June 13, 2013.
9. Chabner BA, Chabner Thomson E. Cellular and molecular basis of cancer. The Merck Manual for Health Care Professionals website. http://www.merckmanuals.com /professional/hematology_and_oncology/overview_of_cancer/cellular_and_molecular _basis_of_cancer.html. Revised February 2013. Accessed June 13, 2013.
10. Cogliano VJ, Baan R, Straif K, et al. Preventable exposures associated with human cancers. *J Natl Cancer Inst*. 2011; 103:1827–1839.
11. National Cancer Institute. Endometrial cancer prevention (PDQ). http://www .cancer.gov/cancertopics/pdq/prevention/endometrial/HealthProfessional /page3#Section_159. Revised February 15, 2013. Accessed June 13, 2013.

12. Ruddon RW. *Cancer Biology.* 4th ed. New York, NY: Oxford University Press; 2007:78–94.

13. Zatonski WA, Lowenfels AB, Boyle P, et al. Epidemiologic aspects of gallbladder cancer: a case-control study of the SEARCH Program of the International Agency for Research on Cancer. *J Natl Cancer Inst.* 1997;89:1132–1138.

14. Oxnard GR, Lo PC, Nishinio M, et al. Natural history and molecular characteristics of lung cancers harboring EGFR exon 20 insertions. *J. Thorac Oncol.* 2013;8(2):179–184.

15. Munshi NC, Avet-Loiseau H. Genomics in multiple myeloma. *Clin Cancer Res.* 2011;17:1234–1242.

16. National Cancer Institution at the National Institutes of Health. Understanding cancer series. http://www.cancer.gov/cancertopics/understandingcancer/cancergenomics/AllPages. Accessed June 13, 2013.

17. Riley GJ, Marks J, Pao W. KRAS mutations in non–small cell lung cancer. *Proc Am Thor Soc.* 2009;6:201–205.

18. Weinberg RA. How cancer arises. *Sci Am.* 1996;275:62–71.

19. Medina PJ, Shord SS. Cancer treatment and chemotherapy. In: DiPiro JT, Talbert RL, Yee GC, et al, eds. *Pharmacotherapy: A Pathophysiologic Approach.* 8th ed. New York, NY: McGraw-Hill; 2011:2191–2228.

20. Yap TA, Sandhu SK, Workman P, de Bono JS. Envisioning the future of early anticancer drug development. *Nat Rev Cancer.* 2010;10:514–523.

21. Griggs J, Mangu P, Anderson H, et al. Appropriate chemotherapy dosing for obese patients with cancer: American society of clinical oncology clinical practice guideline. *J Clin Oncol.* 2012;30(13):1553–1561.

22. Liesveld J, Asselin B. It's all in the liposomes: vincristine gets a new package. *J Clin Oncol.* 2013;31:657–659.

23. Gligorov J, Lotz JP. Preclinical pharmacology of the taxanes: implications of the differences. *The Oncologist.* 2004;9(suppl 2):3–8.

24. Rowinsky E. Microtubule-targeting natural products. In: Kufe DW, Bast RC, Hait WN, et al, eds. *Cancer Medicine.* 7th ed. Hamilton, Ont, Canada: BC Decker; 2006:699–721.

25. Verweij J, Clavel M, Chevalier B. Paclitaxel (Taxol) and docetaxel (Taxotere): not simply two of a kind. *Ann Oncol.* 1994;5:495–505.

26. Lexi-Comp Online. Lexi-Drugs Online. Hudson, OH: Lexi-Comp, Inc. http://online.lexi.com/. Accessed June 13, 2013.

27. DRUGDEX System [Internet database]. Greenwood Village, CO: Thomson Healthcare. Accessed June 13, 2013.

28. National Comprehensive Cancer Network templates. Available at: http://www.nccn.org/ordertemplates/default.asp. Accessed June 13, 2013.

29. Eberly AL, Anderson GD, Bubalo JS, Mccune JS. Optimal prevention of seizures induced by high-dose busulfan. *Pharmacotherapy.* 2008;28(12):1502–1510.

30. Richards D, Coleman J, Reynolds J, Coleman J. *Oxford Handbook of Practical Drug Therapy.* New York, NY: Oxford University Press; 2011:576.

31. Lam MS. The need for routine bleomycin test dosing in the 21st century. *Ann Pharmacother.* 2005;39(11):1897–1902.

32. Santoso JT, Lucci JA III, Coleman RL, Schafer I, Hannigan EV. Saline, mannitol, and furosemide hydration in acute cisplatin nephrotoxicity: a randomized trial. *Cancer Chemother Pharmacol.* 2003;52:13–18.

33. Lenz HJ. Management and preparedness for infusion and hypersensitivity reactions. *Oncologist.* 2007;12:601–609.

34. Preston JN, Trivedi MV. Eribulin: a novel cytotoxic chemotherapy agent. *Ann Pharmacother.* 2012;46:802–811.

35. Dahllof B, Billstrom A, Cabral F, Hartley-Asp B. Estramustine depolymerizes microtubules by binding to tubulin. *Cancer Res.* 1993;53:4573–4581.

36. Dorr RT, Von Hoff DD. *Cancer Chemotherapy Handbook.* 2nd ed. Norwalk, CT: Appleton & Lange; 1994.

37. Hensley ML, Hagerty KL, Kewalramani T, Slack JA. American Society of Clinical Oncology clinical practice guideline update: use of chemotherapy and radiation therapy protectants. *J Clin Oncol.* 2009;27:127–145.

38. Cheson BD, Rummel MJ. Bendamustine: rebirth of an old drug. *J Clin Oncol.* 2009;27:1492–1501.

39. Tsang LLH, Farmer PB, Gescher A, et al. Characterization of urinary metabolites of temozolomide in humans and mice and evaluation of their cytotoxicity. *Cancer Chemother Pharmacol.* 1990;26:429–436.

40. Rixe O, Ortuzar W, Alvarez M, et al. Oxaliplatin, tetraplatin, cisplatin, and carboplatin: spectrum of activity in drug-resistant cell lines and in the cell lines of the National Cancer Institute's Anticancer Drug Screen panel. *Biochem Pharmacol.* 1996;52:1855–1865.

41. Calvert AH, Newell DR, Gumbrell LA, et al. Carboplatin dosage: prospective evaluation of a simple formula based on renal function. *J Clin Oncol.* 1989;7:1748–1756.

42. Grothey A, Goldberg RM. A review of oxaliplatin and its clinical use in colorectal cancer. *Expert Opin Pharmacother.* 2004;5:2159–2170.

43. Brundage D. Cancer chemotherapy and treatment. In: Chisolm-Burns MA, Schwinghammer TL, Wells BG, et al, eds. *Pharmacotherapy: Principles & Practice.* 2nd ed. New York, NY: McGraw-Hill; 2010:1445–1474.

44. Keefe DL. Anthracycline-induced cardiomyopathy. *Semin Oncol.* 2001;28:2–7.

45. Emadi A, Gore SD. Arsenic trioxide—an old drug rediscovered. *Blood Rev.* 2010; 24:191–199.

46. Holle LM. Pegaspargase: an alternative? *Ann Pharmacother.* 1995;29:1042–1044.

47. Kavanaugh SA, White LA, Kolesar JM. Vorinostat: a novel therapy for the treatment of cutaneous T-cell lymphoma. *Am J Health-Syst Pharm.* 2010;67:793–797.

48. American Medical Association. Monoclonal antibodies. http://www.ama-assn.org//ama/pub/physician-resources/medical-science/united-states-adopted-names-council/naming-guidelines/naming-biologics/monoclonal-antibodies_page. Accessed June 13, 2013.

49. Paul M, Mukhopadhyay AK. Tyrosine kinase—role and significance in cancer. *Int J Med Sci.* 2004;1:101–115.

50. Wood LS. Managing the side effects of sorafenib and sunitinib. *Comm Oncol.* 2006;3:558–562.

51. FDA Approved Drugs.http://www.centerwatch.com/drug-information/fda-approvals/. Accessed June 13, 2013.

52. Thyrell L, Hjortsberg L, Arulampalam V, et al. Mechanisms of Interferon-alpha induced apoptosis in malignant cells. *Oncogene.* 2002;21:1251–1262.

53. Michaud LB, Barnett CM, Esteva FJ. Breast cancer. In: DiPiro JT, Talbert RL, Yee GC, et al, eds. *Pharmacotherapy: A Pathophysiologic Approach.* 8th ed. New York, NY: McGraw-Hill; 2011:2229–2270.

54. Weckermann D, Harzmann R. Hormone therapy in prostate cancer: LHRH antagonists versus LHRH analogues. *Eur Urol.* 2004;46:279–283.

55. Ryan CJ, Cheng ML. Abiraterone acetate for the treatment of prostate cancer. *Expert Opin Pharmacother.* 2013;14:91–96.

56. Ryan CJ, Smith MR, de Bono JS, et al. Abiraterone in metastatic prostate cancer without previous chemotherapy. *N Engl J Med.* 2013;368:138–148.

57. De Bono JS, Logothetis CJ, Molina A, et al. Abiraterone and increased survival in metastatic prostate cancer. *N Engl J Med.* 2011;364:1995–2005.

58. Therasse P, Arbuck SG, Eisenhauer EA, et al. New guidelines to evaluate the response to treatment in solid tumors. *J Natl Cancer Inst.* 2009;92:205–216.

59. Eisenhauer EA, Therasse P, Bogaerts J, et al. New response evaluation criteria in solid tumours: revised RECIST guideline (version 1.1). *Eur J Cancer.* 2009;45:228–247.

60. National Comprehensive Cancer Network Clinical Practice Guidelines in Oncology. http://www.nccn.org/clinical.asp. Accessed June 13, 2013.

61. Karnofsky DA, Burchenal JH. The clinical evaluation of chemotherapeutic agents in cancer. In: Macleod CM, ed. *Evaluation of Chemotherapeutic Agents.* New York, NY: Columbia University Press. 1949;199–205.

62. Oken MM, Creech RH, Tormey DC, et al. Toxicity and response criteria of the Eastern Cooperative Oncology Group. *Am J Clin Oncol.* 1982;5:649–655.

63. Schag CC, Heinrich RL, Ganz PA. Karnosky performance status revised: reliability, validity and guidelines. *J Clin Oncol.* 1994;2:187–193.

SUGGESTED READING

- Perry MC, Doll DC, Freter CE. *Chemotherapy Source Book.* 5th ed. Philadelphia, PA: Lippincott Williams & Wilkins; 2012.
- Skeel RT, Khleif SN. *Handbook of Cancer Chemotherapy.* 8th ed. Philadelphia, PA: Lippincott Williams & Wilkins; 2011.
- Package inserts for individual drugs.

CHAPTER 2

Basics of Systemic Anticancer Therapy Prescribing and Verification

Trinh Pham
Joan Rivington

LEARNING OBJECTIVES

Upon completion of the chapter, the reader will be able to:

1. Write clear and concise anticancer therapy prescriptions that reduce the risk of errors.
2. Effectively review anticancer therapy prescriptions with the recognition of essential elements that should be included in the prescription.
3. Identify the components that should be included in a prescription for oral cancer therapy.
4. Identify the potential risks for errors with intrathecal drug prescribing, verification, and administration.
5. Identify supportive care measures and ancillary drugs that should be considered in anticancer therapy prescriptions.

INTRODUCTION

Over the last decades, systemic anticancer therapy options have expanded and improved significantly, resulting in the development of more complex treatment regimens. Many of the anticancer regimens include traditional cytotoxic chemotherapy in conjunction with biologic, immunologic, and targeted therapy in some combination or sequence to inhibit cancer cell growth at various steps. Because of the complexity of the treatment regimens, the narrow therapeutic window of the anticancer agents, and the potential for serious and fatal consequences of anticancer therapy medication errors, it is essential that oncology practices have in place a systematic approach in prescribing and verifying anticancer therapy that prevents medication errors when providing treatment for cancer patients. The goal of cancer therapy is to ensure the delivery of the right drug in the right dose and dosage form at the right time to the right patient.[1] The achievement of this goal requires establishing and implementing specific policies and procedures for the process of cancer therapy prescribing, verification, dispensing, and administration with the involvement of a multidisciplinary team (physicians, physician assistants, nurses, and pharmacists). The purpose of this chapter is to provide recommendations that ensure safe prescribing, dispensing, and administration of anticancer therapies. Cancer therapy drug administration is provided to patients both in the outpatient and inpatient settings; thus, the recommendations provided in this chapter will refer to both of these settings inclusively as the practice site. The following topics will be addressed in this chapter:

- The role of education and training of oncology healthcare providers
- Anticancer therapy prescribing (role of the prescriber) and verification (role of pharmacists and nurses)
- Strategies to prevent errors in anticancer therapy prescriptions including parenteral, oral, and intrathecal orders
- Precautions with intrathecal anticancer regimens
- Supportive care and ancillary agents for anticancer therapy

ONCOLOGY TRAINING

An unrestricted registered nurse license qualifies a nurse to practice anywhere in the United States; however, individual hospitals and oncology practices may stipulate additional chemotherapy competency requirements in order to practice in an oncology specialty. The Oncology Nursing Society (ONS) offers a chemotherapy and biotherapy program to prepare nurses to administer chemotherapy to patients and fulfills the continuing education requirement of the basic oncology nursing certification exams. The Oncology Nursing Certification Corporation (ONCC) offers the following five certification examinations in the field of oncology: (1) Oncology Certified Nurse (OCN), (2) Certified Pediatric Hematology Oncology Nurse (CPHON), (3) Certified Breast Care Nurse (CBCN), (4) Advanced Oncology Certified Nurse Practitioner (AOCNP), and (5) Advanced Oncology Certified Clinical Nurse Specialist (AOCNS). The certification program allows nurses to gain professional credentials in the field of oncology.

For a pharmacist to become licensed and registered he/she must pass the North American Pharmacist Licensure Examination (NAPLEX) and the Multistate Pharmacy Jurisprudence Exam (MPJE) for the state in which he/she wishes to practice. The license qualifies the pharmacist to practice in all areas of pharmacy; however, residency training in different specialty areas is offered after completion of pharmacy school and attainment of a registered pharmacist license. In oncology, a 1-year oncology specialty residency (postgraduate year 2, PGY2) is available to licensed pharmacists after completion of a general practice pharmacy residency (postgraduate year 1, PGY1). Furthermore, board certification in oncology pharmacy (BCOP) is available for all licensed pharmacists (completion of a residency is not a prerequisite) and is provided by the Board of Pharmacy Specialties. The American College of Clinical Pharmacy, the American Society of Health-System Pharmacists, and the Hematology/Oncology Pharmacy Association provides oncology preparatory and recertification courses, and information about these programs is available at their respective websites. As with nursing, a registered pharmacist license allows the practitioner to practice anywhere in the United States, but certain hospitals and oncology practices may require BCOP or residency training as a stipulation for employment to practice in the oncology specialty area.

For physicians, 3-year oncology and hematology fellowships are offered through many schools of medicine in affiliation with major cancer centers and hospitals to provide clinical and basic research training for MDs or MD/PhDs. Physicians are also eligible for board certification in oncology, hematology, or both through the American Board of Internal Medicine (ABIM). At the time of application for certification in hematology or oncology, the physician has to be previously certified in internal medicine by ABIM; satisfactorily complete the requisite graduate medical education fellowship training; demonstrate clinical competence, procedural skills, and moral and ethical behavior in the clinical setting; hold a valid, unrestricted, and unchallenged license to practice medicine; and pass the hematology or oncology certification examination.

Table 2-1 Recommended Websites for Oncology Education and Oncology Certification Information

Nurses

Education program	www.ons.org/CNECentral/Chemo
Certification program	www.oncc.org

Pharmacists

Education programs	www.accp.com/education/oncologyCourses.aspx www.ashp.org/menu/Education/Certifications /OncologyCourse.aspx www.hoparx.org/education/default/bcop-recert.html
Certification program	www.bpsweb.org

Physicians

Certification program	www.abim.org

Physician Assistants

Certification program	Currently, no certificate of added qualifications in oncology

A physician assistant (PA) is a graduate of an accredited PA educational program who is nationally certified and state licensed to practice medicine with the direction and responsible supervision of a doctor of medicine or osteopathy. All 50 states and the District of Columbia allow PAs to practice and prescribe medications. Practicing PAs must complete 100 hours of continuing medical education every 2 years. PAs must be authorized by the state (licensed, certified, or registered) before they can begin practice. All the states and the District of Columbia require that applicants meet the following criteria: (1) graduation from an accredited PA program; and (2) passage of the National Commission on Certification of physician assistant Physician Assistant National Certifying Exam (PANCE). Currently, there is no certification with added qualifications in oncology for physician assistants and no formal training requirements for PAs to work in oncology. The majority of PAs specializing in the field of oncology receive training through direct mentorship by their supervising physician and self-study.[2] There are few postgraduate PA oncology programs available in the United States, and 2 example programs include the MD Anderson Cancer Center Postgraduate PA Program in Oncology and the Mayo Clinic Postgraduate PA Fellowship in Hospital Internal Medicine with an optional hematology/oncology track. See **Table 2-1** for websites with oncology training information.

EDUCATION

Knowledge is empowering, and the maintenance of continuing education by healthcare professionals involved in cancer treatment encourages active engagement and critical thinking in the prescribing and assessment of anticancer therapies. Before healthcare professionals are allowed the privilege of prescribing, dispensing, or administering anticancer therapy they should undergo training, certification, and orientation to gain competency to perform these functions. Institutions that treat cancer patients should have a process that confirms staff and trainees have been appropriately educated and are qualified to prescribe, dispense, or administer anticancer therapy. Furthermore, professional continuing education (CE) opportunities should be available, proof of annual completion of CE should be required, and annual reassessment of basic competencies should be performed so that employers can ascertain that healthcare professionals are up to date with their knowledge base of anticancer therapy. Lastly, policies and procedures should be reviewed periodically to ensure that the oncology practice has incorporated technological advances or contemporary information on newly approved anticancer agents to ensure that the healthcare professionals are performing their responsibilities with current information.

Healthcare providers practicing in the field of oncology should be knowledgeable and have current information available about the following aspects of the anticancer therapies:

1. The principles involved in treating patients with cancer
2. The basics of anticancer therapy:
    a. Names of the anticancer therapy formulations
    b. Mechanisms of action
    c. Appropriate dosages (maximum dose when applicable)
    d. Routes of administration
    e. Administration schedules
3. Indications for the anticancer therapy, which may be clarified from:
    a. Food and Drug Administration (FDA) –approved indication
    b. Standard anticancer therapy protocols commonly used for specific diagnosis
    c. Data from clinical trials
    d. Investigational drug protocols
4. Preparation, storage, and transportation of anticancer therapy
5. Appropriate and safe handling of anticancer therapy

6. Potential adverse effects:
   a. Principles of prevention and management
   b. Early identification of adverse events
   c. Ongoing monitoring
7. Potential drug interactions

CANCER THERAPY PRESCRIBING

The prescription for an anticancer regimen is initiated by a physician or a non-physician healthcare provider, such as nurse practitioners or physician assistants, with prescribing privileges. The prescribing of cancer therapy should be restricted to providers with appropriate oncology education and clinical privileges. At least one other medically responsible individual who is knowledgeable about medical oncology should countersign cancer therapy orders prescribed by physicians in training and nonphysician healthcare providers. The verification by the countersigner should include confirmation that the correct treatment is being initiated along with checking the appropriateness of the dose, administration schedule, and any modifications from planned or expected treatment.[3] Because of the inherent risk of misinterpretation and circumvention of a checkpoint in the order-verification process, oral communication of cancer therapy prescription orders (verbal orders) by the prescriber should not be permitted by the practice site except to hold or stop anticancer therapy.[3-5]

There are many factors involved in choosing the best cancer therapy for a particular patient, and these factors include the patient's cancer diagnosis, stage of the disease, comorbidities, performance status, and organ function. Furthermore, cancer therapy prescribing is a complex process because in addition to standard anticancer regimens for a specific cancer diagnosis, in some instances, the treatment regimens may be derived from preliminary research reports (published abstracts), published studies, and clinical trials. In these instances the indications, dosages, and administration schedules may differ amongst the varying publications or from FDA-approved product labeling. Thus, in prescribing cancer therapy, it is crucial that the chosen treatment regimen is clearly communicated to the patient and all members of the healthcare team to prevent medication errors and ensure safe preparation, dispensing, and administration of the anticancer drugs. Documentation of the cancer therapy prescription should include why a regimen was chosen for a patient, and a reference source for the chosen regimen should be readily available. When a patient's treatment deviates from the standard of care or a referenced source, the rationale for the change should be documented to facilitate the verification process and prevent misinterpretation of the prescribed regimen by other members of the healthcare team. The following section provides recommendations on factors to consider and policies to implement to ensure safe treatment of cancer patients.

Computerized Provider-Order-Entry for Anticancer Agents

In order to prevent anticancer therapy errors, the *American Society of Clinical Oncology/Oncology Nursing Society Chemotherapy Administration Safety Standards Including Standards for the Safe Administration and Management of Oral Chemotherapy* recommend that practice sites maintain and use standardized, regimen-level, preprinted or electronic forms for all parenteral anticancer prescription writing.[4] Standardized forms simplify and expedite anticancer prescribing because well-designed, organized forms prompt prescribers to approach anticancer therapy in a clear, consistent, and uniform manner and reduce errors that may occur in the transcription process. The standardized forms should contain information such as the following:

- The patient's name and unique identifying number (date of birth or medical record number)
- The date the order was written
- The diagnosis
- The regimen name and cycle number
- Protocol name and number (if applicable)
- Appropriate criteria to treat (eg, based on relevant laboratory results and toxicities)
- Allergies
- Reference to the methodology of dose calculation or standard practice equations (eg, calculation of creatinine clearance)
- Height, weight, and any other variables used to calculate the dose
- Dosage (doses do not include trailing zeros; use a leading zero for doses less than 1 mg [eg, 0.5 mg])
- Route and rate (if applicable) of administration
- Length of infusion (if applicable)
- Supportive care treatments appropriate for the regimen (including premedications, hydration, growth factors, and hypersensitivity medications)
- Sequence of administration (if applicable).[4]

Additional information that may be helpful includes the date and time the treatments are to be administered, patient-specific laboratory values from which the dosage is calculated, and lastly, the prescriber's name, signature, and contact information. These standardized forms may be incorporated into e-prescribing software or electronic health records.[4] If available, computerized provider-order entry (CPOE) provides the same safety and convenience features as preprinted, standardized order forms with additional advantages such as eliminating illegible and incomplete orders, ensuring completeness in prescribing fields, and facilitating efficient prescription order processing through simultaneous, instantaneous transmission of the prescription order to various members of the healthcare team, such as pharmacy or nursing, or to geographically distant sites.[6] In addition to medication prescribing, CPOE systems may include other built-in functions such as diagnostic test ordering along with clinician alerts to prevent errors and to assist with adherence to current clinical practice guidelines.

A discussion on the process of implementing a CPOE system is beyond the scope of this chapter. The following readings are recommended for a thorough review on CPOE: *ASHP Guidelines on Pharmacy Planning for Implementation of Computerized Provider-Order-Entry Systems in Hospitals and Health Systems; A Consensus Statement on Considerations for a Successful CPOE Implementation;* and *CPOE Configuration to Reduce Medication Errors: A Literature Review on the Safety of CPOE Systems and Design Recommendations.*[6-8]

Strategies to Prevent Errors in Cancer Therapy Prescribing

Application of some practical strategies in writing cancer therapy prescriptions can prevent medication errors. When cancer therapy drugs are ordered, the full name of the drug should be used, and the generic name is preferred over brand names, nicknames, or abbreviations. The exception to this rule may apply in instances when there is potential for confusion between different formulations of the same drug.[5] The *ASCO/ONS Chemotherapy Administration Safety Standards* recommend that all medications within cancer therapy order sets and prescriptions are listed using full generic names and follow Joint Commission standards regarding abbreviations.[4] The standards further state that brand names should be included with the generic name only in orders where there are multiple products or including the brand name otherwise assists in identifying a unique drug formulation.[4] See **Clinical Pearl 2-1**.

In the field of oncology, the use of acronyms and abbreviations to designate cancer therapy regimens is pervasive (**Table 2-2**). However, because of the possibility of confusion and misinterpretation, this practice is not recommended when prescribing systemic anticancer therapy or for clinical documentation.[3]

Cancer therapy orders should inclusively list all chemotherapy agents in the regimen and their individual dosing parameters.[4] When writing the frequency of administration of a cancer regimen, abbreviations should not be used (eg, write *daily,* not *QD* or *every other day,* not *QOD,* because this may be mistaken as *QID* and patients may receive 4 doses a day instead of the intended once daily or every other day schedule).

CLINICAL PEARL 2-1
Abbreviations, Brand Name, Class Name, or Chemical Name

Some examples of when errors may occur when abbreviations, brand names, or nicknames are used:

- Does **Paraplatin** refer to cisplatin or carboplatin?
- Does **CDDP** refer to carboplatin or cisplatin?
- Does **CPT-11** refer to cisplatin or irinotecan?
- Does **Taxol** refer to paclitaxel or docetaxel?
- Does **vinca alkaloid** refer to vincristine, vinblastine, or vinorelbine?
- Does **anthracycline** refer to doxorubicin, daunorubicin, idarubicin, or epirubicin?
- **Adria** (doxorubicin) may be misunderstood for **Aredia** (pamidronate)
- **G-CSF** is the abbreviation for *"granulocyte colony-stimulating factor"*

  - Filgrastim and pegfilgrastim are both **G-CSF** products with different doses and schedules
  - Filgrastim (**Neupogen**) is a short-acting agent and is administered on a daily basis
  - Pegfilgrastim (**Neulasta**) is a long-acting agent and is dosed only once per cycle of cancer therapy
  - The use of the abbreviation *G-CSF* should be avoided because of ambiguity of which CSF is indicated, filgrastim or pegfilgrastim.
  - The generic name or brand name should be used to avoid confusion and ensure that the intended, ordered drug is dispensed and administered.

Exceptions to the Rule—When Brand Name May Be More Appropriate

- **Abraxane** is the trade name for *paclitaxel protein-bound particles for injectable suspension (albumin bound)*

  - The dose for conventional paclitaxel and **Abraxane** is not the same.
  - Using the generic name, *albumin-bound paclitaxel,* may lead to the conventional paclitaxel being erroneously dispensed or administered instead of **Abraxane** or vice versa.
  - Add the trade name **Abraxane** to the generic name, *albumin-bound paclitaxel,* in prescription orders to ensure that the correct drug is dispensed.

- **Doxil** is the trade name for *liposomal doxorubicin*

  - The dose for conventional doxorubicin and **Doxil** is not the same.
  - Using the generic name, *liposomal doxorubicin,* to order **Doxil** may lead to the conventional doxorubicin being erroneously dispensed.
  - Add the trade name **Doxil** to the generic name, *liposomal doxorubicin,* in prescription orders to ensure that the correct drug is dispensed.

- **Kadcyla** is the trade name for *ado-trastuzumab emtansine.*

  - The dose for trastuzumab (Herceptin) and **Kadcyla** is not the same.
  - Using the generic name for *ado-trastuzumab emtansine* to order **Kadcyla** may lead to trastuzumab (Herceptin) erroneously being dispensed.
  - Add the trade name **Kadcyla** to the generic name, *ado-trastuzumab emtansine,* in prescription orders to ensure that the correct drug is dispensed.

Abbreviations for Common Cancer Agents
(*Do Not* Use Abbreviations to Order Cancer Therapy)

Abbreviation	Generic Name
Anti-CD20	Rituximab
Ara-C	Cytarabine
BCNU	Carmustine
C-225	Cetuximab
CDDP	Cisplatin
CPT-11	Irinotecan
ESA	Erythropoiesis-stimulating agents • Epoetin (Procrit, Epogen) • Darbepoetin (Aranesp)
5-FU	Fluorouracil
Folinic acid	Calcium leucovorin
G-CSF	Granulocyte colony-stimulating factor • Filgrastim (Neupogen) • Pegfilgrastim (Neulasta)
MTX	Methotrexate
VCR	Vincristine
VP-16	Etoposide

Table 2-2 Abbreviations for Commonly Used Anticancer Regimens

Abbreviation	Regimen	Disease
ABVD	Adriamycin (doxorubicin) Bleomycin Vinblastine Dacarbazine	Hodgkin's lymphoma
BEACOPP	Bleomycin Etoposide Adriamycin (doxorubicin) Cyclophosphamide Oncovin (vincristine) Procarbazine Prednisone	Hodgkin's lymphoma

(*continues*)

Table 2-2 Abbreviations for Commonly Used Anticancer Regimens (*continued*)

Abbreviation	Regimen	Disease
R-CHOP	Rituximab Cyclophosphamide Hydroxydaunorubicin (another name for doxorubicin) Oncovin (vincristine) Prednisone	Non-Hodgkin's lymphoma **Note:** R-CHOP: every 21 days R-CHOP-14: every 14 days
CVP	Cyclophosphamide Vincristine Prednisone	Non-Hodgkin's lymphoma
R-FCM	Rituximab Fludarabine Cyclophosphamide Mitoxantrone	Non-Hodgkin's lymphoma
EPOCH	Etoposide Prednisone Oncovin (vincristine) Cyclophosphamide Hydroxydaunorubicin (another name for doxorubicin)	Non-Hodgkin's lymphoma
AC-T	Adriamycin (doxorubicin) Cyclophosphamide Taxol (paclitaxel)	Breast cancer
TAC	Taxotere (docetaxel) Adriamycin (doxorubicin) Cyclophosphamide	Breast cancer
TC	Taxotere (docetaxel) Cyclophosphamide	Breast cancer
MVAC	Methotrexate Vinblastine Adriamycin (doxorubicin) Cisplatin	Bladder cancer
EOX	Epirubicin Oxaliplatin Xeloda (capecitabine)	Gastric cancer
ECF	Epirubicin Cisplatin Fluorouracil	Gastric cancer

FOLFOX	Folinic acid (leucovorin) Fluorouracil Oxaliplatin	Colorectal cancer
FOLFIRI	Folinic acid (leucovorin) Fluorouracil Irinotecan	Colorectal cancer
FOLFIRINOX	Folinic acid (leucovorin) Fluorouracil Irinotecan Oxaliplatin	Pancreatic cancer
7+3	Cytarabine for 7 days Idarubicin or daunorubicin for 3 days	Acute myelogenous leukemia
HDAC	High-dose Ara-C (cytarabine, cytosine arabinoside)	Acute myelogenous leukemia

The Prescribing Vocabulary—Anticancer Therapy Regimen Cycle

A cycle of an anticancer regimen is a period of treatment followed by a period of rest before the treatment is repeated again. There are 3 factors to consider in a cycle—the duration, frequency, and number of cycles. The duration is the number of days the anticancer agents are administered within a cycle. The frequency refers to when the cycle is repeated, such as every 7, 14, 21, or 28 days. The number of cycles refers to the length of therapy from start to finish; for example, this may be 4 to 6 cycles for the treatment of breast cancer. When numbering treatment days, day 1 typically describes the day treatment commences. For hematopoietic progenitor-cell transplantation regimens, day 0 refers to the day stem cells are infused and anticancer therapy is typically administered prior to day 0 and is preceded by a negative sign (see **Clinical Pearl 2-2**).

Within a cycle of an anticancer regimen it is critical to write prescriptions for intended daily dose instead of total dose over a period of time to minimize the possibility of error. For example, the order, *cisplatin 100 mg/m² over 4 days,* is ambiguous, may lead to overdosing error, and cause severe toxicity or fatality. The intention of the order is to administer 25 mg/m² daily for 4 days (total of 100 mg/m² for the cycle). As written, the order may be misinterpreted, dispensed, and administered as 100 mg/m² daily for 4 days (total of 400 mg/m² for the cycle). To avoid errors, anticancer therapy prescriptions should be written with the specified dose per meter squared for *each* day instead of the total dose for the cycle. The route, rate, and duration of administration should also be indicated. Healthcare

CLINICAL PEARL 2-2
Numbering of Treatment Days of High Dose Cancer Therapy with Stem Cell Transplant

The labeling of the days of treatment for a high-dose B̲CNU (carmustine), e̲toposide, A̲ra-c, m̲elphalan (BEAM) regimen for autologous peripheral stem cell transplant is shown below. The days prior to stem cell transplant are referred to as negative days and the days post–stem cell transplant are positive days.

Day −6	Day −5	Day −4	Day −3	Day −2	Day −1	Day 0	Day +1	Day +2
BCNU	Etoposide Ara-C	Etoposide Ara-C	Etoposide Ara-C	Ara-C	Melphalan	Stem cell infusion		

providers involved with anticancer drug therapy should be aware of the usual maximum dose limits for individual agents per dose and cycle along with the maximum lifetime cumulative dose for specific agents (eg, anthracyclines and bleomycin). Additionally, when communicating dosing schedules, a dash mark should not be used (eg, day 1 *through* 8 or day 1 *and* 8 should be used; *not* days 1-8). Thus, to minimize the risk of errors, the correct order for a patient with a BSA of 2 m^2 should read, "cisplatin IV 25 mg/m^2/day (dose = 50 mg) in 500 mL 0.9% sodium chloride injection to run over 2 hours day 1 through 4. Start on 4/1/2013."

Care should also be taken to distinguish the same protocol with different cycle frequency such as CHOP (cyclophosphamide, hydroxydaunorubicin [doxorubicin], Oncovin [vincristine], prednisone) versus CHOP14, where CHOP is administered every 21 days and CHOP14 is administered every 14 days.

Dose Calculation

A priori, the institution/clinical practice should establish criteria for whether a dose should be routinely calculated based on ideal body weight, adjusted body weight, or actual body weight, and which equation will be used to calculate body surface area (BSA) for dosing (refer to the *Dosing Calculations* chapter elsewhere in this text). When the dose of an anticancer agent is calculated based on a weight different from established criteria, the prescription order should indicate which weight was used in calculating drug dosages.[3] If the dose or administration schedule of an anticancer agent is modified due to a specific toxicity or organ pathology, the cancer therapy prescription should explicitly indicate the factor that prompted the treatment modification.[3] It is essential to note that doses for anticancer agents can vary tremendously for different disease states or even the same tumor type that is treated by different protocols, and this difference in dosing is a potential source of medication errors (**Clinical Pearl 2-3**).[9] This emphasizes the need for clear documentation and reference citation of the prescribed regimen against which the order will be verified. Finally, all doses should be calculated independently by the prescriber who writes the order, the pharmacist who prepares the drug, and the nurse who administers it.[1]

CLINICAL PEARL 2-3
Variations in Dosing of Anticancer Drugs
Metastatic Colorectal Cancer

There are many variations of the FOLFOX regimen for the adjuvant treatment of colorectal cancer. Clinicians should be aware of these differences since the dosing and schedule of administration is different depending on the regimen. Furthermore, when writing prescription orders for these regimens, the clinician should document the specific regimen that is intended for the patient and the reference source. The FOLFOX4 and FOLFOX6 regimens that follow are only 2 examples of many possible variations for this specific regimen.

FOLFOX4

Leucovorin 200 mg/m^2 IV over 2 hours before fluorouracil, day 1 and 2

Fluorouracil 400 mg/m^2 IV bolus and then 600 mg/m^2/day IV over 22 hours, day 1 and 2

Oxaliplatin 85 mg/m^2 IV day 1

Every 2 weeks × 12 cycles

FOLFOX6

Leucovorin 400 mg/m^2 IV over 2 hours before fluorouracil day 1

Fluorouracil 400 mg/m^2 IV bolus day 1 followed by 2400 mg/m^2/dose IV over 46 hours

Oxaliplatin 100 mg/m^2 in 500 mL dextrose 5% IV over 2 hours day 1

Every 2 weeks × 12 cycles

Once the dose of an anticancer agent has been calculated, excessive attempt at precision in dose ordering should be avoided, and doses greater than 5 mg should be rounded to the nearest integer or nearest reasonable amount. For example, for oxaliplatin, write for a dose of 130 mg when the calculated dose is 127.5 mg; or write for a dose of 525 mg for a calculated dose of 521.6 mg for fluorouracil.[5] Consider rounding to certain percentage changes from the actual calculated dose. For instance, policies and procedures from the institution may allow rounding between 5% and 10% to allow dosing that can be more accurately measured. There is a lack of data regarding appropriateness of dose rounding, but clinically, many institutions allow rounding within this range. Additionally, whether the therapy is curative or noncurative may help to guide dose rounding. Use a leading zero, *not* a leading decimal, when the dose is *less* than 1 mg or 1 g (eg, write *0.1 mg* to prevent reading .1 mg as 1 mg). *Do not* use a trailing zero when writing orders (eg, write *10 mg*, not *10.0 mg* to prevent misinterpretation as 100 mg).[3–5]

References

Orders for noninvestigational anticancer medications should be verified against published standards (eg, published primary reference in professional journals or meeting proceedings, validated standard reference texts, investigational drug treatment protocol). In order for nonprescribing personnel to be able to independently verify the prescriber's orders for a cancer therapy, all members of the healthcare team should have access to complete, up-to-date copies of published articles for a referenced regimen, validated reference texts for standard anticancer therapy regimens by diagnosis, institutional review board– (IRB-) approved clinical research protocols or guidelines for investigational studies, and drug information references.[3,4] When a primary reference is not available for verification of a cancer therapy regimen, 2 alternative publications, such as a tertiary reference (textbook) and secondary reference (review article), may be used. Two alternative references are recommended because of the possibility of errors that may occur in the publication process.

Investigational Anticancer Regimens or Medications

Cancer patients often receive investigational anticancer agents as part of their treatment. Institutions that have an active cancer clinical trials program should apply the same safety precautions for the prescribing, verifying, preparing, and administration of investigational cancer regimens/agents as for standard FDA-approved agents. Prior to the implementation of a new IRB-approved investigational study protocol, all healthcare professionals involved should receive protocol-specific information through an educational in-service and an up-to-date copy of the protocol should be readily available for review by all involved with the study protocol. A more in-depth discussion on the policies and procedures related to management and maintenance of an investigational drug service is discussed in the *Investigational Drugs* chapter, elsewhere in this text.

CANCER THERAPY VERIFICATION

The process of cancer therapy verification requires the pharmacist and nurse to independently double check the original anticancer therapy regimen written by the prescriber against published standards. The prescribed anticancer therapy regimen should be evaluated for completeness, agreement with the planned regimen, and deviations from previous treatments for repeated cycles of the regimen. A checklist of the verification process is included in **Table 2-3** and potential sources of errors are illustrated in **Clinical Pearl 2-4**.[3,4,10] For other potential sources of errors, see the *Drug Safety and Risk Management* chapter, elsewhere in this text. The practice site should establish guidelines for the frequency of obtaining a patient's weight and specifications for when a dose should be adjusted based on the percentage of weight fluctuation. The anticancer therapy treatment plan should also indicate regimen-specific laboratory tests, including the time interval, to obtain based upon existing evidence-based national guidelines (eg, the American Society of Clinical Oncology [ASCO], the National Comprehensive Cancer Network [NCNN], and the Children's Oncology Group [COG]). When no evidence-based guideline exists, the practice site should determine best practice for its specific institution.[3,4] There are multiple risk points in the process of anticancer therapy prescribing, verification, dispensing, and administration. The implementation of a double checking policy serves as a safeguard to ensure accuracy and appropriateness of an anticancer regimen prior to completion of the prescription order for dispensing and administration. At the prescribing level, double checking occurs when a second prescriber countersigns a prescription that is written by a physician in training or a nonphysician healthcare provider. The pharmacy double checks by verifying that the regimen is accurate against an appropriate reference, then the anticancer agents are reviewed another time against the original order after the drugs are compounded and prior to dispensing. At the drug administration level, the anticancer regimen is first verified by a nurse against an appropriate reference, then the anticancer regimen is checked one more time against the original order by 2 nurses prior to administration of the drug. Overall, the anticancer prescription is verified at many levels by multiple healthcare professionals providing different types of healthcare services with the goal of maintaining patient safety.

Table 2-3 Checklist for Cancer Therapy Prescribing and Verification[3,4]

---

1. Confirm that the prescriber is authorized to prescribe systemic anticancer therapy as per the practice site's policies, procedures, and/or guidelines

2. Confirm the patient's full name and second patient identifier (eg, medical record number, date of birth)

3. Confirm the patient's cancer diagnosis and stage of the disease from the medical records

4. Confirm the date and time the order is written

5. Confirm the date the anticancer regimen is to be administered

6. When indicated, obtain finance approval prior to preparation, dispensing, or administration of the cancer therapy regimen

7. Verify the cancer therapy regimen against validated reference text for standard regimens, IRB-approved research protocols for investigation regimens, or primary literature for nonstandard regimens

8. Verify that the regimen is appropriate based on:

   a. Patient's diagnosis (including pharmacogenomics if applicable)

   b. Performance status

   c. Organ function status

   d. Chemotherapy history and, if applicable, radiation therapy history

   e. Goal of therapy (prevention, improvement in time to progression, prolong survival, cure, palliation)

   f. Response to last cycle

9. On the first cycle, confirm that the ordered cancer therapy is the intended treatment regimen for the patient as documented in the medical records

10. For subsequent cycles, the date the patient was last treated and the next planned treatment date should be compared to ensure that it is the appropriate scheduled time for the next dose (ie, current cycle and day)

11. Check for allergies, drug hypersensitivity reactions, drug sensitivity

12. Check for a complete medication history to assess for potential drug–drug interactions with the planned cancer therapy regimen

    a. The medication history should include over-the counter, complementary, and alternative medications

13. Review the patient's complete medical history and physical examination data from the medical records. At a minimum, the following information should be obtained and the data should be checked for accuracy in measurement and calculation:

    a. Age, height, weight, body surface area (BSA), performance status (PS)

        i. Height and weight should be remeasured, BSA recalculated, and PS reassessed as indicated to determine if dosage modification is necessary when there is significant difference with baseline measurements

    b. Assessment of organ-specific organ function (renal, hepatic, cardiac, pulmonary, etc.) and bone marrow function as appropriate for the planned regimen

        i. If abnormal laboratory values or organ dysfunction is present, primary references or standard references should be consulted to determine if the abnormality is within acceptable ranges for treatment continuation or if treatment modification is indicated

14. Check for accuracy of dose calculation and correctness of dose unit, frequency, number of doses, and scheduled days of therapy

15. If the dose is different from the referenced protocol, check for the reason for the dose adjustment and ensure the reason is documented (eg, renal or hepatic dysfunction, experienced toxicities)

16. Check maximum individual dose as appropriate (eg, 2 mg for vincristine)

17. Check cumulative dose as indicated (eg, lifetime dose limit for bleomycin, doxorubicin)

18. Check route of administration (and rate if applicable) is appropriate

19. Check that supportive care is prescribed and it is appropriate for the patient and regimen

20. Sign and date the prescription as a record of verification. Digital signature/record is sufficient for electronic prescribing systems

CLINICAL PEARL 2-4
Potential Sources of Errors in Anticancer Therapy Prescriptions

Incorrect Name

Two different identifiers should be used to identify a patient (name *and* birthdate or medical record number).

  Example: A father and son with the same name are being treated for different cancers at the same institution. The use of 2 identifiers can avoid a mix-up in prescribing, dispensing, and administration of chemotherapy regimens.

Incorrect Height and Weight

Example 1: A person is weighed in pounds but the information was documented as kilograms. A child weighing 80 pounds had information recorded as 80 kg (about 175 pounds), resulting in a possible 2-fold overdose.

Example 2: Failure to update height information and unfamiliarity with the metric system may lead to errors. If the height for a 16-year-old has not been updated since she was 4 years old in the chart and was recorded as 109 cm, using this data to calculate the body surface area for dosing would result in underdosing. This is because 109 cm equals to 3 feet and 7 inches (1 inch = 2.54 cm), which would be obviously incorrect for a normal 16-year-old.

ORAL ANTICANCER THERAPY

Oral anticancer therapy is an emerging option for the treatment of cancer in selected patients and disease states, and it is expected that the use of oral anticancer therapy and the number of available oral anticancer agents will continue to expand.[11] Oral anticancer therapy has the same potential for error and harmful side effects as with anticancer therapy administered by the parenteral route. **Table 2-4** outlines information that a complete prescription for oral anticancer therapy should include as recommended by the *ASCO/ONS Chemotherapy Administration Safety Standards Including Standards for the Safe*

Table 2-4 Information That Should Be Included in a Prescription for Oral Chemotherapy

1. Patient's full name and second identifier (eg, date of birth)

2. Prescriber's name

3. Date

4. Diagnosis[a]

5. Allergies[a]

6. Drug name

7. Dosage[b] and quantity

8. Route and frequency of administration

9. Administration instructions

10. Duration of therapy (days of rest, if applicable)

11. Number of refills (if applicable)

12. Reference to methodology of dose calculation, height, weight, and other applicable variables

[a] Although not listed in the ASCO/ONS guidelines as a requirement, this information may be useful for clinicians dispensing or administering the medications.

[b] Doses may be rounded to the nearest tablet size or specify alternating doses each day to obtain the correct overall dosage. Do not include trailing zeros and use a leading zero for doses less than 1 mg.

Administration and Management of Oral Chemotherapy.[4] Patients should also receive education regarding their anticancer agents, and information should include side effects to expect and what side effects may require immediate suspension of therapy and seeking medical attention, how to take the medication with regards to meals, the plan for management of missed doses, instructions regarding any associated supportive care medications or measures, possible drug–drug or drug–food interactions, safe handling, storage, and disposal. Refer to the chapter titled *Oral Cancer Therapy,* elsewhere in this text, for more in-depth discussion.

INTRATHECAL ANTICANCER THERAPY

In oncology, intrathecal anticancer therapy is used to treat cancers that have reached the central nervous system, including some types of leukemia and lymphoma. The anticancer agents are delivered into the cerebrospinal fluid (CSF) by injection into the subarachnoid space of the spinal cord (lumbar puncture or spinal tap) or through an Ommaya reservoir (a soft plastic dome attached to a catheter, the tip of which sits in the lateral ventricle) that is placed subcutaneously under the scalp.[12] Safe prescribing and administration of intrathecal anticancer agents involves education of all staff involved with intrathecal anticancer therapy along with implementation of policies and procedures that describes the role of all involved healthcare professionals and delineation of procedures to follow when intrathecal anticancer therapy is administered to patients.

Anticancer Agents for Intrathecal Administration and Dosing Considerations

Only a few anticancer agents are used for intrathecal administration. The 2 most commonly prescribed agents are methotrexate and cytarabine, either alone or in combination with hydrocortisone.[12] Cytarabine is available in 2 formulations—standard cytarabine and slow-release liposomal cytarabine, which produces prolonged cytarabine CSF exposure up to 40 times that of standard cytarabine.[13] Thiotepa, dexamethasone, or methylprednisolone are less commonly prescribed agents for intrathecal administration.

The dose of intrathecal anticancer therapy and the volume for administration are important factors for consideration. The dosing of intrathecal anticancer therapy is based on age because there is not a correlation between CSF volume and BSA; meaning, there is not a consistent relationship between drug dose and CSF concentration if the dose is based on BSA.[12,14] The CSF volume of children after the first 3 years of age is equivalent to the CSF volume of adults because CSF volume of an infant increases more rapidly than its BSA.[14] **Table 2-5** provides common doses for intrathecal anticancer agents based on patient age.[12,14–17] The volume of drug for intrathecal administration should always be of the most minimal volume to avoid increase in intracranial pressure and compromise patient safety. The maximum volume for intrathecal administration is 10 mL; however, in practice, the preferred volume is 5 mL because prior to installation of the intrathecal drug, the same volume of CSF has to be removed as the amount of fluid that will be administered intrathecally. For the Ommaya reservoir, a volume of 3–5 mL of anticancer drug is instilled followed by 5 mL of preservative-free

Table 2-5 Common Intrathecal Anticancer Therapy Dosing[12,14–16]

	Patient Age (Years)					
Anticancer Agent	< 1	1	> 2	≥ 3–9	≥ 10	Adult
Methotrexate dose (mg)	6	8	10	12	15	$10–15 \text{ mg/m}^2$ 15 mg
Cytarabine (mg)	12	16	20	24	30	30 mg/m^2
Hydrocortisone (mg)	No Data	8	10	12	12	15–25 mg
Liposome cytarabine dose (mg)	20	25	35	35	35–50	50

normal saline to flush the drug through the reservoir and into the lateral ventricle. It is also important to note that all drugs for intrathecal administration should be *preservative free* to prevent the risk of inflammatory reactions resulting in effects such as arachnoiditis and sterile meningitis.

Avoid Intrathecal Vincristine Injection

Oncology healthcare professionals should be aware of the catastrophic consequences of accidental administration of intrathecal vincristine. Deaths have occurred worldwide due to the inadvertent administration of vincristine via the intrathecal route; thus, it is essential that appropriate precautions are taken when prescribing, dispensing, and administering vincristine to prevent fatal errors.[18–21] Unintentional intrathecal vincristine administration occurs when a syringe containing vincristine is mistaken as either methotrexate or cytarabine for intrathecal administration. Mistakes may also occur when a syringe of vincristine is placed in proximity to a syringe containing intrathecal anticancer drugs and the healthcare provider picks up vincristine after incorrectly assuming that it is an additional intrathecal drug. Other reasons for error include mislabeling, unfamiliarity with anticancer therapy, and failure to check medication orders. To avoid inadvertent intrathecal vincristine administration, the United States Pharmacopeial Convention recommends that the dispensed vincristine must be enclosed in an overwrap bearing the statement "Do Not Remove Covering Until Moment of Injection. • For Intravenous Use Only—Fatal If Given By Other Routes•."[22] There are recommendations from the Joint Commission that vincristine should be diluted for intravenous infusion in a minibag that would preclude administration via the intrathecal route with a syringe.[23] When intrathecal anticancer agents are prescribed, it should be ordered separately from IV anticancer therapy; furthermore, intrathecal drugs should be packaged and transported immediately before administration. Intrathecal medications should also be separate from other IV drugs and should not be stored in a patient care area.[23]

SUPPORTIVE CARE AND ANCILLARY MEDICATIONS

An anticancer therapy prescription is not complete without supplemental orders for ancillary medications that prevent or alleviate side effects. Without the proper supportive care orders, patients may not be able to tolerate or complete their anticancer therapy. Supportive medications are divided into the following categories: premedications to prevent infusion-related or hypersensitivity reactions and medications to prevent side effects such as nausea and vomiting, febrile neutropenia, tumor lysis syndrome, and nephrotoxicity. **Table 2-6** provides a checklist to ensure that appropriate supportive care medications are considered, and **Table 2-7** lists the recommendations for prevention of nephrotoxicity associated with anticancer therapy.[24-26] An in-depth discussion for each of these supportive care issues is beyond the scope of this chapter; however, recommended readings for each of these topics are listed in the *Suggested Reading* section at the end of this chapter.

Table 2-6 Checklist of Ancillary Medications to Consider

- Are premedications indicated?
- Is there a need for IV hydration to prevent nephrotoxicity?
- What is the emetogenic potential of the anticancer regimen and are antiemetics necessary?
- Is there a need for IV hydration and medications to prevent complications from tumor lysis syndrome?
- Are chemoprotectants necessary (eg, mesna for ifosfamide or cyclophosphamide, leucovorin for methotrexate)?
- Is there a need for urine alkalinization to prevent toxicity from methotrexate?
- Does the patient need an order for a colony-stimulating factor (eg, filgrastim, pegfilgrastim)?
- Are prophylactic antibiotics necessary (eg, immunosuppressive regimens such as high-dose chemotherapy, fludarabine, alemtuzumab)?
- Does the patient need anticoagulants to prevent the risk of thromboembolism (eg, lenalidomide and corticosteroids for multiple myeloma)?

Table 2-7 Prevention of Nephrotoxicity[24-26]

Nephrotoxicity: Clinicians should be aware of anticancer drugs that induce nephrotoxicity and be well versed in the preventive measures available for the anticancer agents.

Preventive Measures for Drugs Commonly Known to Cause Nephrotoxicity

Cisplatin: Saline based IV hydration maintained at 3–4 L/24 hours, 12 hours prior to and for at least 1 day after cisplatin administration. Potassium and magnesium supplementation as needed. Monitor renal function and reduce dose as indicated based on renal function.

Methotrexate: IV hydration with sodium bicarbonate to achieve urine alkalinization and maintain urine pH at 7 to prevent precipitation of the methotrexate in the renal tubules and collecting ducts. Begin hydration 12 hours before infusion of methotrexate and continue for 48–72 hours.

Bevacizumab: Monitor for proteinuria with a dipstick urinalysis and if result is 2+ or higher, it should be confirmed with a timed 24-hour urine collection. Hold bevacizumab if 24-hour urine collection shows protein amount greater than 2.

Infusion-Related Reactions

Some anticancer agents or the vehicles in which they are formulated may interact with mast cells and basophils producing anaphylactoid responses that are not true type 1 IgE-mediated hypersensitivity reactions. Mild-to-moderate infusion-related reactions are manifested as flushing, dyspnea, fever, rigors, chills, mild hypotension, and rash. Severe reactions are associated with bronchospasms, hypotension requiring treatment, cardiac dysfunction, and anaphylaxis. Infusion-related reactions may occur with all the monoclonal antibodies; however, the incidence varies among the different agents. Rituximab (77%) and trastuzumab (40%) produce the highest incidence rate, followed by cetuximab (12%), panitumumab (4%), and bevacizumab (3%). Infusion-related reactions predominantly occur with the first infusion, and the incidence declines with subsequent infusions. Premedications are recommended to prevent or reduce the severity of infusion-related reactions.[27,28] Another chapter in this text, *Overview of Cancer Therapy*, provides a table of anticancer agents and recommendations for premedications as indicated to prevent infusion-related reactions for specific agents, including monoclonal antibodies.

Tumor Lysis Syndrome

Tumor lysis syndrome (TLS) is a set of metabolic complications that can arise from treatment of rapidly proliferating malignancies causing tumor cells to release their intracellular contents of potassium, phosphorus, and uric acid leading to the characteristic findings of hyperkalemia, hyperphosphatemia, hypocalcemia, hyperuricemia, and acute kidney injury.[29,30] TLS may occur spontaneously prior to administration of anticancer therapy in tumors with high proliferative rates, or it may occur after anticancer therapy administration in tumors with high sensitivity to cytotoxic therapy. **Table 2-8** summarizes the risk factors for the development of TLS.[29,30] The successful prevention and management of TLS involves maintaining a high index of suspicion and identifying patients who are at high risk for TLS along with the implementation of prophylactic strategies that prevent complications from TLS development (Table 2–8).[29-31]

Chemotherapy-Induced Nausea and Vomiting

Chemotherapy-induced nausea and vomiting (CINV) can have negative effect on patients' quality of life and lead to poor compliance with anticancer therapy. It is essential that antiemetics are a component of anticancer treatment regimens for patients at risk of experiencing CINV to prevent metabolic imbalances, nutrient depletion, decline in performance status, and other complications that occur as a result of CINV. Criteria used to determine if antiemetics are necessary and the appropriate antiemetics to administer include: (1) the emetogenic potential of the specific anticancer agents, (2) the dose, schedule, and route of administration of the anticancer agent, (3) individual patient characteristics (eg, age, sex, history of alcohol use, CINV experience with prior anticancer therapy), (4) the side effect profile of the antiemetics, and (5) patient preference. Drugs commonly used to prevent and treat CINV include the 5-HT3 receptor antagonists (eg, ondansetron, granisetron, dolasetron, palonosetron), neurokinin-1 (NK-1) receptor antagonists (eg, aprepitant, fosaprepitant), corticosteroids (eg, dexamethasone), and antidopaminergic agents (eg, haloperidol, prochlorperazine, promethazine, and metoclopramide). Treatment recommendations for CINV are available at the following organizations' websites: the National Comprehensive Cancer Network (NCCN), the Multinational Association of Supportive Care in Cancer (MASCC), and ASCO (**Table 2-9**).

Table 2-8 Identifying Risk Factors for Developing Tumor Lysis Syndrome[29-31]

Cancer Diagnosis

Hematologic Cancers

Common	High-grade non-Hodgkin's lymphoma (eg, Burkitt's lymphoma), acute lymphocytic leukemia
Less common	Acute myeloid leukemia, chronic lymphocytic leukemia, multiple myeloma, chronic myeloid leukemia in blast crisis

Solid Tumors With High Proliferative Rates and High Response Rate to Anticancer Therapy

Breast cancer, small lung cancer, testicular cancer

Tumor-related Risk Factors

High tumor cell proliferation rate, tumor size, tumor sensitivity to anticancer therapy

Patient Risk Factors

Preexisting chronic renal insufficiency, decreased urinary flow, acidic urine, dehydration, preexisting hyperuricemia, hypotension, receiving concomitant nephrotoxic drugs

Laboratory Risk Factors

High white blood cell (WBC) count, high lactate dehydrogenase (LDH) level (greater than 2 × upper limit of normal range), elevated uric acid level

Recommendations for Prevention of Complications From Tumor Lysis Syndrome

Hydration	Intravenous hydration with 2.5-3 L/day of fluids to maintain urine output of 2 mL/kg/hour. Initiate 24 hours prior to and continue for up to 72 hours after anticancer therapy. The addition of a diuretic may be necessary.
Hyperuricemia	Initiation of prophylactic allopurinol prior to anticancer therapy is recommended for patients at low risk (normal uric acid level, WBC $\leq 50 \times 10^9$/L, normal LDH) of developing TLS. Rasburicase is recommended for patients with high risk (uric acid level > 8 mg/dL, WBC $\geq 50 \times 10^9$/L, high LDH, receiving intensive anticancer therapy) factors for TLS.
Electrolytes	Unless it is medically necessary, discontinue potassium and phosphate electrolyte supplementations.
Laboratory monitoring	Obtain laboratory tests (serum creatinine, LDH, uric acid, potassium, phosphorus, calcium) daily for patients at low risk for TLS, every 8-12 hours for high-risk patients, and every 4-6 hours for patients who have established TLS.

Table 2-9 Oncology Professional Organizations, Websites, and Resources

American Society of Clinical Oncology (ASCO)   www.asco.org

Examples of some available guidelines or clinical opinions:

- *Appropriate Chemotherapy Dosing for Obese Adult Patients With Cancer*
- *Antiemetics*
- *Update on the Use of Epoetin and Darbepoetin in Adult Patients With Cancer*
- *Chronic Hepatitis B Virus Infection Screening in Patients Receiving Cytotoxic Chemotherapy for Treatment of Malignant Diseases*
- *Use of Chemotherapy and Radiation Therapy Protectants*
- *Update of Recommendations for the Use of White Blood Cell Growth Factors: An Evidence-Based Clinical Practice Guideline*
- *Venous Thromboembolism Prophylaxis and Treatment in Patients With Cancer*
- *Testing for KRAS Gene Mutations in Patients with Metastatic Colorectal Carcinoma to Predict Response to Anti-Epidermal Growth Factor Receptor Monoclonal Antibody Therapy*
- *Epidermal Growth Factor Receptor (EGFR) Mutation Testing for Patients With Advanced Non–Small Cell Lung Cancer Considering First-Line EGFR Tyrosine-Kinase Inhibitor (TKI) Therapy*

Chemoregimen Website   www.chemoregimen.com

- Lists the most common anticancer regimens organized by disease state. The regimens include drug, dosage, and schedule with links to the primary references
- Links to dosing of anticancer therapy in renal and hepatic impairment

Children's Oncology Group (COG)   www.childrensoncology group.org

- Access to protocols used in the treatment of childhood cancers
- Long-term follow-up guidelines for screening and management of late effects of cancer and cancer therapy

The Gynecologic Oncology Group (GOG) www.gog.org

Access to the website is available for members. Information regarding the treatment of pelvic malignancies such as cancer of the ovary, cervix, and uterus.

Hematology/Oncology Pharmacy Association (HOPA) www.hoparx.org

Newsletter that provides a review of the most recent FDA-approved anticancer therapies and timely topics.

Multinational Association of Supportive Care in Cancer (MASCC) www.mascc.org

Some example guidelines provided include:

- Antiemetics, mucositis, EGFR inhibitor skin toxicity, oral agent teaching tool

National Cancer Institute (NCI) www.cancer.gov

- List of NCI clinical trials

- General overview of different cancers and cancer treatment

National Comprehensive Cancer Network (NCCN) www.nccn.org

- Guidelines for the treatment of the major cancers

- Guidelines for age-related recommendations (adolescent, young adult, and senior adult)

- Guidelines for supportive care. Examples include:
  - Antiemesis, myeloid growth factors, chemotherapy and cancer-induced anemia, prevention and treatment of cancer-related infections, venous thromboembolic disease, pain and palliative care management, distress management, survivorship

- Guidelines for screening

The Oncology Nursing Society (ONS) www.ons.org

- Review of the major common cancers
- Clinical practice resources for chemotherapy-induced nausea and vomiting, oral mucositis, safe handling, oral therapies, and vincristine

This list is not all inclusive and is intended only as a point of reference.

Febrile Neutropenia and Colony-Stimulating Growth Factors

Neutropenia (defined as < 500 neutrophils/microliter or < 1000 neutrophils/microliter with a predicted decline to ≤ 500 neutrophils/microliter over the next 48 hours) and the possibility of febrile neutropenia (defined as temperature ≥ 38.3°C or ≥ 38°C over 1 hour) development is a consequence of myelosuppressive anticancer therapy. Febrile neutropenia (FN) is a dose-limiting toxicity of anticancer therapy that requires hospitalization and broad-spectrum antibiotic administration. Furthermore, FN may cause treatment delays and dose reductions that can adversely affect clinical outcomes. The administration of granulocyte colony-stimulating factors (G-CSFs) with each cycle of anticancer therapy can reduce the risk of developing FN or the severity and duration of FN. It is essential to consider if patients require the addition of a granulocyte colony-stimulating factor to their anticancer treatment regimen to prevent chemotherapy-induced FN and help patients stay on track with their treatment schedule. The most commonly prescribed granulocyte colony-stimulating factors are filgrastim and pegfilgrastim, and updated guidelines for the use of these agents are available at the NCCN website (Table 2-9).

NONONCOLOGY INDICATIONS FOR ANTICANCER THERAPY

Anticancer therapies are indicated for ectopic/molar pregnancies and many autoimmune disorders such as rheumatoid arthritis, systemic lupus erythematosus, Sjögren's syndrome, Crohn's disease, Wegener's granulomatosis, and multiple sclerosis. The anticancer agents most commonly used to treat autoimmune disorders include cyclophosphamide, mitoxantrone, methotrexate, and rituximab. Utilizing anticancer therapy for nononcology indications requires the same evaluation and monitoring as for oncology indications. Anticancer therapy for nononcology patients is administered in cancer centers because they are equipped and have staff that are qualified and experienced in providing cytotoxic therapy. It is important to establish good communication channels between nononcology practices and the oncology treatment center so that treatment plans can be verified and adhered to correctly. The oncology treatment center needs to have access to the patient's chart and laboratory data to be able to determine if it is safe and appropriate for the patient to be treated. In addition, many of these agents are expensive, and treatment centers need to be able to predict patient need to manage inventory. When verifying orders for nononcology indications, it is important to know the diagnosis, the correct dose for the indication, and follow the same steps to verify the prescription as for oncology indications (see Table 2-3).

RESOURCES

There are many professional organizations and cooperative groups dedicated to promoting the delivery of high-quality care for oncology patients; cancer prevention, research, and advocacy; and ongoing education and professional development of oncology healthcare providers. These organizations have online resources that provide access to clinical guidelines and recommendations developed by expert panels based on best available evidence, educational events, and newsletters or journals that publish the latest data on the advances in the treatment of cancers. The online sites for these professional organizations and cooperative groups are excellent resources to stay current in the field of oncology. Oncology healthcare professionals should investigate these various websites to identify situations in which they will be beneficial in the course of providing care for the cancer patients. Table 2-9 provides a listing of key oncology professional organizations and resources along with a brief summary of guidelines/information that are available at the website.

In addition to the resources listed in Table 2-9, package inserts are often overlooked, valuable resources. They provide preparation, dosing, and administration guidelines as well as a comprehensive list of adverse events. Micromedex is a web-based resource that is available via subscription in many institutions. It provides valuable drug information on individual systemic anticancer agents and answers many questions regarding drug interactions along with IV drug and solution compatibility.

SUMMARY

The field of oncology is rapidly changing and improving to provide patients with better treatment outcomes. The improved treatment plans are often much more complex and errors can cause serious harm to patients. The prescribing and verification process must include a systematic approach that is provided in policies and procedures to ensure patients are treated both safely and effectively. All healthcare professionals involved in oncology should be vigilant in following standard of practice when prescribing, verifying, dispensing, and administering anticancer agents. Healthcare providers should also communicate with each other openly in order to facilitate correction of errors when they are identified.

REFERENCES

1. Cohen M, Anderson R, Attilio R, Green L, Muller R, Pruemer J. Preventing medication errors in cancer chemotherapy. *Am J Health-System Pharm.* 1996;53(1):737–746.
2. Ross A, Polansky M, Parker P, Palmer J. Understanding the role of physician assistants in oncology. *J Oncol Pract.* 2010;6:26–30.
3. ASHP Council on Professional Affairs. ASHP guidelines on preventing medication errors with antineoplastic agents. *Am J Health-System Pharm.* 2002;59:1648-1668.
4. American Society of Clinical Oncology. Neuss MN, Polovich M, McNiff K, et al. 2013 *Updated American Society of Clinical Oncology/Oncology Nursing Society Chemotherapy Administration Safety Standards Including Standards for the Safe Administration and Management of Oral Chemotherapy.* http://www.asco.org/sites/www.asco.org/files/oral_standards_jop_article.pdf. Accessed May 29, 2013.
5. Kloth D. *Guide to the prevention of chemotherapy medication errors.* 2nd ed.:New York, New York; McMahon Publishing,2010:48.
6. ASHP Section of Pharmacy Informatics and Technology. ASHP guidelines on pharmacy planning for implementation of computerized provider-order-entry systems in hospitals and health systems. *Am J Health-Syst Pharm.* 2011;68:e9–e31.
7. Ash J, Stavri P, Kuperman G. A consensus statement on considerations for a successful CPOE implementation. *J Am Med Inform Assoc.* 2003;10:229–234.
8. Sengstack P. CPOE configuration to reduce medication errors: A literature review on the safety of CPOE systems and design recommendations. *J Healthc Inf Manage.* 2010;24:26–32.
9. Tournigand C, Andre T, Achille E, et al. FOLFIRI followed by FOLFOX6 or the reverse sequence in advanced colorectal cancer: a randomized GERCOR study. *J Clin Oncol.* 2004;22(2):229–237.
10. British Oncology Pharmacy Association. Williamson S. *Guidance to support BOPA standards for clinical pharmacy verification of prescriptions for cancer medicines.* Updated 2010. http://www.bopawebsite.org/contentimages/publications/verification.pdf. Accessed May 29, 2013.
11. Weingart S, Brown E, Bach P, et al. NCCN task force report: Oral chemotherapy. *JNCCN.* 2008;6:S1-S14.
12. Kerr J, Berg S, Blaney S. Intrathecal chemotherapy. *Crit Rev Oncol Hematol.* 2001;37:227–236.
13. Kwong Y, Yeung D, Chan J. Intrathecal chemotherapy for hematologic malignancies: Drugs and toxicities. *Ann Hematol.* 2009;88:193–201.
14. Ruggiero A, Conter V, Milani M, et al. Intrathecal chemotherapy with antineoplastic agents in children. *Paediatr Drugs.* 2001;3:237–246.
15. Benesch M, Sovinz P, Krammer B, et al. Feasibility and toxicity of intrathecal liposomal cytarabine in 5 children and young adults with refractory neoplastic meningitis. *J Pediatr Hematol Oncol.* 2007;29:222–226.
16. Lassaletta A, Lopez-Ibor B, Mateos E, et al. Intrathecal liposomal cytarabine in children under 4 years with malignant brain tumors. *J Neurooncol.* 2009;95:65–69.
17. Navajas A, Lassalatta A, Morales A, et al. Efficacy and safety of liposomal cytarabine in children with primary CNS tumours with leptomeningeal involvement. *Clin Transl Oncol.* 2012;14:280–286.

18. al Fawaz I. Fatal myeloencephalopathy due to intrathecal vincristine administration. *Ann Trop Paediatr.* 1992;12:339–342.

19. Alcaraz A, Rey C, Concha A, Medina A. Intrathecal Vincristine: fatal myeloencephalopathy despite cerebrospinal fluid perfusion. *Clin Toxicol.* 2002;40:557–561.

20. Fernandez C, Esau R, Hamilton D, Fitzsimmons B, Pritchard S. Intrathecal vincristine: an analysis of reasons for recurrent fatal chemotherapeutic error with recommendations for prevention. *J Pediatr Hematol Oncol.* 1998;20:587–590.

21. Hennipman B, de Vries E, Bokkerink J, Ball L, Veerman A. Intrathecal vincristine. 3 fatal cases and a review of the literature. *J Pediatr Hematol Oncol.* 2009;31:816-819.

22. U.S. Pharmacopeial Convention. Vincristine_sulfate_for_injection.pdf. Revision Bulletin Official July 1, 2011. http://www.usp.org/sites/default/files/usp_pdf/EN/USPNF/revisions/vincristine_sulfate_for_injection.pdf. Accessed August 5, 2013.

23. Schulmeister L. Preventing vincristine administration errors: does evidence support minibag infusions? *Clin J Oncol Nurs.* 2006;10:271–273.

24. de Jonge M, Verweij J. Renal toxicities of chemotherapy. *Semin Oncol.* 2006;33:68-73.

25. Launay-Vacher V, Rey J, Isnard-Bagnis C, Deray G, Daouphars M. Prevention of cisplatin nephrotoxicity: state of the art and recommendations from the European Society of Clinical Pharmacy special interest group on cancer care. *Cancer Chemother Pharmacol.* 2008;61:903–909.

26. Shord S, Bressler L, Tierney L, Cuellar S, George A. Understanding and managing the possible adverse effects associated with bevacizumab. *Am J Health-Syst Pharm.* 2009;66:999–1013.

27. Lenz H. Management and preparedness for infusion and hypersensitivity reactions. *The Oncologist.* 2007;12:601–609.

28. Chung C. Managing premedications and the risk for reactions to infusional monoclonal antibody therapy. *The Oncologist.* 2008;13:725–732.

29. Cairo M, Bishop M. Tumour lysis syndrome: A new therapeutic strategies and classification. *Br J Haematol.* 2004;127:3–11.

30. Howard S, Jones D, Pui C. The tumor lysis syndrome. *NEJM.* 2011;364:1844-1854.

31. Wilson F, Berns J. Onco-nephrology: Tumor lysis syndrome. *Clin J Am Soc Nephrol.* 2012;7:1730–1739.

SUGGESTED READING

- American Society of Clinical Oncology. Neuss MN, Polovich M, McNiff K, et al. 2013. *Updated American Society of Clinical Oncology/Oncology Nursing Society Chemotherapy Administration Safety Standards Including Standards for the Safe Administration and Management of Oral Chemotherapy.* http://www.asco.org/sites/www.asco.org/files/oral_standards_jop_article.pdf. Accessed May 29, 2013.

- Ash J, Stavri P, Kuperman G. A consensus statement on considerations for a successful CPOE implementation. *J Am Med Inform Assoc.* 2003;10:229–234.

- ASHP Section of Pharmacy Informatics and Technology. ASHP guidelines on pharmacy planning for implementation of computerized provider-order-entry systems in hospitals and health systems. *Am J Health-Syst Pharm.* 2011;68:e9–e31.

- Chung C. Managing premedications and the risk for reactions to infusional monoclonal antibody therapy. *The Oncologist*. 2008;13:725-732.
- de Jonge M, Verweij J. Renal toxicities of chemotherapy. *Semin Oncol*. 2006;33:68–73.
- Howard S, Jones D, Pui C. The tumor lysis syndrome. *NEJM*. 2011;364:1844–1854.
- ASHP Council on Professional Affairs. ASHP guidelines on preventing medication errors with antineoplastic agents. *Am J Health-System Pharm*. 2002;59:1648–1668.
- Launay-Vacher V, Rey J, Isnard-Bagnis C, Deray G, Daouphars M. Prevention of cisplatin nephrotoxicity: state of the art and recommendations from the European Society of Clinical Pharmacy special interest group on cancer care. *Cancer Chemother Pharmacol*. 2008;61:903–909.
- Lenz H. Management and preparedness for infusion and hypersensitivity reactions. *The Oncologist*. 2007;12:601-609.
- Sengstack P. CPOE configuration to reduce medication errors: a literature review on the safety of CPOE systems and design recommendations. *J Healthc Inf Manage*. 2010;24:26–32.
- Shord S, Bressler L, Tierney L, Cuellar S, George A. Understanding and managing the possible adverse effects associated with bevacizumab. *Am J Health-Syst Pharm*. 2009;66:999–1013.
- Wilson F, Berns J. Onco-nephrology: tumor lysis syndrome. *Clin J Am Soc Nephrol*. 2012;7:1730–1739.

Dosing Calculations

Trinh Pham
Man Yee Merl
Jia Li

LEARNING OBJECTIVES

Upon completion of the chapter, the reader will be able to:

1. Calculate body surface area (BSA) and understand the limitations of determining anticancer drug doses based on the BSA.
2. Calculate dosing of anticancer agents in special populations such as obese, underweight, and amputee patients.
3. Understand the role of genotyping in dosing consideration of anticancer agents.
4. Calculate carboplatin dosing using the Calvert formula.
5. Calculate estimated renal function and understand its role in dosing of anticancer agents.
6. Calculate the dose of an anticancer agent taking into consideration the patient's liver or kidney function.
7. Recommend dosing of anticancer agents for patients who are on hemodialysis.

INTRODUCTION

Cytotoxic anticancer agents are considered to be high-risk medications because they have a narrow therapeutic index in which there is a small difference between the dose that provides maximum antitumor effect and the dose that causes unwanted toxicity. In order to ensure safe prescribing, preparation, and administration of anticancer agents, it is essential that clinicians practicing in the field of oncology are knowledgeable with the nuances of anticancer therapy dosing and are competent in math calculations. The process of determining the dose of an anticancer agent for a patient is complex. Comprehension of the methods utilized to calculate the dose (eg, body-surface area [BSA] vs. pharmacokinetic dosing), the pharmacokinetic predisposition of the anticancer agents (eg, absorption, distribution, metabolism, and excretion), and patient-specific characteristics (eg, height, weight, age, organ function, performance status, and genotype) are necessary to perform dose calculations. In order to maintain consistency in dose computation by all involved healthcare professionals, institutions should assemble a multidisciplinary team composed of physicians, nurses, physician associates, and pharmacists to establish guidelines that address issues such as policies and procedures for the dose verification process (eg, independent dose calculation by the prescribers who write the order, the pharmacists who prepare the dose, and the nurses who administer the dose), the agreed-upon weight (ideal weight vs. actual weight vs. adjusted weight) and formula to use to calculate the BSA and creatinine clearance, the criteria for consideration of dose adjustments (eg, organ function, genotyping, toxicity), the policies for rounding doses and percentage of acceptable variance (eg, 5%–10%), and agreed-upon supporting references to use to verify a dose or anticancer regimen. This chapter will review the major principles involved in the process of calculating an anticancer drug dose for patients and factors to consider prior to final dose determination for optimal patient outcome.

METHODS FOR DOSE CALCULATION

In oncology, it is standard practice to individualize the dose of an anticancer agent with the aim of optimizing antitumor effect while minimizing toxicity. Many different methods exist to calculate the dose of an anticancer agent for a patient. No one universal dose calculation strategy applies for every drug or patient due to the complexity of drug metabolism and elimination and wide disparity in individual patient characteristics. Currently, the most common methods utilized to calculate an anticancer drug dose in clinical practice include BSA-based dosing for most agents, pharmacokinetic-based dosing for specific agents such as carboplatin, fixed-dose dosing most commonly applied for oral anticancer therapy, and weight-based (mg/kg) dosing. Recently, genotype-based dosing has also been introduced for drugs such as irinotecan and mercaptopurine. The following sections will provide a brief review of each of these dose calculation methods.

BSA-BASED DOSING

BSA-based dosing is the most common method used to individualize anti-cancer therapy. The dose is determined by multiplying the patient's BSA by a constant derived for each drug from phase I and II studies or by convention[1] (**Clinical Pearl 3-1**). The calculated doses are frequently empirically reduced in cases of toxicity, organ impairment, older age, or obesity. The rationale for using the BSA as the factor to calculate the dose of an anticancer agent is based on the observation that there is some correlation between body size and physiologic characteristics (eg, glomerular filtration rate, blood volume, basal metabolic rate).[1,2] Furthermore, in phase I studies, when the starting dose of a drug is based on data derived from animal models (where the dose is calculated relative to mg/kg or BSA) the BSA is useful for scaling between species or between infants and adults.[1,2] Lastly, studies published in the 1950s suggested a role for BSA in the calculation of anticancer drugs.[1,2]

Many formulas have been derived for estimating the BSA from body weight and height, and there is no clear evidence that one BSA formula is superior over another. Different formulas (**Table 3-1**) compute significantly different BSA values for the same individual. Therefore, in order to maintain dose consistency, it is recommended that each institution establish consensus on the specific BSA formula that will be used in anticancer therapy dose calculations. The BSA formula established by DuBois and DuBois in 1916 and the formula proposed by Mosteller in 1987 are the 2 most commonly utilized equations.[3,4] Additionally,

CLINICAL PEARL 3-1
Dose Calculation

A 52-year-old Caucasian woman is newly diagnosed with breast cancer with metastasis to the liver. She is scheduled to receive a combination of doxorubicin (60 mg/m^2) and cyclophosphamide (600 mg/m^2) every 3 weeks for 4 cycles for treatment of her cancer. The patient's height is 165 cm and weight is 85 kg. Her serum creatinine is 1.5 mg/dL (non–isotope dilution mass spectrometry [IDMS]), total bilirubin is 1.5 mg/dL, and aspartate aminotransferase (AST) and alanine aminotransferase (ALT) are 120 IU/L and 145 IU/L, respectively. Left ventricular ejection fraction is 50%.

Calculate the patient's BMI:

$$BMI = 85 \text{ kg} \div (1.65 \text{ m})^2 = 31.2 \text{ kg/m}^2$$

(Use BMI equation or go to one of the websites in Table 3-4 to get BMI.)

This patient is considered to be obese based on her BMI.

Calculate the patient's BSA using the DuBois and Mosteller formula:

Dubois: $BSA = 0.007184 \times (165 \text{ cm})^{0.725} \times (85 \text{ kg})^{0.425} = 1.923 \text{ m}^2$

Mosteller: $BSA = \sqrt{[(165 \text{ cm} \times 85 \text{ kg}) / 3600]} = 1.974 \text{ m}^2$

(Use the equations or one of the websites that calculates BSA from Table 3-1.)

The institution has decided to use Dubois as the standard formula for BSA calculation.

Calculate the patient's estimated creatinine clearance:

Cockcroft-Gault: $\{[(140-52 \text{ yr}) \times (85 \text{ kg})] \div (72 \times 1.5 \text{ mg/dL})\} \times 0.85 = 59 \text{ mL/min}$

MDRD: $186 \times (1.5 \text{ mg/dL})^{-1.154} \times (52 \text{ yr})^{-0.203} \times 0.742 = 39 \text{ mL/min/1.73 m}^2$

(Use the equations or one of the websites that calculates glomerular filtration rate (GFR) from Table 3-9.)

This patient has decreased renal function and elevated bilirubin; thus, dosing should be checked to see if dose adjustment is necessary.

Calculate the patient's chemotherapy dose:

Doxorubicin $= 60 \text{ mg} \times 1.923 = 115 \text{ mg}$

- Bilirubin level is 1.5 mg/dL—need to reduce dose by 50%
- 115 mg $\times$ 0.5 $=$ 57.5 mg (round to 60 mg)

Cyclophosphamide $= 600 \text{ mg} \times 1.923 = 1154 \text{ mg}$ (round to 1160 mg)

The patient's actual body weight is used to calculate the dose based on the American Society of Clinical Oncology (ASCO) guidelines.

For both doxorubicin and cyclophosphamide, no recommendation for dose adjustment based on the patient's estimated creatinine clearance exists. However, for doxorubicin, the recommendation is to dose reduce by 50% for bilirubin level of 1.2 to 3 mg/dL, the patient's is 1.5 mg/dL (Note: with the bilirubin being borderline high, some clinicians may not consider dose reduction at this point, depending on the cause for the elevated bilirubin). No dose adjustment for cyclophosphamide is needed until the bilirubin is 3.1 mg/dL or greater. For doxorubicin, the dose should not be given if the left ventricular ejection fraction (EF) is less than 30%–40%; the patient's EF is at 50%, thus she may receive the drug. The total lifetime dose of doxorubicin should not exceed 550 mg/m^2, so the patient's medication history should be checked to see if she has ever received doxorubicin or another anthracycline in the past.

Table 3-1 Formulas for Calculating BSA[3]

DuBois and DuBois Formula[3]

BSA (m^2) = 0.007184 × Height (cm)$^{0.725}$ × Weight (kg)$^{0.425}$

or

BSA (m^2) = 0.20247 × Height (m)$^{0.725}$ × Weight (kg)$^{0.425}$

Mosteller Formula[4]

BSA (m^2) = $\sqrt{\text{Height (cm)} \times \text{Weight (kg)} / 3600}$

OR

BSA (m^2) = $\sqrt{\text{Height (inches)} \times \text{Weight (lbs)} / 3131}$

Haycock Formula[5]

0.024265 × height (cm)$^{0.3964}$ × weight (kg)$^{0.5378}$

Gehan and George[6]

0.0235 × height (cm)$^{0.42246}$ × weight (kg)$^{0.51456}$

Boyd

0.0003207 × height (cm)$^{0.3}$ × weight (grams)$^{0.7285 - [0.0188 \times \log(\text{weight})]}$

[a] Online calculators using these equations can be found at the following websites:
http://www.medcalc.com/body.html
http://www.globalrph.com/bsa2.htm
http://www.chemotherapyadvisor.com/medical-calculators/section/2445/

institutions and practices should establish policies to determine if the patient's actual body weight, ideal body weight, or adjusted body weight (**Table 3-2**) should be used to calculate the BSA. Generally, actual body weight is used for normal weight and underweight patients. However, the dose calculation for obese patients is inconsistent depending on the physician, practice, or patient

Table 3-2 Body Weight Equations

Ideal Body Weight (IBW)[a]
Male: IBW = 50 kg + 2.3 kg for each inch over 5 feet
Female: IBW = 45.5 kg + 2.3 kg for each inch over 5 feet

Adjusted Body Weight (AdjBW)
AdjBW = IBW + [(ABW − IBW) × 25%–40%][b]

ABW, actual body weight

[a] http://www.globalrph.com/ibw_calc.htm
[b] Adjusted body weight—the percentage used for dose adjustment is institution or practitioner specific; 25%–40% is the commonly used range.

condition (this issue is discussed in more depth in the next section on dosing in obese patients).

It is recently recognized that BSA-based dosing is an inaccurate method because it has been found that there is no correlation between the BSA and pharmacokinetic parameters for a number of anticancer drugs.[1] BSA-based dosing does not take into account intra- and interpatient pharmacokinetic or pharmacodynamic variability of anticancer drugs. The systemic exposure after standard doses of anticancer drugs can vary 4- to 10-fold between patients due to differing activity of drug elimination processes related to genetic and environmental factors.[1,7] Furthermore, BSA-based dosing can lead to overdosing (10%) or underdosing (30%) of patients.[8] Despite these limitations, the use of BSA for dose calculation of anticancer agents has been firmly entrenched in oncology practice for more than 50 years, and until validated alternative dosing strategies are available and broadly accepted in clinical practice, the BSA-based dosing system will continue to be used routinely by clinicians. In order to optimize anticancer therapy dosing and minimize toxicity with the BSA dosing method, general principles should be taken into account (**Table 3-3**). These principles are not comprehensive and are meant only as a guide to rationally assist clinicians in the process of determining a dose while performing dose calculations.[8,9]

Dose Calculation in Obese and Underweight Patients

The rise in the rate of obesity is an issue both in the United States and globally. The Centers for Disease Control and Prevention estimates that more than 60% of adult Americans have a body mass index (BMI) of greater than 25 kg/m^2, and this percentage is steadily increasing. An adult who has a BMI between 25 and 29.9 kg/m^2 is considered overweight; an adult with a BMI greater than or

Table 3-3 Guiding Principles for Dose Calculation[8-10]

Principle	Example
Patients with extremes of weight (BSA less than 1.5 or greater than 2)	• Use actual body weight • Do not cap dose at 2 m^2
Know how a drug is eliminated and adjust the dose based on the appropriate test of drug elimination or metabolism	• Creatinine clearance or GFR • Total bilirubin • Transaminases (AST/ALT)
Check for other medications that may inhibit or enhance elimination of anticancer drugs	• Drugs that inhibit or induce CYP450 enzymes
Check for factors that affect normal tissue sensitivity that may require dose reduction	• Prior chemotherapy or radiation • Performance status
Check weight during the course of therapy	• Recalculate BSA when body weight has changed. A lack of data exists regarding appropriate threshold for recalculation, but many institutions use a threshold of more than 5% or 10% weight change
Measure biological endpoints to check effect of the administered dose; the dose may be adjusted down or up accordingly	• Myelosuppression • Thrombocytopenia
Round the calculated dose liberally. Do not order fractional dose size	• 102 mg of doxorubicin can be 100 • 67.6 mg of methotrexate can be 65 or 70 mg • Consider establishing institution-specific protocols that allow rounding somewhere between 5% and 10% to be acceptable for medication compounding purposes. A lack of data exists regarding appropriateness of dose rounding, but clinically, many institutions allow rounding within this range • Whether the therapy is curative or noncurative may help to guide dose rounding
Always have dose calculations double checked	• Doses should be verified by all practitioners independently (physicians, nurses, pharmacists)

ALT, alanine transaminase; AST, aspartate aminotransferase; BSA, body surface area; CYP450, cytochrome P450; GFR, glomerular filtration rate.

equal to 30 kg/m^2 is considered to be obese; and an adult with a BMI greater than 40 kg/m^2 or greater than 35 kg/m^2 with comorbid conditions is considered to be morbidly obese.[11] **Table 3-4** provides the formula for calculating BMI. Overweight or obese cancer patients are at risk of having poorer outcomes from their cancer therapy because oncologists use either ideal body weight or adjusted body weight or cap the BSA at 2 m^2 in performing dose calculations for fear of toxicity.[10] Numerous studies observed that obese patients did not experience excessive toxicity when chemotherapy dose was calculated based on actual body weight (ABW).[10] ASCO recently published practice guidelines on appropriate chemotherapy dosing for obese adult patients with cancer.[10] The ASCO guidelines recommend that actual body weight be used in dose calculation regardless of obesity status, particularly when the goal of treatment is cure, with the caveat that other comorbid conditions should be taken into consideration for the morbidly obese patient. The ASCO panel concludes that there is no evidence that short- or long-term toxicity is increased when obese patients receive full weight-based dosing and that reduced dose may result in poorer disease-free and overall survival rates. If an obese patient experiences high-grade toxicity from the anticancer therapy, the same guidelines for dose

Table 3-4 Calculation of BMI[a]

Measurement Unit	Formula and Calculation Example
Kilograms and meters (m) Since height is commonly measured in centimeters (cm), divide height in centimeters by 100 to obtain height in meters.	**Weight (kg) / [height (m)]^2** The formula for BMI is weight in kilograms divided by height in meters squared. **Example:** Weight = 68 kg Height = 165 cm or 1.65 m **Calculation:** $68 \div (1.65)^2 = 24.98$
Pounds and inches	**Weight (lb) / [height (in)]$^2 \times 703$** The formula for BMI is dividing weight in pounds (lbs) by height in inches (in) squared and multiplying by a conversion factor of 703. **Example:** Weight = 150 lbs Height = 5 feet and 5 inches (5'5") = 65 inches (65") **Calculation:** $[150 \div (65)^2] \times 703 = 24.96$

[a] BMI is calculated the same way for both adults and children. The calculation is based on formulas found at the following websites:
http://www.medcalc.com/body.html
http://www.cdc.gov/healthyweight/assessing/bmi/index.html

reduction used for nonobese patients should be applied.[10] No evidence exists to support one BSA calculation formula over another for obese patients, and any of the standard BSA formulas are acceptable.[10] Fixed dosing of anticancer therapy is recommended only for select agents, such as carboplatin and bleomycin; otherwise, it is not clear that fixed dosing is optimal for any other anticancer agents. The dose of vincristine is generally capped at 2 mg single dose for obese patients, as for nonobese patients, because of neurotoxicity concerns.[10] It is recommended that clinicians review the ASCO guidelines for a more thorough review of chemotherapy dosing in obese adult patients.[10]

There is scant data available for dosing of anticancer therapy in underweight cancer patients. In practice, underweight patients are usually treated based on their actual body weight.[12]

Dose Calculation in Adult Amputees

There is no evidence or guidelines to determine dose modifications in amputee patients. Metabolism and clearance of a drug does not necessarily change in amputee patients, but renal function estimated based on serum creatinine may not be accurate due to loss of muscle mass.[13] To calculate BSA following amputation (BSA_{amp}), the BSA of individual body parts (BSA_{part}) needs to be determined. Colangelo and colleagues proposed 2 methods for estimating BSA_{amp}: They are (1) using regression equations derived from comparison of BSA_{part} with total BSA; and (2) using mean percentage of total BSA contributed by particular body part[14] (**Table 3-5**).

Table 3-5 Calculation of BSA Following Amputation (BSA_{amp})[14]

Method 1: Regression Equations		Method 2: Percentage of Total BSA		
Body Part	Regression Equation	Body Part	% BSA_{part} in Women	% BSA_{part} in Men
Index finger	$BSA_{part} = (0.0027)BSA + 0.0013$	Index finger	0.32	0.34
Hand plus 5 fingers	$BSA_{part} = (0.0243)BSA + 0.0075$	Hand plus 5 finger	2.65	2.83
Lower arm	$BSA_{part} = (0.0414)BSA + 0.0030$	Lower arm	3.80	4.04
Upper arm	$BSA_{part} = (0.0656)BSA + 0.0140$	Upper arm	5.65	5.94
Thigh	$BSA_{part} = (0.0989)BSA + 0.0410$	Thigh	12.55	11.80

(*continues*)

Table 3-5   Calculation of BSA Following Amputation (BSA$_{amp}$)[14] (*continued*)

Method 1: Regression Equations		Method 2: Percentage of Total BSA		
Body Part	**Regression Equation**	**Body Part**	**% BSA$_{part}$ in Women**	**% BSA$_{part}$ in Men**
Lower leg	BSA$_{part}$ = (0.0649)BSA + 0.0093	Lower leg	6.27	5.99
Foot	BSA$_{part}$ = (0.0315)BSA + 0.0008	Foot	2.94	3.15
BSA$_{amp}$ = BSA − BSA$_{part}$		BSA$_{amp}$ = BSA − [(BSA) × (% BSA$_{part}$)]		

BSA, measured or calculated body surface area before amputation; BSA$_{part}$, BSA of individual body parts; BSA$_{amp}$, BSA following amputation.

PHARMACOKINETIC-BASED DOSING—AREA UNDER THE CURVE

Carboplatin Dosing

Carboplatin was the first anticancer drug for which individualized dosing was based on a calculated pharmacokinetic target—the area under the curve (AUC). Carboplatin is mainly eliminated by the kidneys as noted by the fact that 70% of an administered dose is excreted in the urine as intact drug, and its clearance is closely correlated with the glomerular filtration rate (GFR).[15] The nonrenal clearance of carboplatin represents a quarter of the total body clearance when the renal function is normal. In an individual, the AUC of carboplatin is the most important predictor of the degree of thrombocytopenia, leukopenia, and therapeutic effect.[16] Calvert and colleagues have developed a validated formula, referred to in clinical practice as the Calvert equation (**Table 3-6**), which incorporates an estimate of renal function using measured or calculated GFR to determine a carboplatin dose that achieves a specific target AUC (**Clinical Pearl 3-2**).[15] The chosen target AUC of carboplatin is generally empiric and is determined based on factors such as the cancer diagnosis, dosing schedule (eg, weekly vs. every 21 days cycle), concurrent radiation therapy, monotherapy or combination therapy, and previous toxicities. The target AUC for carboplatin may range from as low as 1.5 to as high as 7.5; thus, it is necessary that clinicians refer to specific protocols or supportive literature to verify the appropriate carboplatin dose for specific diagnosis and chemotherapy regimens.

Table 3-6 Carboplatin Dosing

Calvert Equation[15]

Carboplatin dose (mg) = AUC (mg/mL × min) × (GFR + 25)(mL/min)

Cap the dose of carboplatin if standardized IDMS method[a] was used to measure serum creatinine[17]:

Use a maximum GFR of 125 mL/min

Total carboplatin dose (mg) = (target AUC) × (GFR + 25)

For a target AUC = 6, the maximum dose is 6 × 150 = 900 mg

For a target AUC = 5, the maximum dose is 5 × 150 = 750 mg

For a target AUC = 4, the maximum dose is 4 × 150 = 600 mg

Gynecologic Oncology Group (GOG)[b] Recommendations for Carboplatin Dosing[18]

Switch from the Jelliffe to Cockcroft-Gault formula for estimation of GFR

- In patients with abnormally low serum creatinine, use a minimum value of 0.7 mg/dL to reflect the fact that newer IDMS values tend to be lower
- Consider using preoperative serum creatinine values in surgical patients when estimating GFR since surgery and/or aggressive intravenous hydration can lead to artificially low serum creatinine values
- Use adjusted rather than actual body weight in patients with BMI greater than or equal to 25 kg/m²

$$AdjBW = IBW + [(ABW - IBW) \times 40\%]$$

- Use actual body weight for patients with BMI less than 25 kg/m²

Recalculate carboplatin dose for subsequent cycles if a patient has greater than or equal to 10% weight change from baseline or has CTAE grade 2 or greater renal toxicity (SCr greater than 1.5 ULN).

AUC, area under the curve; BMI, body mass index; CTCAE, common terminology criteria for adverse events; GFR, glomerular filtration rate; IDMS, isotope dilution mass spectrometry; SCr, serum creatinine; ULN, upper limit of normal; AdjBW, adjusted body weight; ABW, actual body weight; IBW, ideal body weight

[a] IDMS creatinine value should not be converted back to non-IDMS values to calculate carboplatin dosing since the formulas to calculate this have not been validated.

[b] Members of GOG may access the carboplatin dosing calculator under tools at www.gogmember.gog.org

CLINICAL PEARL 3-2
Carboplatin Calculation With Calvert Equation

A 40-year-old African American female is diagnosed with ovarian cancer and is scheduled to receive a chemotherapy regimen containing carboplatin and paclitaxel. The target AUC for carboplatin is 5 and the paclitaxel dose is 175 mg/m². The patient's height is 160 cm and weight is 83 kg. Her serum creatinine is 0.7 mg/dL (IDMS); total bilirubin is 0.5 mg/dL.

Calculate the patient's BMI:

$$\text{BMI: } 83 \text{ kg} \div (1.60 \text{ m})^2 = 32.4 \text{ kg/m}^2$$

Calculate the patient's BSA using the Dubois formula:

DuBois: $\text{BSA} = 0.007184 \times (160 \text{ cm})^{0.725} \times (83 \text{ kg})^{0.425} = 1.862 \text{ m}^2$

(Use the equations or one of the websites that calculates BSA from Table 3-1.)

Calculate the patient's estimated creatinine clearance:

Cockcroft-Gault:

$$\{[(140 - 40 \text{ yrs}) \times (83 \text{ kg})] \div (72 \times 0.7 \text{ mg/dL})\} \times 0.85 = 140 \text{ mL/min}$$

Modified Cockcroft-Gault:

$$\{[(140 - 40 \text{ yr}) \times 83 \text{ kg}] \div [(72 \times 0.7 \text{ mg/dL}) \times (1.73 \text{ m}^2/1.862 \text{ m}^2)]$$
$$\times 0.85\} = 150 \text{ mL/min}$$

MDRD:

$$175 \times (0.7 \text{ mg/dL})^{-1.154} \times (40 \text{ yrs})^{-0.203} \times 0.742 \times 1.210 = 112$$
mL/min/1.73 m^2 (Use the equations or one of the websites that calculates GFR from Table 3-9.)

(The National Kidney Disease Education Program (NKDEP) presently recommends reporting estimated GFR values **greater than or equal to 60 mL/min/1.73 m^2** simply as "≥ 60 mL/min/1.73 m^2", not an exact number.)

Calculate the patient's carboplatin dosing based on the Calvert equation:

Carboplatin dose (mg) = 5 (mg/mL × min) × (125 + 25)(mL/min)
Carboplatin dose = 5 × 150 = 750 mg
The GFR is maxed at 125 mL/min since IDMS creatinine was used to calculate GFR.

Calculate the patient's paclitaxel dose:

$$\text{Paclitaxel dose} = 175 \text{ mg} \times 1.862 \text{ m}^2 = 326 \text{ mg}$$

The patient's actual weight is used to calculate the BSA based on ASCO dosing guidelines for obese patients. There is no recommendation for dose adjustment based on the patient's renal and liver function. The dose could be rounded up or down within 5%-10% of calculated dose for ease of preparation.

Another factor to consider in carboplatin dosing using the Calvert equation is if the GFR was calculated based on the standardized isotope dilution mass spectrometry (IDMS) method to measure serum creatinine (refer to the *Renal Function Assessment and Anticancer Therapy Dosing* section in this chapter). If a patient's GFR is calculated based on IDMS-standardized serum creatinine, this could result in a higher than desired carboplatin dose and increased toxicity; thus, the National Cancer Institute Cancer Therapy Evaluation Program (NCI CTEP) published an action letter on guidelines for carboplatin dosing in October 2010. The guidelines recommend that oncologists consider capping the dose of carboplatin when IDMS standardized creatinine is used. The maximum dose should be based on a GFR that is capped at 125 mL/min for patients with normal renal function (Table 3-6).[17] The GOG historically uses the Jelliffe equation to estimate the GFR to be used in the Calvert equation. With the publication of the NCI action letter, the GOG switched to the Cockcroft-Gault formula for GFR estimation and made further recommendations for carboplatin dosing to ensure patient safety (Table 3-6).[18]

FLAT FIXED-DOSE DOSING SYSTEM

Flat fixed-dose dosing is not standard in anticancer therapy but has been adopted for a few specific cytotoxic agents (eg, bleomycin, vincristine) and anticancer agents with relatively limited life-threatening toxicities, such as the new oral targeted agents (eg, sunitinib, sorafenib, imatinib). Bleomycin is prescribed at a fixed dose of 30 mg (equal to 30 units) for the BEP (bleomycin, etoposide, cisplatin) regimen in testicular cancer because that was the dose that was used in clinical trials.[19] The normal dose of vincristine is 1.4 mg/m² but is generally capped at 2 mg because of neurotoxicity concerns.[20]

GENOTYPE-GUIDED DOSING

Some enzymes involved in the biotransformation of drugs have polymorphic gene expression. Assessing the polymorphism in genes encoding for these enzymes, referred to as genotyping, may help to predict optimal dose regimens.

Genotyping to identify patients who are at risk for poor outcome and may require dose adjustment can be applied to the following agents: 6-mercaptopurine (mercaptopurine), fluorouracil, and irinotecan.

Azathioprine is a purine analog that interferes with DNA synthesis and it is also a prodrug of mercaptopurine. Mercaptopurine is a widely used anticancer agent for childhood acute lymphoblastic leukemia, and it is inactivated by the enzyme thiopurine methyltransferase (TPMT).[21] Polymorphism in TPMT defines 3 different patient populations: 86%-97% of the population is homozygous for wild-type TPMT expression with 2 functional alleles; thus, these patients have normal TPMT enzyme activity; 3%-14% of the population has 1 TPMT nonfunctional allele (heterozygous) leading to low or intermediate enzyme activity; and 0.03%-0.6% of the population has 2 nonfunctional alleles (homozygous TPMT deficient), which results in low or no detectable enzyme activity.[21,22] Patients who are TPMT deficient are at risk of experiencing significant hematologic toxicity that can be fatal when mercaptopurine is administered at standard doses. Patients with high TPMT expression may be resistant to mercaptopurine therapy. Of the patients who are heterozygous for TPMT expression, 30%-60% show moderate to severe toxicity; therefore, they should be closely monitored, and some patients may require dose reduction.[21,22] Genetic testing for TPMT polymorphism is not required but is recommended by the FDA for patients who receive mercaptopurine, and it should be performed in patients who experience significant toxicity after dosing.[23] The Clinical Pharmacogenetics Implementation Consortium has published guidelines for TPMT genotyping and thiopurine dosing based on genotype.[22] Please refer to the *Suggested Websites and Reading* list at the end of the chapter for websites providing guidelines and dosing recommendations based on genotyping for the thiopurines and other drugs.

Fluorouracil is a fluorinated pyrimidine analog that is commonly used in combination chemotherapy regimens to treat patients with breast, colorectal, and other malignancies. Capecitabine is the oral prodrug of fluorouracil. The rate-limiting step in pyrimidine catabolism is dihydropyrimidine dehydrogenase (DPD), which is encoded by the DPYD gene.[24] Patients who are deficient in DPD experience profound toxicity such as neutropenia, mucositis, and diarrhea with fluorouracil and capecitabine because of decreased catabolism of the drugs and prolonged exposure to the active parent compounds.[24] Mutations or inactivation of the DPYD gene has been characterized as an autosomal recessive disease in the Caucasian and African American population and affects approximately 5% of the overall population.[25] At this time, testing for DPYD mutation and DPD status is not a standard of practice to guide fluorouracil dosing because the correlation between genotype and phenotype is not ideal. Clinical reports based solely on DPYD genetic mutation underestimate the actual effect of DPD deficiency in the severity of toxicities encountered with fluororuracil.[26] Until there is a definitive role of genetic testing for DPYD mutation and DPD deficiency, capecitabine or fluorouracil is contraindicated in patients with known or suspected DPD deficiency. There are guidelines in the package insert for dosing modifications of capecitabine based on the severity of toxicities experienced by patients; refer to the *Suggested Websites and Readings* section in this chapter for dose adjustment recommendations.

Another example of the significance of genotyping in anticancer therapy dosing involves the enzyme UDP glycosyltransferase 1A1 (UGT1A1). Irinotecan is a topoisomerase inhibitor that is commonly used in colorectal cancer chemotherapy regimens, and SN-38 is the active metabolite of irinotecan. SN-38 undergoes UGT1A1 catalyzed glucuronide conjugation to form the inactive SN-38 glucuronide.[27] A microsatellite mutation in the promoter region of the UGT1A1 gene (*UGT1A1*28*) is responsible for life-threatening myelosuppression with a standard irinotecan dose. *UGT1A1*28* is present in 32%-39% of Caucasians and 16%-33% of Asians.[27] Commercial genotype testing for the *UGT1A1*28* variant is available through the following companies ARUP Laboratories, LabCorp, and EntroGen. However, the role of routine testing for the presence of UGT1A1 mutation is unclear. The reason is because in patients who are homozygous for the *UGT1A1*28* variant, toxicity is observed in patients who received high-dose irinotecan (greater than 250 mg/m^2) but not in patients who received lower doses of irinotecan (100–125 mg/m^2).[28] Furthermore, in patients with the *UGT1A1*28* variant, toxicity was observed when irinotecan was administered with oxaliplatin but not with fluorouracil.[27] Thus, genotyping may be considered and is reasonable for patients who are scheduled to receive high-dose irinotecan or irinotecan combined with oxaliplatin, for patients who experience severe toxicity after irinotecan dosing, or for patients who are suspected of having UGT1A1 mutation. The package insert for irinotecan (refer to the *Suggested Websites and Readings* list) recommends that a reduction in the starting dose by at least one level should be considered for patients known to be homozygous for the *UGT1A1*28* allele, and subsequent dose modification may be considered on an individual basis depending on tolerance and specific toxicities.

In general, genotype-guided dosing is beneficial for only a small proportion of individuals with certain genotypes associated with extremes of drug elimination or metabolism. Furthermore, only a few polymorphisms have shown clinical relevance and genotype alone cannot take into account the multiple environmental factors that affect drug disposition. Thus, at this time, genotyping cannot be the sole method used to guide dose calculation of anticancer therapy but should be used in conjunction with other factors such as drug pharmacokinetics and patient characteristics to optimize dosing.[7]

DOSE ROUNDING

Clinicians should be mindful that the formulas (eg, BSA, Calvert equation, Cockcroft-Gault) used to calculate the dose of an anticancer agent are only approximations. Because there is significant variability in the relationship between a drug dose and the pharmacokinetic or pharmacodynamic effect of these drugs in different individuals, it is not necessary to administer the exact dose based on mathematical calculations. This is especially true if considered in the context that 30% of patients are underdosed and 10% are overdosed when the BSA-dose method is utilized.[8] No standard guidelines are available for dose rounding of anticancer agents after a dose has been calculated. In practice, it is reasonable to round the calculated drug dose to the nearest convenient dose that can be accurately measured in the drug preparation process.[8]

ORGAN FUNCTION ASSESSMENT AND ANTICANCER THERAPY DOSING

Cancer patients may present with preexisting hepatic or renal insufficiency due to comorbid conditions or develop organ impairment as a consequence of cancer progression or metastasis. Because the kidney and the liver are essential in the excretion and metabolism of many anticancer drugs, an assessment of renal and hepatic function is vital in the initial workup of all cancer patients before final cancer therapy dose determination. If organ dysfunction is present, patients may have increased exposure to anticancer drugs and potentially excessive toxicity; as a result, dose reduction of anticancer drugs may be necessary. On the other hand, a risk of undertreatment exists with dose reduction because most dose adjustment recommendations are empiric and based on clinical data that are decades old from retrospective observations in small numbers of patients, before the routine use of supportive agents such as colony-stimulating factors.[29] Because hepatic and renal impairment can have unpredictable impact on drug disposition, other factors, such as the patient's performance status, history of treatment, comorbid conditions, goals of therapy, and cancer type should also be taken into account when deciding to apply recommendations for dose adjustments based on organ function.

Suggestions for dose adjustments for most anticancer agents are provided within FDA-approved drug labels (package inserts) and are also available in specific investigational research protocols, oncology reference books, oncology internet resources, and published literature reviews. Clinicians should note that recommendations for dose adjustments vary from source to source. Clinical judgment and individual patient characteristics should be taken into consideration in determining an appropriate dose for a patient. **Table 3-7** cites the available resources for dose adjustments. **Table 3-8** provides dose adjustment recommendations for renal and hepatic dysfunction for specific agents. For anticancer drugs that have been recently approved by the FDA, the National Cancer Institute Organ Dysfunction Working Group is leading an effort to collect pharmacokinetic and clinical toxicity data in phase I dose-escalating studies in different cohorts of patients defined by their degree of organ dysfunction.[30–32]

Renal Function Assessment and Anticancer Therapy Dosing

Many anticancer agents are excreted by the kidneys, and assessing the renal function of a patient is important for adjusting the dose in cases of renal insufficiency. Numerous approaches exist to calculate the GFR as a measure of renal function, and **Table 3-9** lists the different formulas. **Table 3-10** provides the traditional classifications of renal impairment and the Kidney Disease Outcomes Quality Initiative's (KDO/QI) classification for chronic kidney disease. An in-depth discussion on the pros and cons of each method is beyond the scope of this chapter; however, a list of resources that the readers can refer to is available in the *Suggested Websites and Reading* list.

Table 3-7 Recommended Resources for Dose Adjustment Recommendations of Anticancer Therapy[a]

Web-Based Resources

http://chemoregimen.com/Dosage-for-Renal-Dysfunction-c-59-68.html
http://chemoregimen.com/Dosage-for-Hepatic-Dysfunction-c-58-67.html
http://www.childrensoncologygroup.org/ (for members)
Micromedex
UpToDate

Textbooks or Printed Material

Lexicomp's *Drug Information Handbook*
Physician's Cancer Chemotherapy Drug Manual
Package inserts for specific drugs
Investigational drug study protocol for specific agents

[a] This is not intended to be a comprehensive list. It is only a representative list of resources that clinicians may refer to.

Table 3-8 Recommended Dose Adjustment of Selected Anticancer Agents for Hepatic and Renal Dysfunction[29, 33-34;a]

Generic (Brand)	Recommendations in the Presence of Hepatic Impairment	Recommendations in the Presence of Renal Impairment
Bendamustine (Treanda)[33]	Bilirubin greater than 1.5 × ULN or AST/ALT 2.5–10 × ULN: • Avoid	CrCl less than 40 mL/min: • Avoid
Bleomycin (Blenoxane)[29,34]	No dose reduction	CrCl 40-50 mL/min: • Reduce dose by 30% CrCl 30-40 mL/min: • Reduce dose by 40% CrCl 20-30 mL/min: • Reduce dose by 48% CrCl 10-20 mL/min: • Reduce dose by 54%
Bortezomib (Velcade)[30,31]	Bilirubin greater than 1.5 × ULN: • Reduce dose to 0.7 mg/m^2 during first cycle. For subsequent doses escalate to 1 mg/m^2 or reduce to 0.5 mg/m^2 on the basis of patient tolerance	No dose reduction
Capecitabine (Xeloda)[29,34]	No dose reduction	CrCl 30-50 mL/min: • Reduce dose by 25% CrCl less than 30 mL/min: • Avoid --- Mild renal insufficiency: • No dose reduction Moderate renal insufficiency: • Reduce dose by 75% Severe renal insufficiency: • Avoid
Carboplatin (Paraplatin)[34]	No dose reduction	In patients with end-stage renal disease (ESRD): • Set GFR to 0

Carmustine—BCNU (BiCNU)[35,36]	No dose reduction	eGFR 30-60 mL/min: • Reduce dose by 25% eGFR less than 30 mL/min: • Avoid
		CrCl less than 60 mL/min: • Reduce dose by 20% CrCl less than 45 mL/min: • Reduce dose by 25% CrCl less than 30 mL/min: • Reduce dose by 30%
Chlorambucil (Leukeran)[36]	No dose reduction	eGFR 10-50 mL/min: • Reduce dose by 25% eGFR less than 10 mL/min: • Reduce dose by 50%
Cisplatin—CDDP (Platinol)[34,35]	No dose reduction	Not recommended for ovarian cancer patients with renal insufficiency.
		CrCl less than 46-60 mL/min: • Reduce dose by 25% CrCl 31-45 mL/min: • Reduce dose by 50% CrCl less than 30 mL/min: • Consider alternate drug
Cladribine—2-CdA (Leustatin)[36]	No dose reduction	eGFR 10-50 mL/min: • Reduce dose by 25% eGFR less than 10 mL/min: • Reduce dose by 50%
Cyclophosphamide (Cytoxan)[29,34–36,37]	Bilirubin 3.1-5 mg/dL: • Reduce dose by 25% Bilirubin greater than 5 mg/dL: • Avoid • Some references recommend no dose adjustments	eGFR 10-50 mL/min: • No dose reduction eGFR less than 10 mL/min: • Reduce dose by 25%
		Renal insufficiency: • 20%–30% dose reduction
Cytarabine—Ara-C (Cytosar)[35]	No recommendations	Standard doses (100-200 mg/m^2): • No dose reduction Higher doses (*greater than* 2 g/m^2): SCr 1.5-1.9 mg/dL or 0.5-1.2 mg/dL increase from baseline: • Dose reduction to 1 g/m^2

(continues)

Table 3-8 Recommended Dose Adjustment of Selected Anticancer Agents for Hepatic and Renal Dysfunction[29, 33-34;a] (*continued*)

Generic (Brand)	Recommendations in the Presence of Hepatic Impairment	Recommendations in the Presence of Renal Impairment
		High doses (1-3 g/m^2): CrCl less than 46-60 mL/min: • Reduce dose by 40% CrCl 31-45 mL/min: • Reduce dose by 50%
		CrCl less than 30 mL/min: • Avoid full dose
Dacarbazine (DTIC-Dome)[35]	No dose reduction	CrCl less than 46-60 mL/min: • Reduce dose by 20%
		CrCl 31-45 mL/min: • Reduce dose by 25%
		CrCl less than 30 mL/min: • Reduce dose by 30%
Daunorubicin[35] (Cerubidine)	Bilirubin 1.2-3 mg/dL or AST 60-180 IU/L: • Reduce dose by 25%	SCr greater than 2 × ULN • Reduce dose by 50%
	Bilirubin greater than 3.1-5 mg/dL or AST greater than 180 IU/L: • Reduce dose by 50%	
	Bilirubin greater than 5 mg/dL: • Avoid	
Docetaxel (Taxotere)[29,38]	Bilirubin greater than 1 × ULN or AST/ALT greater than 1.5 × ULN and ALP greater than 2.5 × ULN: • Avoid	No dose reduction
Doxorubicin (Adriamycin)[29,37]	Bilirubin 1.2-3 mg/dL: • Reduce dose by 50%	No dose reduction
	Bilirubin 3.1-5 mg/dL: • Reduce dose by 75%	
	Bilirubin greater than 5mg/dL: • Avoid	

Doxorubicin liposome (Doxil)[39]	Bilirubin 1.2-3 mg/dL or AST 60-180 IU/L: • Reduce dose by 50% Bilirubin greater than 3 mg/dL: • Reduce dose by 75%	No dose reduction
Epirubicin (Ellence)[29,34]	AST 150-250 IU/L: • Reduce dose by 25% Bilirubin 1.2-3 mg/dL or AST 250-500 IU/L: • Reduce dose by 50% Bilirubin greater than 3 mg/dL or AST greater than 500 IU/L: • Reduce dose by 75%	SCr greater than 5 mg/dL: • Consider dose reduction
Etoposide (VePesid)[29,35,37]	Bilirubin 1.5-3 mg/dL: • Reduce dose by 50% Bilirubin greater than 3 mg/dL: • Consider dose reduction or omitting Low albumin: • Consider dose reduction	CrCl 10-50 mL/min: • Reduce dose by 25% CrCl less than 10 mL/min: • Reduce dose by 50% ——————————————— CrCl less than 46-60 mL/min: • Reduce dose by 15% CrCl 31-45 mL/min: • Reduce dose by 20% CrCl less than 30 mL/min: • Reduce dose by 25% ——————————————— SCr greater than 1.4 mg/dL: • Consider reduction by up to 30%
Fludarabine (Fludara)[35,36]	No recommendation	eGFR 10-50 mL/min: • Reduce dose by 25% eGFR less than 10 mL/min: • Reduce dose by 50% ——————————————— CrCl 31-45 mL/min: • Reduce dose by 25% CrCl 30-70 mL/min: • Reduce dose by 20% CrCl less than 30 mL/min: • Avoid
Fluorouracil (Adrucil)[29]	No dose reduction	No dose reduction

(continues)

Table 3-8 Recommended Dose Adjustment of Selected Anticancer Agents for Hepatic and Renal Dysfunction[29, 33-34;a] (*continued*)

Generic (Brand)	Recommendations in the Presence of Hepatic Impairment	Recommendations in the Presence of Renal Impairment
Gemcitabine (Gemzar)[37,38]	Mild to moderate liver dysfunction: • Reduce dose by 20%, increase as tolerated	No recommendations
Hydroxyurea (Hydrea)[35]	No dose reduction	CrCl 10-50 mL/min: • Reduce dose by 50% CrCl less than 10 mL/min: • Reduce dose by 80%
Idarubicin (Idamycin)[35]	Bilirubin 2.6-5 mg/dL: • Reduce dose by 50% Bilirubin greater than 5mg/dL: • Avoid	CrCl 10-50 mL/min: • Reduce dose by 25% CrCl less than 10 mL/min: • Reduce dose by 50%
Ifosfamide (Ifex)[34–36]	No dose reduction	eGFR 10-50 mL/min: • No dose reduction eGFR less than 10 mL/min: • Reduce dose by 25% ―――――――――――― Not recommended for ovarian cancer patients with renal insufficiency. ―――――――――――― CrCl less than 46-60 mL/min: • Reduce dose by 20% CrCl 31-45 mL/min: • Reduce dose by 25% CrCl less than 30 mL/min: • Reduce dose by 30%
Imatinib (Gleevec)[29,32,40,41]	Mild liver dysfunction: (Bilirubin greater than 1-1.5 × ULN with any AST or bilirubin less than ULN and AST greater than ULN: • Maximum dose of 500 mg/day	CrCl 40-59 mL/min: • Doses greater than 600 mg not recommended CrCl 20-39 mL/min: • 50% decrease in recommended starting dose and future doses increased as tolerated • Doses greater than 400 mg not recommended

Liver dysfunction on treatment: Bilirubin greater than 3 × ULN or AST/ALT greater than 5 × ULN:

- Hold treatment until bilirubin is less than 1.5 × ULN and AST/ALT is less than 2.5 × ULN and resume at a reduced dose (eg, 400 mg to 300 mg, 600 mg to 400 mg, 800 mg to 600 mg)

Severe renal impairment:
- Use with caution. Dose of 100 mg a day was tolerated in 2 patients

Irinotecan—CPT-11 (Camptosar)[29,42]

Bilirubin 1.5-3 × ULN:
- 200 mg/m^2 every 3 weeks

Bilirubin median 2.1 mg/dL (range, 1-5.5 mg/dL):
- 115 mg/m^2 every 3 weeks

Package insert does not recommend dosing for patients with bilirubin > 2 mg/dL.

No specific dose reduction recommendations
Use with caution in patients with renal impairment

Ixabepilone (Ixempra)[29,43]

Monotherapy:
- AST or ALT ≤ 2.5 × ULN or bilirubin ≤ 1 × ULN: standard dose of 40 mg/m^2
- AST or ALT ≤ 10 × ULN or bilirubin ≤ 1.5 × ULN: dose of 32 mg/m^2
- AST or ALT ≤ 10 × ULN or bilirubin > 1.5 × ULN to ≤ 3 × ULN: dose of 20-30 mg/m^2
- AST or ALT > 10 × ULN or bilirubin > 3 × ULN: not recommended

In combination with capecitabine:
- AST or ALT > 2.5 × ULN or bilirubin > 1 × ULN: contraindicated
- AST or ALT ≤ 2.5 × ULN or bilirubin ≤ 1 × ULN: standard dose of ixabepilone 40 mg/m^2

No recommendations

(continues)

Table 3-8 Recommended Dose Adjustment of Selected Anticancer Agents for Hepatic and Renal Dysfunction[29, 33-34;a] (*continued*)

Generic (Brand)	Recommendations in the Presence of Hepatic Impairment	Recommendations in the Presence of Renal Impairment
Lenalidomide (Revlimid)[35]	No recommendations	For multiple myeloma (MM) and myelodysplastic syndrome (MDS): CrCl 30-59 mL/min: • MM: 10 mg once daily • MDS: 5 mg once daily CrCl less than 30 mL/min: • MM: 15 mg every 48 hours • MDS: 5 mg every 48 hours
Lomustine (CCNU) (CeeNU)[36]	No dose reduction	eGFR 30-60 mL/min: • Reduce dose by 30% eGFR less than 30 mL/min: • Avoid
Melphalan (Alkeran)[36]	No dose reduction	eGFR 10-50 mL/min: • Reduce dose by 25% eGFR less than 10 mL/min: • Reduce dose by 50%
Methotrexate (MTX) (Trexall)[35,36]	Bilirubin 3.1-5 mg/dL or AST greater than 180 IU/L: • Reduce dose by 25% Bilirubin greater than 5mg/dL: • Avoid	eGFR 10-50 mL/min: • Reduce dose by 50% eGFR less than 10 mL/min: • Avoid --- CrCl 61-80 mL/min: • Reduce dose by 25% CrCl 51-60 mL/min: • Reduce dose by 30% CrCl 10-50 mL/min: • Reduce dose by 50% CrCl 10 mL/min: • Reduce dose by 70%
Mitomycin-C (Mutamycin)[44]	No recommendations	No recommendations
Mitoxantrone (Novantrone)[45]	Patients with hepatic impairment should be treated with caution, and dosage adjustment may be required	No recommendations

Nilotinib (Tasigna)[46]	Hepatic impairment (mild, moderate or severe)[b] in newly diagnosed Ph+ CML: • Initial dose 200 mg twice daily, followed by 300 mg twice daily if tolerated Hepatic impairment for patients with resistant or intolerant Ph+ CML in chronic phase or accelerated phase at 400 mg twice daily: • Mild or moderate—an initial dosing regimen of 300 mg twice daily followed by dose escalation to 400 mg twice daily based on tolerability • Severe—a starting dose of 200 mg twice daily followed by a sequential dose escalation to 300 mg twice daily and then to 400 mg twice daily based on tolerability Elevated hepatic transaminases or bilirubin or serum lipase or amylase ≥ Grade 3: • Withhold nilotinib and monitor transaminases, bilirubin, lipase, and amylase • Resume treatment at 400 mg once daily if transaminases, bilirubin, lipase, or amylase returns to ≤ Grade 1	No dose reduction
Oxaliplatin (Eloxatin)[29]	No dose reduction	CrCl less than 20 mL/min: • Avoid
Paclitaxel (Taxol)[29,37]	Bilirubin 1.6-3 mg/dL: • 100 mg/m² over 3 hours Bilirubin greater than 3 mg/dL: • 50 mg/m² over 3 hours Increased AST: • Reduction is required	No dose reduction
Pemetrexed (Alimta)[47]	No dose reduction	CrCl less than 45 mL/min: • Avoid

(continues)

Table 3-8 Recommended Dose Adjustment of Selected Anticancer Agents for Hepatic and Renal Dysfunction[29, 33-34;a] (*continued*)

Generic (Brand)	Recommendations in the Presence of Hepatic Impairment	Recommendations in the Presence of Renal Impairment
Pentostatin (Nipent)[35,36]	No dose reduction	eGFR 30-60 mL/min: • Reduce dose by 25% eGFR less than 30 mL/min: • Avoid CrCl less than 46-60 mL/min: • Reduce dose by 30% CrCl 31-45 mL/min: • Reduce dose by 40% CrCl less than 30 mL/min: • Use alternative drug
Procarbazine (Matulane)[35]	Use with caution in hepatic impairment	Use with caution in renal impairment; may result in increased toxicity
Topotecan (Hycamtin)[29]	No dose adjustment	CrCl greater than 40 mL/min: • No adjustment CrCl 20-39 mL/min: • Reduce dose by 50%
Vinblastine (Velban)[29,48]	Bilirubin 1.5-3 mg/dL: • Reduce dose by 50% Bilirubin greater than 3 mg/dL: • Avoid Package insert: Bilirubin > 3 mg/dL: 50% reduction in dose	No dose reduction
Vincristine (Oncovin)[29]	Bilirubin 1.5-3 mg/dL: • Reduce dose by 50% Bilirubin greater than 3 mg/dL: • Avoid	No dose reduction
Vinorelbine (Navelbine)[29]	Bilirubin 2.1-3 mg/dL: • Reduce dose by 50% Bilirubin 3.1-5 mg/dL: • Reduce dose by 75% Bilirubin greater than 5 mg/dL: • Avoid	No dose reduction

Greater than 75% liver
metastasis:
- Reduce dose by 50%

---

[a] Refer to package insert for additional information regarding dose adjustments for all toxicities
(eg, renal, hepatic, hematologic, cardiac, dermatologic).
[b] Mild hepatic impairment = Child-Pugh Class A; moderate hepatic impairment = Child-Pugh Class
B; severe hepatic impairment = Child-Pugh Class C.

Note: The dose adjustment recommendations contained within the table are not all inclusive, and
recommendations may vary depending on the reference source used. The intent of the table is to
provide recommendations readily available from primary sources. Clinicians should also use clinical
judgment when choosing anticancer therapy doses for patients with hepatic or renal impairment.

Abbreviations: ALT, alanine transaminase; ALP, alkaline phosphatase; AST, aspartate
aminotransaminase; CrCl, creatinine clearance; CML, chronic myeloid leukemia; eGFR, estimated
glomerular filtration rate; Ph+, Philadelphia chromosome positive; SCr, serum creatinine; ULN,
upper limit of normal.

Table 3-9 Commonly Used Equations for Estimation of Renal Function[49-55]

Measured Creatinine Clearance from 24-hour Urine Collection
GFR (mL/min) = [Creatinine $(mg/dL)_{urine}$/Creatinine $(mg/dL)_{serum}$] ×
[Volume $(mL)_{urine}$ /Time (hours) × 60]
Recommended for patients with low body mass index (BMI less than 18.5).

Cockcroft Gault Equation[50]
eCrCl (mL/min) = {[140-age (years)] × weight (kg)} / [72 × SCr (mg/dL)]
For female: multiply results by 0.85.
Comments: Consistent results in patients with stable renal function, average size and
body build. Not adjusted for body surface area. Not revised for use with creatinine
methods standardized to IDMS reference method. There is no evidence that the use of
ideal body weight is a more accurate predictor of GFR or provides better drug-dosing
guidelines compared to actual body weight.

Modified Cockcroft Gault Equation[51]
eCrCl $(mL/min/1.73\,m^2)$ = {[140-age (years)] × weight (kg)} / [72 × SCr (mg/dL)]
$\times (1.73\,m^2/BSA)$

For female: multiply results by 0.85.

Comments: Equation adjusts for body surface area and was found to be more accurate
at estimating renal function when applied to the original Cockcroft-Gault study
population.

BSA was calculated using the DuBois formula (Table 3-1).

Modification of Diet in Renal Disease (MDRD) Study Equation[50]
(For use with creatinine methods that do not have calibration traceable to IDMS)
eGFR $(mL/min/1.73\,m^2)$ = 186 × [SCr $(mg/dL)]^{-1.154}$ × [age $(years)]^{-0.203}$ × (0.742 if
female) × (1.210 if African American)

**Modification of Diet in Renal Disease (MDRD) Study Equation Calibrated to IDMS
Reference Method[50]**
(This equation is for use with creatinine methods calibrated to an
IDMS reference method)   (continues)

Table 3-9 Commonly Used Equations for Estimation of Renal Function[49-55] (*continued*)

eGFR (mL/min/1.73 m²) = 175 × [SCr (mg/dL)]$^{-1.154}$ × [age (years)]$^{-0.203}$ × (0.742 if female) × (1.210 if African American)
Comments: Reasonably accurate in patients known to have chronic kidney disease. Most optimal when renal function is stable. Not recommended for individuals less than 18 years, with abnormal muscle mass (amputees, paraplegia or quadriplegia, severe malnutrition or obesity, pregnant women) and those on extreme diets (vegetarian or low-meat diet, creatine dietary supplements).

Jelliffe Formula[52]
CrCl (mL/min) = (98 − {0.8 × [age (years) − 20]} / SCr (mg/dL) × 0.9 (if female)

Modified-Jelliffe Formula (corrected by BSA)[53]
CrCl (mL/min) = (98 − [0.8 × (age − 20)] / SCr (mg/dL) × Patient's BSA /1.73 m²) × 0.9 (if female)

Original Schwartz Formula:[54]
CrCl (mL/min/1.73 m²) = K × Height (cm) /SCr (mg/mL)
Preterm babies < 1 year: K = 0.33; full-term infants < 1 year: K = 0.45; child or adolescent girl: K = 0.55; adolescent boy: K = 0.7

Revised Schwartz Formula:[55]
GFR (mL/min/1.73 m²) = 0.413 × Height (cm)/SCr (mg/dL)

Web-Based Calculators With Equations to Calculate Estimated Renal Function for the Various Formulas
- http://www.kidney.org/professionals/kdoqi/gfr_calculator.cfm
- http://www.nephron.com/MDRD_GFR.cgi
- http://nkdep.nih.gov/lab-evaluation/gfr-calculators/adults-conventional-unit.shtmL
- http://www.kidney.org/professionals/kdoqi/gfr_calculator.cfm

Notes: eCrCl, estimated creatinine clearance; eGFR, estimated glomerular filtration rate; SCr, serum creatinine.

Table 3-10 Classifications of Renal Impairment[40]

Traditional Classification of Renal Impairment[a,40]

Normal renal function	CrCl greater than or equal to 60 mL/min
Mild renal dysfunction	CrCl 40–59 mL/min
Moderate renal dysfunction	CrCl 20–39 mL/min
Severe renal dysfunction	CrCl less than 20 mL/min

Classification of Chronic Kidney Disease According to Kidney Disease Outcomes Quality Initiative (K/DOQI)

Stage 1 Kidney damage with normal or increasing GFR	GFR ≥ 90 mL/min/1.73 m²

Stage 2   GFR 60-89 mL/min/1.73 m^2
Kidney damage with mild decrease in GFR

Stage 3[b]   GFR 30-59 mL/min/1.73 m^2
Moderate decrease in GFR

Stage 4[b]   GFR 15-29 mL/min/1.73 m^2
Severe decrease in GFR

Stage 5[b]   GFR less than 15 mL/min/1.73 m^2
Kidney failure

Notes: CrCl, creatinine clearance; GFR, glomerular filtration rate.
[a] Some renal function studies may correct for body size by indexing to BSA of 1.73 m^2 by expressing as mL/min/1.73 m^2.
[b] At this level of renal function, drugs cleared by the kidney remain in the body for a longer duration than in those with normal renal function.

A 24-hour urine collection is one method that can be used to calculate creatinine clearance and estimate GFR, but it is time consuming, inconvenient for patients, and is subject to inaccuracies when patients do not collect timed urine samples accurately. A more convenient method of estimating GFR is through the use of validated formulas. The 2 most commonly used formulas to estimate renal function are the Cockcroft-Gault (CG) equation, which estimates creatinine clearance (eCrCl), and the Modification of Diet in Renal Disease (MDRD) Study equation, which estimates GFR (eGFR) (Table 3-9). Stevens and colleagues conducted a large simulation study comparing CG and MDRD to each other and to the gold-standard measurement of GFR using urinary clearance of iothalamate. The results suggest that for the majority of patients and for most drugs tested, there was little difference in the drug dose using either eCrCl or eGFR.[56] Based on this data, the National Kidney Disease Education Program (NKDEP) suggests that either the eGFR or eCrCL may be utilized to calculate drug dosing.[50] Lastly, trends in serum creatinine changes should be considered when doses are based on renal function, not just the actual numerical values of serum creatinine, creatinine clearance, or GFR.

In an effort to standardize serum creatinine assays, in 2010 all clinical laboratories in the United States implemented the new standardized isotope dilution mass spectrometry (IDMS) method to measure serum creatinine.[54] This standardization will allow for less variability in creatinine values used for managing patients; thus, leading to less variation in estimating kidney function and consequently, more consistent drug dosing.[50] An effect of the IDMS method is that it generates a lower creatinine value than older methods of measuring creatinine in patients with normal renal function, and it is also more likely to generate creatinine levels that are below the lower limit of normal.[50] The use of IDMS creatinine for calculation of creatinine clearance has only been evaluated with the MDRD study equation and is not validated with the Cockcroft-Gault or Jelliffe formula.[50] The use of an IDMS-creatinine value in the Cockcroft-Gault equation will lead to a higher eCrCl value in some patients with normal renal function and overestimates eCrCl when the serum creatinine values are relatively low. It is not possible to have a single, uniform conversion factor or formula to relate IDMS standardized creatinine values back to non-IDMS traceable values. Formulas utilizing a conversion factor to translate IDMS creatinine to a corrected (non-IDMS) creatinine have been proposed, but none have been adequately validated; thus, corrected IDMS creatinine should not be used to calculate carboplatin dosing.[50] It is recommended that clinicians ascertain if the standard IDMS traceable creatinine is utilized and reported in their institution or laboratory when using serum creatinine to calculate creatinine clearance.

In children, the best equation for estimating GFR is the Schwartz equation (Table 3-9) for use with creatinine methods with calibration traceable to IDMS.[54,55]

Dose and Administration Modification in Hemodialysis Setting

It is difficult to determine the optimal anticancer therapy dose in cancer patients with end-stage renal disease on long-term hemodialysis (HD) because high-level evidence and pharmacokinetic data for this patient population is lacking. Guidelines for dose adjustment in HD patients are available for only a few anticancer drugs, and existing recommendations are mainly derived from case reports or case series. Dosing considerations in HD patients include dose adjustments, timing of drug administration in relation to the dialysis session, and knowledge of the fraction of the drug that is removed by HD. The goal of anticancer drug dosing in HD patients is to avoid nonrenal toxic effects through appropriate dose reduction and prevent early drug elimination during dialysis that may result in subsequent lower dose intensity and efficacy. In general, if the primary elimination pathway of an anticancer drug is via the kidneys and the drug is not significantly removed by dialysis, the drug can be administered at any time, before or after HD sessions. On the other hand, if the drug is partially removed by dialysis, it should be administered after HD sessions to avoid loss of efficacy.[57] A summary of dosing recommendations of anticancer drugs in HD patient is listed in **Table 3-11**, and **Clinical Pearl 3-3** provides an example of anticancer therapy dose determination in a patient on hemodialysis.

Table 3-11 Recommendations for Dosage Adjustment in Patients Receiving Hemodialysis[57,58]

Drug (Grade Level of Evidence)[a]	Recommendations	
	Dosing	Administration of Cancer Therapy in Relation to Hemodialysis (HD)
Carboplatin[57,58] (B)	AUC-directed calculation where GFR is set equal to zero	• After HD or on nondialysis days • A delay of 16 hours is recommended between administration and hemo-dialysis
Cisplatin[57,58] (B)	• Partially cleared by hemodialysis • Reduce dose by 50%	Conflicting recommendations: • After HD or on nondialysis days • HD immediately after administration
Cyclophosphamide[57,58] (B)	Reduce by 25%	• After HD or on nondialysis days • Dialysis should not be initiated earlier than 12 hours after cyclophospha-mide infusion
Docetaxel[57] (C)	• Start dose at 65 mg/m^2 and adjust according to tolerance and efficacy	• Before or after HD
Doxorubicin, daunorubicin, epirubicin[57,58] (C)	• Not dialyzed • No dose adjustment	• After HD or on nondialysis days
Etoposide[57,58] (B)	Reduce dose by 50%–60%	• Before or after HD
5-Fluorouracil[57,58] (C)	No dose adjustment	• After HD
Gemcitabine[57] (B)	No dose adjustment	• Start HD 6–12 hours after gemcitabine administration
Ifosfamide[58]	Avoid in HD patients	
Irinotecan[57]	Reduce initial weekly dose at 50 mg/m^2; can escalate dose to 80 mg/m^2 as tolerated	After HD or on nondialysis days

(continues)

Table 3-11 Recommendations for Dosage Adjustment in Patients Receiving Hemodialysis [57,58](*continued*)

Drug (Grade Level of Evidence)[a]	Recommendations	
	Dosing	Administration of Cancer Therapy in Relation to Hemodialysis (HD)
Methotrexate[57,58] (C)	• If mandatory for cancer, reduce dose by 75% • Monitor closely for adverse effects • Prolonged rescue with leucovorin recommended	• Administer after HD
Oxapliplatin[57] (C)	• If mandatory, reduce dose by 30% • Limited data	• After HD
Paclitaxel[57,58] (B)	• No dose adjustment	• Before or after HD
Vinorelbine, vincristine[57,58] (C)	• Not dialyzed	• After HD or on nondialysis days

[a] **Grade A:** Scientific evidence on the basis of randomized clinical trials with significant population; and meta-analysis of clinical trials.
Grade B: Scientific evidence on the basis of randomized clinical trials but with a weak power; nonrandomized clinical trials; and cohort studies.
Grade C: Low level of scientific evidence based on case-control studies; comparative trials with historical data; retrospective studies; and case series or case reports.

CLINICAL PEARL 3–3
Dosing of Anticancer Therapy in a Patient on Hemodialysis

A 45-year-old male with end-stage renal disease is scheduled for HD on Mondays, Wednesdays, and Fridays. He was also recently diagnosed with extensive small cell lung cancer and is scheduled to receive carboplatin and etoposide. The dose of carboplatin is an AUC of 5 on day 1 and the etoposide dose is 100 mg/m^2 on days 1, 2, and 3.

His height is 175 cm, weight is 70 kg, and liver function tests and bilirubin are within normal limits.

> **Calculate the patient's BSA using the Mosteller formula:**
>
> **Mosteller:** $BSA = \sqrt{[(175\ cm \times 70\ kg)/3600]} = 1.845\ m^2$
>
> (Use the equation or one of the websites that calculates BSA from Table 3-1.)
>
> **Calculate the patient's carboplatin dose using the Calvert equation:**
>
> Carboplatin dose (mg) = 5 (mg/mL × min) × (0 + 25)(mL/min)
>
> Carboplatin dose = 5 × 25 = 125 mg
>
> Using the recommendations from Table 3-11, the patient's GFR is set to 0 and the dose should be administered after each HD.
>
> **Calculate the patient's etoposide dose:**
>
> Etoposide dose = 1.845 m² × 100 mg = 185 mg
>
> 50% of etoposide dose = 185 mg divided by 2 = 92 mg
>
> Using the recommendations from Table 3-11, the dose should be decreased by 50% and may be administered before or after dialysis. The dose could be rounded up or down within 5%-10% of calculated dose for ease of preparation.

Hepatic Function Assessment and Anticancer Therapy Dosing

Many anticancer agents undergo hepatic metabolism resulting in drug activation, degradation, and excretion. In cancer patients, liver dysfunction may occur from liver metastasis or preexisting diseases such as hepatitis, cirrhosis, or Gilbert's disease. The effect of liver disease on drug kinetics include changing intrinsic hepatic clearance of drugs, altering biliary excretion of drugs, reducing hepatic metabolism capacity, reducing albumin production resulting in increased fraction of free drugs, and altering absorption of drugs from the gastrointestinal tract in cases of severe hepatic portal hypertension.[59]

The outcome of administering anticancer agents to patients with liver impairment is the decreased production of active metabolites for prodrugs or decreased detoxification of drugs that undergo hepatic biotransformation. Subsequently, patients may experience decreased effectiveness of anticancer therapy or increased toxicity in the presence of liver dysfunction. Unfortunately, for many anticancer agents, there is a paucity of data on drug disposition in patients with liver dysfunction. Patients with abnormal liver function are usually excluded from phase I, II, and III clinical trials. Dose reduction recommendations for individual agents are based on small retrospective studies or empirical guidelines, and there is a lack of reliable dose modification scheme based on detailed studies.[37,59] More recently, the National Cancer Institute Organ Dysfunction Working Group has evaluated some recently FDA-approved drugs in clinical trials with the aim of developing specific dosing guidelines on the basis of standard biochemical tests of liver function.[31,32] Table 3-8 provides dose adjustment recommendations in patients with liver dysfunction for specific agents. The recommendations for dose adjustment in patients with liver dysfunction differ among the various sources, as with dosing recommendations in patients with renal impairment. Clinicians should be cautious in administering anticancer agents in patients with impaired hepatic function and use clinical judgment, patient-specific factors, and goals of therapy to guide in determining which recommendations to apply.

No standardized system that defines liver dysfunction in patients with cancer exists. Total serum bilirubin level, transaminase levels (AST or ALT) are the markers most commonly used to assess the need for anticancer therapy dose adjustments. An excellent review on the function of these biomarkers, their roles, and their limitations as markers of liver function can be found in the review article by Field and colleagues.[60]

SUMMARY

The process of calculating the dose of an anticancer agent to be administered to a patient is involved and requires clinicians to consider many factors. A checklist that includes the minimum necessary information prior to computing an anticancer therapy dose should include:

- Patient diagnosis, height and weight, age, gender, and comorbidities
- Anticancer regimen and supporting reference to verify the dosage
- Patient's organ function (serum creatinine, total bilirubin, AST/ALT)
- Method for calculating BSA, renal function
- Method for calculating dose: mg/m^2, mg/kg, AUC, flat dose

A multidisciplinary approach involving physicians, pharmacists, and nurses each performing independent verification of the calculated dose will ensure accurate and safe prescribing, preparation, and administration of anticancer therapy agents. The implementation of policies and procedures that standardize the process of anticancer therapy dose verification, delineate agreed-upon formulas for BSA and renal function calculation, and define criteria for dose adjustments will ascertain dose agreement among clinicians involved in the dose calculation process. When doses are not in agreement with independent practitioners' calculations, a policy on how to address the situation should be in place. The chapter titled, *Basics of Systemic Anticancer Therapy Prescribing and Verification* and the *Pediatric Oncology* and *High-Dose Cancer Therapy* chapters in this text will provide more detailed information in ensuring appropriate prescribing and verification of anticancer drugs for all healthcare providers involved with prescribing, admixing, or administering anticancer agents.

REFERENCES

1. Gurney H. Dose calculation of anticancer drugs: a review of the current practice and introduction of an alternative. *J Clin Oncol.* 1996;14(9):2590–2611.
2. Felici A, Verweij J, Sparreboom A. Dosing strategies for anticancer drugs: the good, the bad and body-surface area. *Eur J Cancer.* 2002;38:1677–1684.
3. DuBois D, DuBois EF. A formula to estimate the approximate surface area if height and weight be known. *Arch Int Med.* 1916;17:863–871.
4. Mosteller RD. Simplified calculation of body surface area. *N Engl J Med.* 1987;317:1098.
5. Haycock G, Schwartz G, Wisotsky D. Geometric method for measuring body surface area: a height, weight formula validated in infants, children, and adults. *J Pediatr.* 1978;93:62–66.
6. Gehan E, George S. Estimation of human body surface area from height and weight. *Cancer Chemother Rep.* 1970;54:225–235.
7. Gao B, Klumpen HJ, Gurney H. Dose calculation of anticancer drugs. *Expert Opin Drug Metab Toxicol.* 2008;4(10):1307–1319.
8. Gurney H. How to calculate the dose of chemotherapy. *Br J Cancer.* 2002;86: 1297–1302.
9. Kaestner SA, Sewell GJ. Chemotherapy dosing part I: scientific basis for current practice and use of body surface area. *Clin Oncol.* 2007;19:23–37.
10. Griggs J, Mangu P, Anderson H, et al. Appropriate chemotherapy dosing for obese patients with cancer: American society of clinical oncology clinical practice guideline. *J Clin Oncol.* 2012;30(13):1553–1561.
11. Centers for Disease Control and Prevention. Overweight and obesity. http://www .cdc.gov/nchs/data/hestat/obesity_adult_07_08/obesity_adult_07_08.htm. Accessed October, 2012.
12. Field K, Kosmider S, Jefford M, et al. Chemotherapy dosing stategies in the obese, elderly, and thin patient: results of a nationwide survey. *JOP.* 2008;4(3):108–113.
13. Duong C, Loh J. Laboratory monitoring in oncology. *J Oncol Pharm Pract.* 2006;12:223–236.
14. Colangelo P, Welch D, Rich D, Jeffrey L. Two methods for estimating body surface area in adult amputees. *Am J Hosp Pharm.* 1984;41:2650–2655.

15. Calvert A, Newell D, Gumbrell L, et al. Carboplatin dosage: Prospective evaluation of a simple formula based on renal function. *J Clin Oncol.* 1989;7(11):1748–1756.
16. Canal P, Chatelut E, Guichard S. Practical treatment guide for dose individualisation in cancer therapy. *Drugs.* 1998;56(6):1019–1038.
17. NCI Cancer Therapy Evaluation Program. Carboplatin dosing. US Food and Drug Administration website. http://www.fda.gov/AboutFDA/CentersOffices/OfficeofMedicalProductsandTobacco/CDER/ucm228974.htm. Accessed October 10, 2012.
18. O'Cearbhaill R. New guidelines for carboplatin dosing. Gynecologic Oncology Group website. http://www.gog.org/Spring2012newsletter.pdf. Accessed October 5, 2012.
19. Culine S, Kramar A, Theodore C, et al. Randomized trial comparing bleomycin/etoposide/cisplatin with alternating cisplatin/cyclophosphamide/doxorubicin and vinblastine/bleomycin regimens of chemotherapy for patients with intermediate- and poor-risk metastatic nonseminomatous germ cell tumors: Genito-urinary group of the French federation of cancer centers trial T93MP. *J Clin Oncol.* 2008;26:421–427.
20. Coiffer B, Lepage E, Briere J, et al. CHOP plus rituximab compared with CHOP alone in elderly patients with diffuse large B-cell lymphoma. *N Engl J Med.* 2002;346:235–242.
21. McLeod H, Krynetski E, Relling M, Evans W. Genetic polymorphism of thiopurine methyltransferase and its clinical relevance for childhood acute lymphoblastic leukemia. *Leukemia.* 2000;14:567–572.
22. Relling M, Gardner E, Sandborn W, et al. Clinical pharmacogenetics implementation consortium guidelines for thiopurine methyltransferase genotype thiopurine dosing. *Clin Pharmacol Ther.* 2011;89(3):387–391.
23. Mercaptopurine (purethinol) [package insert]. Teva Pharmaceuticals; 2011. Greeville, NC.
24. Longley D, Harkin D, Johnston P. 5-fluorouracil: mechanism of action and clinical strategies. *Nat Rev Cancer.* 2003;3:330–338.
25. Lee A, Ezzeldin H, Fourie J, Diasio R. Dihydropyrimidine dehydrogenase deficiency: impact of pharmacogenetics on 5-fluorouracil therapy. *Clin Adv Hematol Oncol.* 2004;2:527–532.
26. Ciccolini J, Gross E, Dahan L, Lacarelle B, Mercier C. Routine dihydropyrimidine testing for anticipating 5-FU-related severe toxicities: hype or hope? *Clin Colorectal Cancer.* 2010;9(4):224–228.
27. McLeod HL, Sargent DJ, Marsh S, et al. Pharmacogenetic predictors of adverse events and response to chemotherapy in metastatic colorectal cancer: results from North American gastrointestinal intergroup trial N9741. *J Clin Oncol.* 2010;28:3227–3233.
28. Swen J, Nijenhuis M, de Boer A, et al. Pharmacogenetics: from bench to byte–an update of guidelines. *Clin Pharmacol Ther.* 2011;89:662–673.
29. Superfin D, Iannucci A, Davies A. Commentary: Oncologic drugs in patients with organ dysfunction: a summary. *Oncologist.* 2007;12:1070–1083.
30. Leal T, Remick S, Takimoto C, et al. Dose-escalating and pharmacological study of bortezomib in adult cancer patients with impaired renal function: a National Cancer Institute organ dysfunction working group study. *Cancer Chemother Pharmacol.* 2011;68:1439–1447.
31. LoRusso P, Venkatakrishnan K, Ramanathan R, et al. Pharmacokinetics and safety of bortezomib in patients with advanced malignancies and varying degrees of liver dysfunction: Phase I NCI organ dysfunction working group study NCI-6432. *Clin Cancer Res.* 2012;18(10):2954–2963.

32. Ramanathan R, Egorin M, Takimoto C, et al. Phase I and pharmacokinetic study of imatinib mesylate in patients with advanced malignancies and varying degrees of liver dysfunction: a study by the National Cancer Institute organ dysfunction working group. *J Clin Oncol.* 2008;26:563–569.

33. Bendamustine (Treanda) [package insert]. Teva Pharmaceuticals; 2012. Frazer, PA.

34. Li Y, Fu S, Liu J, Finkel K, Gershenson D. Systemic anticancer therapy in gynecological cancer patients with renal dysfunction. *Int J Gynecol Cancer.* 2007;17:739–763.

35. Bondanini F, Brunetti G, Cartoni C, Cupelli L, de Fabritiis P, Del Poeta G. Management of hematological malignancies in patients affected by renal failure. *Expert Rev Anticancer Ther.* 2011;11:415.

36. Sahni V, Choudhury D, Ahmed Z. Chemotherapy-associated renal dysfunction. *Nature.* 2009;5:450–460.

37. Eklund J, Trifilio S, Mulcahy M. Chemotherapy dosing in the setting of liver dysfunction. *Oncology.* 2005;19:1057–1063.

38. Field K, Michael M. Part II: Liver function in oncology: towards safer chemotherapy use. *Lancet Oncol.* 2008;9:1181–1190.

39. Doxil (doxorubicin HCL liposome injection) [package insert]. Janssen; 2013. Bedford, OH.

40. Gibbons J, Egorin M, Ramanathan R, et al. Phase I and pharmacokinetic study of imatinib mesylate in patients with advanced malignancies and varying degrees of renal dysfunction: a study by the National Cancer Institute organ dysfunction working group. *J Clin Oncol.* 2008;26(4):570–576.

41. Gleevec (imatinib mesylate) [package insert]. Novartis Oncology; 2013. East Hanover, NJ.

42. Camptosar (irinotecan) [package insert]. Pfizer; 2012. New York, NY.

43. Ixempra (ixabepilone) [package insert]. Bristol-Myers Squibb; 2011. Germany.

44. Mutamycin (mitomycin for injection) [package insert]. Bristol-Myers Squibb Oncology; 2001. Princeton, NJ.

45. Food and Drug Administration. *Novantrone (mitoxantrone for injection).* http://www.accessdata.fda.gov/drugsatfda_docs/label/2009/019297s030s031lbl.pdf. Accessed June 3, 2013.

46. Tasigna (nilotinib) [package insert]. Novartis Oncology; 2013. Switzerland.

47. Alimta (pemetrexed) [package insert]. Lilly Pharmaceuticals; 2012. Indianapolis, IN.

48. Vinblastine sulfate [package insert]. APP Pharmaceuticals; 2012. Schaumburg, IL.

49. Centers for Disease Control and Prevention website. Body mass index. http://www.cdc.gov/healthyweight/assessing/bmi/index.html. Accessed October 10, 2012.

50. CKD and drug dosing: information for providers. National Kidney Disease Education Program website. http://www.nkdep.nih.gov/resources/CKD-drug-dosing.shtml. Accessed October 2, 2012.

51. Shoker A, Hossain MA, Koru-Sengal T, Raju DL, Cockcroft D. Performance of creatinine clearance equations on the original Cockcroft-Gault population. *Clin Nephrol.* 2006;66:89–97.

52. Jelliffe R. Estimation of creatinine clearance when urine cannot be collected. *Lancet.* 1971;1:975–976.

53. Jelliffe R. Creatinine clearance: bedside estimate. *Ann Intern Med.* 1973;79:604–605.

54. Schwartz G, Gauthier B. A simple estimate of glomerular filtration rate in adolescent boys. *J Pediatr.* 1985;106:522–526.

55. Schwartz G, Schneider M, Mak R, Kastel F, Warady B, Furth S. New equation to estimate GFR in children with CKD. *J Am Soc Nephrol.* 2009;20:629–637.

56. Stevens L, Nolin T, Richardson M, et al. Comparison of drug dosing recommendations based on measured GFR and kidney function estimating equations. *Am J Kidney Dis*. 2009;54(1):33–42.

57. Janus N, Thariat J, Boulanger H, Deray G, Launay-Vacher V. Proposal for dosage adjustment and timing of chemotherapy in hemodialyzed patients. *Ann Oncol*. 2010;21:1395–1403.

58. Tomita M, Aoki Y, Tanaka K. Effect of haemodialysis on the pharmacokinetics of antineoplastic drugs. *Clin Pharmacokinet*. 2004;43(8):515–527.

59. Donelli M, Zucchetti M, Munzone E, D'Incalci M, Crosignani A. Pharmacokinetics of anticancer agents in patients with impaired liver function. *Eur J Cancer*. 1998;34(1):33–46.

60. Field K, Dow C, Michael M. Part I: Liver function in oncology: biochemistry and beyond. *Lancet Oncol*. 2008;9:1092–1101.

SUGGESTED WEBSITES AND READINGS

Genotyping
- http://www.pharmgkb.org
- http://www.pharmgkb.org/drug/PA450379/drug/PA450379 (mercaptopurine)
- http://www.gene.com/gene/products/information/xeloda/pdf/pi.pdf
- http://www.arupconsult.com/Topics/Irinotecan.html
- http://www.entrogen.com/web2/ugt1a1-genotyping-reagents-irinotecan-toxicity
- https://www.labcorp.com/wps/portal/
- http://patient.cancerconsultants.com/druginserts/Irinotecan.pdf

Assessment of Renal Function
- National Kidney Disease Education Program:
  http://nkdep.nih.gov/
  http://nkdep.nih.gov/lab-evaluation/gfr.shtml
  http://www.kidney.org/professionals/kdoqi/guidelines.cfm
- Aapro M, Launay-Vacher V. Importance of monitoring for renal function in patients with cancer. *Cancer Treat Rev*. 2012;38:235–240.
- Stevens LA, Coresh J, Greene T, Levey AS. Assessing kidney function—measured and estimated glomerular filtration rate. *N Engl J Med*. 2006;354:2473–2483.

Assessment of Hepatic Function
- Field K, Dow C, Michael M. Part I: Liver function in oncology: biochemistry and beyond. *Lancet Oncol*. 2008;9:1092–1101.

Cancer Therapy Preparation

Michele Rice
Jeanne Adams
James G. Stevenson

LEARNING OBJECTIVES:

Upon completion of the chapter, the reader will be able to:

1. Explain the regulations that apply to cancer therapy preparation and be able to adopt compliant procedures appropriate to assure safety of the patient and the healthcare worker.
2. List and describe appropriate personal protective equipment and environmental controls for use in the cancer therapy preparation area and outline a process for safe cancer therapy spill cleanup.
3. Compare types of storage and inventory management devices and distinguish between these based on features that are key to outpatient oncology.
4. Review issues in product preparation and dispensing and advocate solutions that produce a safe, accurate product, as well as improve work flow.
5. Construct for cancer therapy preparation personnel a training program that will advocate aseptic technique, safe handling of hazardous medications, and appropriate disposal of hazardous waste.

INTRODUCTION

Historically, there was nothing formal or organized about chemotherapy preparation in a hospital, cancer center, or physician office. Nearly any seasoned oncology nurse or pharmacist can tell a story about mixing chemotherapy without any personal protective equipment (PPE), on a countertop, at the bedside, or while multitasking. Extreme stories might include mixing in a bathroom sink, eating or drinking while mixing cancer therapy, or squirting unused drug at a wall, at the ceiling, or into a plant. These stories all sound outrageous now, but these practices were not really unusual. Mixing the drugs was just part of the ordinary workday, and no extra precautions were routinely taken while preparing the cancer therapies. Knowledge of the potential negative impact of environmental exposure to healthcare workers, as well as an appreciation of the need for high-quality sterile product preparation to assure patient safety, has resulted in significant changes in the practices around the preparation of chemotherapy and other hazardous drugs.[1-5]

Oncology practices and health systems continue to purchase, prepare, and administer cancer medications on site. In many states, this office practice activity takes place under the jurisdiction of the physician license, without requiring the presence of a pharmacist. Whether or not a pharmacy license is required, many cancer centers have begun to acknowledge the clinical and financial benefits of employing a pharmacist to create appropriate sterile product preparation practices, manage drug inventory, develop standardized treatment guidelines, and provide clinical patient interventions, among other tasks.[6]

Because of concerns for healthcare worker exposure as well as for aseptic preparation, cancer therapy preparation practices have changed. Cancer therapy preparation should be planned based on 3 key principles: protect the patient by producing a sterile product, protect the staff by preventing exposure to cytotoxic material, and protect the environment through appropriate disposal of hazardous materials. Having a separate production area for preparation of cancer therapy—a cleanroom—helps accomplish all of these goals and is called for in the standards of the United States Pharmacopeia (USP), which may be enforceable as regulations in some states.[7] All cleanrooms, whether in a hospital or a clinic, should be designed with these primary functions as the highest priority.

CANCER THERAPY PREPARATION AREA: THE CLEANROOM

Producing a sterile product requires controlling the environment and the process of preparation. The environment in the production area is regulated because this is the first source of bacterial contamination. Bacteria can enter the finished product via particles (dust, skin cells, hair, clothing fibers, etc.) in the air, from the surfaces of the counter, or directly from the staff handling the compounded sterile preparation. Bacteria and viruses are small enough to ride on particles that are not always visible to the naked eye. Particles from the air settle on surfaces, are spread around the room by personnel, and are potentially introduced into the patient via the intravenous (IV) administration of the medication.

Environmental Controls

Environmental controls are implemented to minimize this particle count and minimize contamination in the preparation area. Hazardous drugs (both IV and oral) should be stored separately from other inventory to prevent contamination and personnel exposure. When chemotherapy is received from the wholesaler, the personnel unpacking the products should wear PPE, and the outside of chemotherapy vials should be wiped. Since several chemotherapy agents have vapor pressures that allow volatilization at room temperature; cleanrooms with buffer areas and anterooms are recommended, with chemotherapy prepared in a negative pressure environment to allow containment in the event of a spill or aerosolization.[7] In these cases, an ISO Class 5 device such as a biological safety cabinet (BSC) or compounding aseptic containment isolator (CACI) that is vented to the outside through high-efficiency particulate air (HEPA) filtration should be used (**Box 4-1**). Horizontal laminar flow hoods should not be used because the air flow increases exposure of the healthcare worker to the hazardous compounds. These devices should be placed in a buffer area in which there is minimal traffic and particulate matter from boxes and other sources is minimized. Chemotherapy preparation (including oral drugs) should not occur on a countertop.[7,8] These units, commonly called *hoods*, maintain sterility by creating a pattern of air flow to prevent particle settling. Air flow is also HEPA filtered and, if the hood is properly installed, cytotoxic vapors are vented to the outside. The air in the room should have a HEPA filter to remove particles large enough to carry bacteria and other contaminants. All nonhazardous medications (such as premedications) should be compounded in a separate hood and ideally in a separate room from hazardous medications. (See the chapter called *Oral Cancer Therapy* for more information about handling of oral hazardous cancer therapy agents).

BOX 4-1

Biologic Safety Cabinet Versus Isolator[7,8]

Chemotherapy preparation should take place inside a controlled environment, to prevent bacterial contamination of the product and to protect the operator from exposure to hazardous material. There are several types of pharmacy equipment called *hoods*, but only biological safety cabinets (BSCs) and barrier isolators (also known as glove boxes) can accomplish both.[7] The common laminar flow hood used in pharmacies for preparation of nonhazardous compounds maintains sterility by creating a pattern of airflow toward the operator, which would cause unacceptable hazardous drug exposure with chemotherapy agents.

US Center for Disease Control Class II, type A2 BSCs are appropriate for chemotherapy preparation. These BSCs recirculate some of the air within the cabinet through a HEPA filter and vent the rest to a facility exhaust system. Barrier isolators are totally enclosed, with all operations being performed through the attached gloves. All material to be placed into the sterile interior must pass through a vented side chamber; items must remain in the side chamber long enough for the air inside to completely pass through the filter, to maintain the closed system.

Barrier isolators can be compounding aseptic isolators (CAIs) or compounding aseptic containment isolators (CACIs). CAIs may be used for products that are not considered hazardous, but CACIs should be used for compounding hazardous sterile products. CAIs operate under positive pressure and must be used in a fully compliant cleanroom, while CACIs create a negative pressure environment and some have been certified and tested to be placed in an area separate from other production without a full facility remodel.

A disadvantage of barrier isolators is the need for built-in gloves to access the chamber. These gloves are expensive to replace and are often not long enough to allow most operators to reach the back wall of the chamber for cleaning. Special tools are needed to perform routine cleaning, making noncompliance common. Also, the side chamber is fixed, making use by left-handed individuals awkward. Some side chambers can be configured to accommodate left-handedness, but the configuration cannot easily be changed back, making it essentially permanent. Some operators consider the working position required by isolators to be awkward and the gloves cumbersome, while others make the adjustment with little difficulty. Discomfort and additional steps may cause noncompliance with manufacturer instructions, which can defeat the mechanisms that maintain sterility and provide protection from exposure.

The decision to use a barrier isolator over a standard BSC should incorporate the needs of the personnel who will be operating it and the quantity of products and throughput needs of the infusion clinic. For a busy oncology practice or service, barrier isolators are typically only a consideration when renovations to accommodate a BSC are not feasible. In these cases, a CACI for hazardous drug preparation will still require external ducting and connection to a facility exhaust system.

Biological Safety Cabinets		Barrier Isolators	
Advantages	Disadvantages	Advantages	Disadvantages
Easy cleaning	Requires cleanroom	Complete barrier protects staff from exposure	Hard to clean and maintain
Easy access		Production occurs in closed, sterile environment	Access to work area is cumbersome and awkward
Fewer steps in mixing process		Option with less extensive cleanroom remodel	Additional steps added to process, slowing production speed
Lower cost, more ideal for high volume clinics		CACI acceptable for low-volume clinics	Noncompliance with manufacturer instructions for use; cleaning may defeat barrier

United States Pharmacopeia (USP) Chapter 797, Pharmaceutical Compounding—Sterile Preparation,[7] the current cleanroom guidelines, also makes specific recommendation for flooring, ceiling tiles, doors, light fixtures, and wall paint, all intended to minimize particle shedding and maximize the ability to keep a clean environment. The Controlled Environment Testing Association (CETA) guidelines provide additional guidance on design/remodel of clean rooms, such as exhaust methodology.[9] These documents should be reviewed thoroughly when planning a cleanroom design or remodel, and it is a good idea to provide a copy to your contractor, particularly Appendix 1, which contains the principle competencies, conditions, practices, and quality assurances that are required ("shall") and recommended ("should") in Chapter 797 of the USP.[7] Note the difference in meaning between *shall* and *should,* as these terms are used throughout the document. Consultants can be very helpful with engineering of a cleanroom and well worth the cost. At a minimum, BSC certifiers will be able to review construction and equipment purchase plans and provide advice.

Aseptic technique refers to the process used by personnel to avoid introducing bacterial contamination to the final product. This includes not touching anything that needs to remain sterile, not blocking the airflow pattern in the hood, and the use of proper washing, garbing, and gowning, which will be addressed in a later section. Anyone mixing cancer therapy should be trained in proper sterile technique using approved resources.[7]

Protection of the patient by creating and maintaining a sterile final product is part of any IV medication preparation. We now know that minimizing exposure of cytotoxic medications to healthcare staff requires special handling of cancer therapy medications. Several agents (eg, alkylators) have been associated with the development of secondary malignancies; thus, it is hypothesized that occupational exposure could result in cancer. Damage to chromosomes, miscarriages, and infertility are among the conditions that have been associated with chronic occupational chemotherapy exposure.[10-12] Although there is no definition of safe or unsafe exposure or evidence for a causal correlation, reduction of exposure is a prudent precaution.

Protection of the staff requires minimizing exposure to cytotoxic medications. However, for simplicity, it is easier to apply safe handling principles to all medications used to treat cancer than to set up sets of procedures for different drugs based on mechanism of action. Minimizing exposure to staff can include environmental controls, use of PPE, use of closed system transfer devices (CSTDs), and special handling of every aspect of cancer therapy, including packaging.

Environmental controls used to create and maintain sterility by minimizing particles circulating in the air were discussed in the previous sections. The same controls, with modifications, are use in cleanrooms for cancer therapy preparation to minimize contamination in the remainder of the facility (**Clinical Pearl 4-1**). The first controllable environmental feature is exhaust. The properly installed containment device (BSC or CACI) has a mechanism to prevent aerosols or vapors from being recirculated into the room air. Usually this is accomplished by venting exhaust air through HEPA filtration to the outside of the building.[7,8] CSTDs may also be employed to minimize vapor release and exposure of health-care workers. CSTDs are disposable devices that create a barrier between the chemotherapy in the vial and the syringe, preventing the aerosolization or release of cytotoxic vapor, which usually occurs any time these volatile agents are reconstituted or injected (see **Box 4-2**).[7,13] CSTDs are intended to be used in combination with, and not as a replacement for, a BSC or CAI.

CLINICAL PEARL 4-1

It is important to remember that environmental controls use airflow to create and maintain a clean mixing area. Traffic through the cleanroom and even excessive body movement creates turbulence that disrupts the airflow. Movement also increases the numbers of particles released into the room. Therefore, unnecessary movement through the cleanroom should be discouraged.

BOX 4-2
Closed System Transfer Devices[7,13]

Closed system transfer devices (CSTDs) represent recent technology intended to create a mechanical barrier between the chemotherapy vial and the syringe used for reconstitution. A CSTD product traps chemotherapy spray and vapors that are released when vials of volatile compounds are accessed. The whole closed system may include multiple pieces to allow for adapting to different vial sizes, as well as components to allow addition of chemotherapy to bags of IV fluid and for use in administration.

Advantages of CSTDs

- Usually needleless, preventing unnecessary exposure from contaminated needle sticks
- The closed system prevents hazardous vapor from being released and potentially spread throughout the facility
- Provide an additional barrier to contaminants to the sterile preparation
- The presence of a CSTD on the vial minimizes the chance of chemotherapy spill due to poor technique

Disadvantages of CSTDs

- Often require the purchase of multiple pieces, increasing the total expense for their use and requiring additional storage space
- Pieces may be awkward, involve multiple steps, or require perfect technique to assemble
- Additional time for assembly slows down production
- The system must be used correctly to provide a completely closed system
- Storage space for all additional pieces may be difficult in small clinics
- Rushing, skipping steps, or only using some of the pieces could allow exposure anyway

The largest barrier to implementation of CSTDs in community oncology is the expense. All systems require purchase of disposable parts that integrate into a closed system. Yet, CSTDs are not yet reimbursable by any payer. Few practices can justify such a large, continuing, unreimbursed expense at a time when some drugs barely recoup their purchase cost.

Controversy also exists regarding the definition of *unsafe exposure*. While it is common sense that minimizing exposure to hazardous medications is beneficial to cancer center personnel, the actual amount of exposure that should be considered unacceptable is unknown. Most studies validating CSTDs show reduction in urinary excretion of chemotherapy by workers after implementation. However, as laboratory monitoring becomes increasingly sophisticated, new methods may be able to detect the presence of chemotherapy at that point, despite use of CSTDs. Opponents of CSTDs say that chasing this number is impossible and perhaps clinically insignificant, until there is data to suggest safety parameters.

Another main source of environmental protection is the creation of negative pressure within the preparation area. Air circulation by exhaust in the hood, combined with HEPA air filtration (preferably driven by fan filter units), sets up a pressure gradient between the cleanroom and the preparation room outside—USP 797 calls this the *anteroom*.[7] The anteroom should have HEPA filtered air that is ISO 7 compliant. The negative pressure in the cleanroom holds any toxic vapor in the room where chemotherapy drugs are stored and handled, protecting the rest of the facility. A clean (meaning HEPA-filtered air), positive pressure anteroom is necessary, because this will be the source of air flowing across the gradient into the negative pressure cleanroom. If the anteroom is full of particles, the cleanroom will not be clean. If a negative pressure room is not available for the preparation of hazardous drugs, USP 797 recommends a 2-tier approach to containment, including a BSC or CACI used in conjunction with CSTDs.

The most underrecognized source of cancer therapy contamination in a facility comes from drug packaging. Detectable levels of cytotoxic drugs have been found to be present on the surface of drug vials and external packaging.[14] It is important for all clinic staff to be aware that preparing, administering, and even handling the packaging of cancer therapy drugs can cause enough absorption to result in the measurable presence of cancer therapy agents in the urine. Everyone should use the recommended PPE appropriate to the task. Personnel working in chemotherapy storage areas should be educated about the potential contamination of the vials and be instructed to use PPE when appropriate. Outer packaging that has come into contact with hazardous drug containers should be disposed of as trace-contaminated hazardous waste in the same waste stream as chemotherapy gowns, gloves, and wipes used to prepare antineoplastic drugs (**Clinical Pearl 4-2**).

CLINICAL PEARL 4-2

Corrugated cardboard boxes must not be kept in the cleanroom. Cardboard releases a large number of particles, particularly when it is torn in the process of opening boxes. Supplies and drugs should be unpacked outside the anteroom and wiped down with alcohol before transport into the cleanroom. Cardboard boxes should be discarded. Plastic bins come in a variety of sizes and shapes and make a cleanable alternative to storage in cardboard.

While all of this seems overwhelming, the most important rule for cleanrooms can be taught to anyone from any background. The basic underlying principle for cancer center personnel is, "Don't take anything into a cleanroom that doesn't need to be there." Approaching cleanroom design and training from that standpoint will allow the cleanroom to be safe for both patients and staff.

CANCER THERAPY PRODUCTION: CLEANROOM PROCESSES

After a clean and safe environment is established, preparation of chemotherapy requires a specific set of processes to maintain sterility and safety. These processes include a process for storage and inventory, a cleaning regimen for the preparation environment and containment devices, and the use of PPE in the actual preparation of the products.

Personal Protective Equipment

Particles in the air or on work surfaces are a vehicle for microorganisms to be introduced into sterile product. Environmental controls limit the introduction and circulation of particles through the air. Shielding employees in the compounding area with PPE limits spread of particles between work areas and also limits their environmental exposure to the hazardous drugs. USP Chapter 797 recommends proper hand hygiene (**Box 4-3**) and appropriate garbing (**Box 4-4**) to minimize contamination of sterile preparations during the preparation of cancer therapy.[7] Compounding personnel should not wear cosmetics or artificial nails in the cleanroom because of the high rate of particle shedding from these products.[2] Employees who are ill should not work in the cleanroom.

BOX 4-3
Hand-Washing Procedure

Hand cleaning should be performed in the anteroom and prior to donning the nonshedding gown. Jewelry should be removed before hand washing and should not be worn into the cleanroom, even if it would be covered by gloves or sleeves. Nails should be natural, short, and free of polish. Jewelry and long nails can cause tears in gloves, allowing contamination to penetrate.

- Remove debris from underneath fingernails with a nail cleaner and warm water.
- Vigorously wash hands and forearms to the elbow for at least 30 seconds with soap and water.
- Completely dry the hands and forearms using a nontouch or low-lint process.
- Continue with the garbing process.

Antimicrobial scrub brushes should not be used on the skin, as the skin damage they cause can increase skin cell shedding. Drying can be done by an electronic HEPA-filtered, hands-free dryer or using lint-free disposable wipes. Products should be chosen for lint-free or nonshedding properties.

Proper cleanroom garb for IV medication preparation should include gown, hair cover, shoe covers, mask, and gloves. Polyethylene-coated polypropylene gowns should be worn during compounding, administration, spill control, and waste removal of hazardous drugs. Face and eye protection with a mask and glasses/goggles or face shield should be worn whenever there is a spill or the possibility of aerosolization of hazardous drugs. For chemotherapy, double gloving is ideal for minimizing exposure, since the outer layer of gloves can be removed at any time if too much exposure is suspected, without compromising sterility. The outer layer of gloves should be sterile. Dexterity may be decreased with double gloving. If double gloving is not possible, double-thickness gloves intended for chemotherapy preparation must be used. Gloves should be changed often when prolonged mixing is performed. No glove has been found to be impermeable to chemotherapy for longer than 30 minutes in normal use.[15] Gloves should never be reworn. All staff who prepare chemotherapy should be able to demonstrate proper garbing and hand hygiene. The best training plan includes annual competency assessment with documentation and direct observation.

BOX 4-4
Garbing Procedure

Outer garments (including coats, hats, scarves, etc.), cosmetics, and jewelry should be removed before entering the anteroom. The garbing process begins before hand washing and proceeds in a direction from dirtiest to cleanest (i.e., shoes up to head, finishing with hands). Scrubs, due to their lightweight nature, are recommended for comfort but are not required.

- Cover feet with disposable shoe covers or dedicated shoes. Shoe covers should be worn only once and discarded after exiting the cleanroom. If dedicated shoes are used, they should not be worn outside the cleanroom/anteroom area and should be cleaned on a regular basis
- Cover hair with disposable head cover and facial hair cover (if needed)
- Cover face with surgical mask and eye shield
- Clean hands using proper hand hygiene method
- Cover clothing with a chemotherapy-approved, nonshedding gown. Gowns should have sleeves that fit snugly around the wrists and an enclosure at the neck
- Sterile, powder-free gloves should be donned last, after hand washing and before compounding begins. A second set of sterile gloves is donned, with the outer glove covering the sleeve opening of the gown
- Sterile outer gloves should be changed after removing hands from the hood, after any tear or contamination with cancer therapy, and at least every 30 minutes. Sterile alcohol can be kept in the hood for decontaminating the outer layer of gloves between each chemotherapy mix

All garbing items should be removed in the anteroom before leaving the compounding area. Except for gowns, all PPE should be discarded after one use. Disposable gowns may be reused throughout the day if not soiled and kept in the anteroom. Gowns and shoe covers should never be worn outside the cancer therapy preparation area to avoid hazardous drug contamination of the rest of the facility.

Cleaning Regimens

A cleanroom requires a specific cleaning process and plan. Unless routine housekeeping services are trained on the importance of keeping organisms out of the cleanroom, they are likely to contaminate the room via transfer from other areas of the building. To maintain a cleanroom, housekeeping should be using designated cleaning tools, proper cleaning technique, and a designated cleaning schedule. Cleanroom staff must take responsibility for assuring that appropriate cleaning of the environment takes place as general housekeeping staff may be unaware of the requirements. Cleaning and disinfecting the cleanroom, including both negative and positive pressure areas, must be done on a regular schedule using specific types of cleaning products and disinfectants. Bacteria mutate frequently and easily develop resistance to disinfectants. To minimize resistance, brands/manufacturers of cleaning products should be switched regularly. Combinations of at least 2 disinfectants, 1 of which has activity against spores, should be used.[16] Cleaning equipment for the cleanroom should include nonshedding wipes, plastic or stainless steel buckets, and a HEPA-filtered vacuum. The equipment used to clean the cleanroom must be dedicated equipment. It should be kept in a designated area, near the cleanroom but away from the compounding supplies. Wipes should be discarded after each use.

Each hood used for mixing chemotherapy or hazardous drugs should be cleaned at the beginning of each shift, before each batch, every 30 minutes throughout the shift, after a spill, or if surface contamination occurs. It should be recognized that the use of alcohol for disinfecting the BSC or CACI will not deactivate any hazardous drugs and may actually spread the substance rather than clean it. For certain compounds, decontamination of BSCs or isolators should be conducted according to manufacturer recommendations. The material safety data sheets for specific hazardous drugs may recommend sodium hypochlorite, detergents, or thiosulfate neutralizer.

The cleanroom, including the anteroom, should be cleaned at the end of each day. The cleaning process should begin in the cleanest area, the cleanroom, then proceeding toward the dirtiest area, the anteroom. Within the cleanroom, start with the cleanest place (inside the hood) and move to the counters and other work surfaces, then the dirtiest (the floors). Start on the floor at the far corner from the door and move towards the door, so the parts already cleaned do not have to be crossed to exit.

Every month the ceilings, tops of the hoods, walls, and shelves need to be cleaned. Because disinfectants used may irritate the eyes or skin, safety goggles should be worn when cleaning the ceilings and walls. USP 797 requires written standard operating procedures and cleaning logs for all cleaning activities.[7] These cleaning logs should give the frequency of cleaning and procedure for cleaning. The best source for disinfectants and supplies used for cleaning are wholesalers specializing in USP 797–compliant cleaning products.

Chemotherapy Spills

In the event of an accidental chemotherapy spill, a chemotherapy spill kit should be available in each preparation and administration area, and the staff should have adequate education on how to use the kit (see **Box 4-5**). Spills should be contained and cleaned up immediately by trained personnel with appropriate PPE, including respirators. Generally, spills are contained by the use of spill pads. The area should be rinsed with water and then cleaned with detergent, sodium hypochlorite solution, and neutralizer. The areas should be rinsed again several times and glass fragments and all contaminated materials, including the PPE used by the worker managing the spill, should be disposed of in appropriate disposal containers and treated as hazardous waste. The worker should thoroughly wash his or her hands with soap and water after cleaning up the spill. Housekeeping staff should then be instructed to reclean the area. **Figure 4-1** shows an example of a spill kit and **Clinical Pearl 4-3** provides an example of how a chemotherapy spill can be avoided.

Storage and Dispensing

The level of contamination present in packaging of chemotherapy drugs has been discussed previously in this chapter. To prevent the dispersal of cytotoxic drugs to the rest of the facility, all cytotoxic drugs should be stored under negative pressure, if possible. Unpacking the drug order should be considered a hazardous process, during which personnel should wear protective gloves at minimum. Vials may be removed from boxes and wiped down with alcohol before being placed into the drug inventory. Many cancer therapy drugs should be protected

CLINICAL PEARL 4-3

Chemotherapy should be dispensed for administration with primed tubing. The practice of priming tubing with neutral solution before adding chemotherapy is common. Dispensing with primed tubing is considered best practice by the Occupational Safety and Health Administration (OSHA), the National Institute for Occupational Health and Safety (NIOSH), the American Society of Health-System Pharmacists (ASHP), and the Oncology Nursing Society (ONS).[8,13,17] This practice prevents the need for priming with hazardous drug in the treatment area, where chemotherapy released into waste receptacles or onto the floor would present an exposure risk.

BOX 4-5
Elements of a Spill Kit

A chemotherapy spill kit may contain:
- Chemo gown and shoe covers to protect clothing during the cleaning process.
- Chemical safety glasses to protect eyes from volatile compounds dispersed in the spill.
- Gloves, including chemo gloves and/or heavy duty gloves; heavier gloves may be necessary when handling broken glass.
- Absorbent material, including toweling, chemotherapy pads; many kits contain an absorbent compound to soak up large liquid volumes. Clay-based, nonclumping kitty litter may also be used.
- Dust pan and whisk broom to collect broken glass and dry powder spills. Both the pan and broom should be disposed with chemotherapy waste after use.
- Disposal bag to contain contaminated material for transport to chemotherapy waste.

Several manufacturers market commercial spill kits that are complete with most of the aforementioned items. Items from the list could also be purchased separately and assembled into kits by the cancer center.

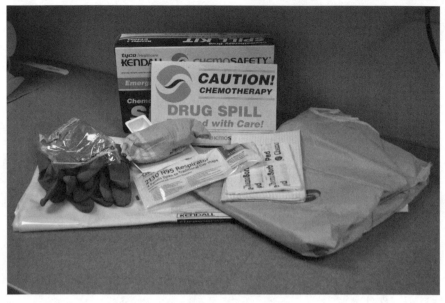

FIGURE 4-1 Chemotherapy Spill Kit

from light during storage. However, sunlight is seldom a concern in inventory areas and cleanrooms, and ambient room light does not penetrate most drug storage cabinets or drawers.[8] Vials should be left in cartons when cartons contain labeling intended for prevention of look-alike/sound-alike errors and to prevent breakage (see the *Drug Safety and Risk Management* chapter in this text for more information about look-alike/sound-alike errors).

One way to address the storage of drugs in the oncology clinic pharmacy or oncology pharmacy drug processing area in a hospital is the use of automated dispensing cabinets (ADCs). Examples of ADCs are displayed in **Figure 4-2**. The most basic features of an automated dispensing system make it little more than a locked cabinet, and many hospitals find loss prevention sufficient reason to implement a cabinet. Used properly, automated dispensing can also facilitate inventory control, billing, reports, and investigational drug services.

ADCs or vertical rolling shelving (carousels), with or without ordering capability, are an excellent system of inventory control. If the institution works exclusively with one wholesaler, an automatic ordering system may be set up. Maximum and minimum inventory levels can be set for each item in a location; an order is created when the wholesaler polls the machines via data or phone line at a set time. No one has to "walk the shelves" to create a manual order.

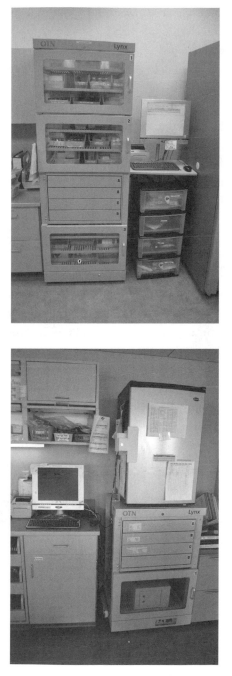

FIGURE 4-2 Automated Dispensing Cabinets

This allows maintenance of a very low stock inventory, a cost-effective system of just-in-time ordering, including for very large, very complicated practices. Even without ordering capability, inventory control allows for early identification and correction of discrepancies. A policy of close inventory control has a multitude of advantages when dealing with expensive cancer agents.

Automated dispensing facilitates any billing system. Charges can be submitted directly from most automated dispensing systems. If charges are submited from another system (like your electronic medical record), the automated dispensing system may be used for auditing, to minimize missed charges. Another way automated dispensing can facilitate billing is the use of kits. Commonly used anticancer regimens can be built as kits, including the infusion charge codes, charges for bags, and any other ancillary charges that have to be entered manually and are often missed. When the kit is pulled, the codes get charged automatically with the drugs.

Another benefit of automated dispensing systems is the ability to generate reports. Because each transaction is recorded and associated with a password, there is improved accountability. Reports can be generated for drug utilization and total inventory for any given time, item auditing to track discrepancies, patient treatment history, pharmacy drug cost for budgeting, and expiration date or lot number tracking. Some vendors offer customized reports to solve problems unique to the setting. The type of automated dispensing system is almost always determined by the drug wholesaler, and many wholesalers will work with the institution to create the reports needed on a one-time or recurring basis.

Practices that have an active research or investigational drug service can take advantage of automated dispensing in another way. A wholesaler can set up a separate cabinet for provided research drugs, meeting the National Cancer Institute (NCI) requirement for separate, locked conditions, and improving accountability for provided investigational drugs. Naming the provided drugs by the corresponding study title or protocol number will minimize the chance of mistaking them for commercial agents, and each transaction will be recorded. The reports from the automated dispensing system may be compared to written logs, or the electronic records could potentially replace written logs.

Refrigeration

Automated or not, drug storage will have to include a plan for maintaining the integrity of drugs requiring refrigeration. Full-size refrigerators are much more reliable and durable than bar-size or dorm-size refrigerators. If possible, frost-free refrigerators should be purchased. The most important aspect of refrigeration is avoiding accumulation of ice in refrigerators. Ice causes the temperature range to be inconsistent, puddles of water from melting ice can saturate packaging, and large ice blocks may block the door seal.[18] If the refrigerator has a freezer compartment, a strict defrosting schedule must be implemented.

Several options for monitoring refrigerator temperatures to maintain drug quality exist. The standard system includes a thermometer with manual log entry. Staff noncompliance or forgetfulness may occur with manual log entries, making this a less than ideal monitoring system. Furthermore, many cancer centers are not open 7 days per week. A power failure could occur on a Friday evening with a full return to normal temperatures by Sunday afternoon and an in-range temperature could be noted on Monday, without awareness of how the drug was compromised. Thus, a manual log entry system for monitoring refrigerator temperatures is not recommended. Monitoring options that include digital range thermometers, data-collecting thermometers, and 24-hour continuous monitoring systems with notification capability improve temperature consistency, drug quality, and are the preferred methods. While these methods are more expensive than manual monitoring, the cost of drug waste when a refrigerator and/or freezer failure occurs and is not quickly recognized can be significant.

Digital range thermometers are the least expensive option. They allow the setting of a maximum and minimum temperature range. The display shows the current temperature and most models record any alarms or extreme temperatures reached since the last time the thermometer was set. They are very simple to use but do not tell how long or when the temperature was out of range and have no reporting capability.

Data collection thermometers are more expensive but they provide useful information about the actual temperatures over time. They usually consist of a graphing thermometer attached to the refrigerator, and the graphs can then be collected and filed. The best role for data collection thermometers is for situations where documentation of temperature monitoring is required (eg, research protocols). The downside of data collection thermometers is that response to out-of-range temperatures is limited to when the temperature graph is being read. This is less useful for sites that are not open daily, because someone must be on-site to collect and read the graph.

The most useful and relevant refrigeration monitoring method is a 24-hour continuous monitoring system. While continuous monitoring is the most expensive method, its notification capability more than compensates for the cost. All other refrigeration monitoring systems only report that a temperature deviation has occurred in the past; whereas, notification capability allows the chance to save drugs, thus, preventing waste and financial loss. An electronic continuous monitoring system will likely consist of a probe, usually set in a vial of glycol, wires, and an electronic box. The box may connect to a telephone system or a computer. Several systems are on the market, and prices vary widely. The cost is almost always worth the high price; often the cost is less than the total cost of the inventory in most clinic or pharmacy refrigerators at any given time. See **Case 4-1** for an example in managing a refrigerator failure.

CASE 4-1
Refrigerator Failure

Statement of the problem: The 24-hour continuous refrigerator monitoring system was activated, generating a cell phone call to the pharmacy manager on a Saturday afternoon. The automated system reported a temperature of 58°F at the main pharmacy refrigerator probe 2 at 2 PM. A dial-in check revealed that the temperature at probe 1 was also high and approaching alert level.

Possible causes of the problem: Power outage, refrigerator failure, door left open, or probe malfunction.

Decision criteria: The main clinic building was equipped with a generator, so facility-wide power failure was ruled out as a cause. Settings on the monitoring system allow the refrigerator to be outside of desired range for 3 hours before generating a call. The temperature at 3 hours was more consistent with a door left open or refrigerator being shut down than with a maladjustment of the refrigerator setting, which is usually closer to the acceptable range. A pharmacy employee who was expected to be near the clinic on Saturday was contacted to check doors and placement of probes. The refrigerator was found to be running, with doors closed, but the interior air was warm. The probes were found to be connected and unobstructed (no objects blocking the airflow around the probes). Refrigerator failure was suspected, so building maintenance was called.

Recommended solution with implementation: The employee was able to move all drugs to secure, refrigerated conditions. The lab's commercial refrigerator had been recently replaced. With the help of maintenance, the employee was able to activate the old laboratory refrigerator, move all drugs, and allow the temperature to equilibrate. A maintenance visit was scheduled for the pharmacy refrigerator. **Outcome**: The main coil was found to have failed, and a new one was ordered. The integrity of all commercial- and research-provided drugs were maintained in the temporary refrigerator. No patients needed to be rescheduled due to wasted drugs. Determining the total cost avoided by monitoring the temperature should include taking inventory of the contents of refrigerator plus costs associated with being unable to treat patients had that occurred.

Implementing a 24-hour continuous temperature monitoring system is complex. These systems make apparent the normal variation in temperatures that occur with refrigerators and freezers, which is often not appreciated in noncontinuous monitoring systems. A written policy should delineate how temperature deviations will be handled, what constitutes an emergency that requires notification (often both an actual temperature deviation and a duration of time), and what constitutes a reasonable response time. Designated staff must be available to make temperature adjustments or rescue the drugs. The policy should address how the clinic will be accessed after hours, including weekends. The larger the practice, the more complicated the policy is likely to be.

Safe Disposal of Hazardous Drug Waste

An increasing concern about pharmaceuticals in the environment, including water and air, exists. The US Environmental Protection Agency (EPA) has very complex regulations that dictate the appropriate disposal of pharmaceutical and hazardous compounds.[19] However, these regulations were written broadly and they apply to manufacturers as well as to hospitals and medical clinics and offices. To comply with these regulations, healthcare providers need to evaluate each drug at each dosage to determine the types of waste that occur and calculate the total weight of all hazardous waste generated each month. This then determines the site's legal disposal options. It only takes 1 kg of hazardous waste pharmaceuticals each month for a healthcare site to be subject to full hazardous waste regulation. Each type of waste has its own unique set of handling and disposal requirements. It has been estimated that approximately 15% of a typical pharmacy's inventory

WASTE SEGREGATION GUIDE

Pharmaceutical Waste

Solid medications	Any medication remaining in a container that is to be discarded, containers include:
• Pills	• Vials
• Powders	• IV bags
• Patches	• Tubing
• Lozenges	• Syringes
	• Ampules
	• Bottles

Pharmaceutical contaminated items

Empty or partially empty containers of:

• Blue pads   • Arsenic Trioxide
• Gauze   • Nicotine
• Gloves   • Physostigmine
• Gowns   • Warfarin
• Packaging

Regulated Medical Waste

SHARPS CONTAINERS
• Syringes with attached needle
• Guide wires
• Needles
• Razors
• Scalpels or Lancets
• Small empty glass vials

RED BAGS
• Blood saturated dressings
• Blood bags with attached tubing
• Bloody tubing
• Pleuravacs
• Suction canisters

BIOHAZARD BUCKETS
• Blood culture vials
• Body tissues
• Blood tubes
• Organs
• Specimen transport vials
• Placentas
• May also be used for sharps disposal

Blood products and body fluid containers that cannot be securely sealed and have the potential to leak more than drips or drops, must be discarded in a biohazard bucket.

Hazardous Waste

• EPA listed waste
• Characteristic waste
  – Flammable
  – Corrosive
  – Reactive
  – Toxic
• Liquid industrial waste
• Mercury

Clean up spills only if you have been trained in the proper procedure and have the appropriate spill kit. If the spill is beyond your capacity or you are not sure how to properly dispose of the cleanup material contact Safety Management Services at 764-4427.

Controlled Substances

Drug Enforcement Administration (DEA) Scheduled Controlled Substances

• Schedule I
• Schedule II
• Schedule III
• Schedule IV
• Schedule V

Liquids are wasted into kitty litter

Solids (i.e. pills, patches are placed into an irretrievable sharps container

Special Disposal and Recycling

• Batteries

• Electronics

• Electric lamps & bulbs

• Paper
• Cardboard
• Plastics

• Toner and printer cartridges

• Beverage containers including: aluminium cans, glass bottles and #1, 2, 4, 5, 6, &7 plastic bottles

General Trash and Glass

• Empty IV bags and tubing (sharps must be removed and spikes cannot be exposed)
• Empty syringes without attached needles
• Food waste
• Non-recyclable plastics
• Paper (recycle)
• Packaging
• Used supplies

• Empty glass only
• Use impervious receptacles
• Keep glass out of general trash receptacles to protect Environmental Service employees from being injured from broken glass.

FIGURE 4-3 Example of Simplified Pharmaceutical Waste Stream with Universal Waste Approach.

meets the definition of hazardous waste. This percentage would be much higher for cancer centers and clinics. Medical waste is subject to completely different handling and disposal requirements. Pharmaceutical waste should not be mixed with medical waste.

Given the complexity of the current EPA regulations and difficulties in compliance, the EPA has proposed a new approach that is currently being tested in several states.[20] This approach advocates handling all waste pharmaceuticals (regardless of whether they are hazardous, nonhazardous, liquid, or solid) under a streamlined standard called *universal waste*. The advantages are that it greatly simplifies the management of pharmaceutical waste materials, eliminating the need to segregate hazardous and nonhazardous compounds and the required record keeping.

General handling and disposal requirements for universal waste are relatively simple. In the universal waste system, all pharmaceutical waste is placed in a universal waste container that is closed and in good condition. The container is then shipped to a universal waste handler or destination facility. These universal waste handlers then use high-temperature incineration to destroy most of the hazardous chemicals and prevent them from cycling into water resources. The commingling of hazardous and nonhazardous pharmaceutical waste is generally expected to be more cost-effective for sites with relatively small amounts of pharmaceutical waste because of the decreased regulatory burden. An example of the simplified waste stream is displayed in **Figure 4-3**.

It is important to note that spill clean-up from hazardous waste drugs can't be managed as universal waste, nor can PPE contaminated with hazardous waste pharmaceuticals. These need to be handled separately as hazardous waste.

CANCER THERAPY PREPARATION PERSONNEL: THE MULTIDISCIPLINARY TEAM

Dispensing and administering drugs in an oncology clinic involves more than just having a pharmacy area or hiring a pharmacy technician or pharmacist. Best practices require planning for the cleanroom environment, personnel protection, maintenance of sterility, drug storage and inventory, handling cancer therapy spills, and safe disposal of hazardous waste. Without these policies and procedures, the cancer center pharmacy is just another room in the clinic.

In hospital-based clinics, all IV medications must be prepared, or at least checked, by a pharmacist. However, private physician practices usually purchase, dispense, and administer medications under the physician license. Without a pharmacy license, private practices in most states do not comply with all of the elements required by the local pharmacy practice act, the way hospitals with hospital pharmacy licenses must. Historically, private practices have used nursing staff for nearly every aspect of care in the cancer clinic. In a small practice, this practice may be based on economic considerations. Larger practices, however, can often support more staffing specialization. Hiring someone solely to mix cancer therapy or process billing makes sense only when that person can be kept busy doing that job and is trained to do other tasks, such as supply ordering, policy and procedure development. Cancer therapy preparation, like every other part of the work flow in a community cancer center, has become a multidisciplinary function. One of the biggest challenges in supervising this process is the diversity in backgrounds and educations that might be encountered in cancer therapy preparation staff; however, this can be overcome with consistent and continual training and competency assessment. For each profession that might be found participating in cancer therapy preparation, prior education/training, the profession's role in the clinic, and possible barriers encountered will be discussed in the following sections.

The Pharmacist

Pharmacists are the members of the team most associated with chemotherapy orders/treatment plans and IV admixture. All pharmacists must be licensed to practice in the state in addition to possessing expertise in drug distribution systems and the clinical use of medications. The entry-level pharmacy degree has been a doctorate (PharmD) since 2000; however, pharmacists with a bachelor of science degree have completed at least 5 years of college, with coursework incorporating medicinal chemistry, pathophysiology, pharmacokinetics, pharmacology, and pharmacotherapeutics. State licensure requires completion of an accredited pharmacy program, a passing score on the North American Pharmacist Licensure Examination (NAPLEX), and meeting the pharmacy law exam requirements of that state. Pharmacy training also includes clinical rotations, usually broken into approximately 1 year's worth of 4- to 6-week blocks. Clinical rotations allow student pharmacists to learn from experienced pharmacist preceptors and encounter practice in multiple different settings. Many pharmacists also have additional clinical training through residencies. A first-year residency (PGY1) includes rotation through various areas of the hospital, multiple projects, participation in clinical research, and staffing experience in the institution.

A second-year residency (PGY2) may be completed in an area of specialization, such as oncology. Pharmacists may also complete board certification in oncology pharmacy (BCOP). This credential is achieved through examination, for which only experienced oncology pharmacists may sit.

The pharmacist's role in the oncology clinic may include order verification, order entry, and/or cancer therapy preparation, as well as clinical or administrative functions. A pharmacist may be responsible for supervision of pharmacy technicians. Barriers to having a pharmacist for cancer therapy preparation in a private practice are primarily financial, due to pharmacist salary requirements. Hospital-based outpatient cancer centers are often able to use a combination of pharmacists and pharmacy technicians for staffing based on their large patient volumes. Whenever possible, it is desirable to have dedicated pharmacists to help assure the safety of the medication use system as well as to provide clinical pharmacy services to optimize the safe and appropriate use of medications by patients. Pharmacists in some settings play a significant role in symptom management programs, oral chemotherapy programs, patient education, and research protocol review.

The Nurse

Nurses will make up the largest part of the multidisciplinary team in any oncology practice. While there are a number of educational tracks that result in the final designation, *registered nurse*, oncology nurses have usually completed a bachelor's degree program and have some clinical experience postgraduation. Oncology certified nurses (OCNs) have passed an examination and maintain this credential with continuing education or repeat examination. Nurses who have experience in oncology may have worked at a physician office practice where nurses mixed all the cancer therapy. Nurses with only hospital experience have no opportunity to develop this skill.

Nurses or personnel with a nursing background may play any role in the cancer center. If no pharmacist is employed in the cancer therapy preparation area, it is most likely nurses who verify orders and mix cancer therapy. If pharmacy technicians mix cancer therapy, nurses will perform the double checks normally performed by a pharmacist in a hospital setting. The barriers encountered in a nurse-driven cancer therapy preparation system include time limitations and a high variability in training and experience. Nursing time is a valuable commodity in the outpatient setting. Assigning a nurse to the cancer therapy preparation area may require pulling a nurse from a treatment room. Depending on patient volume, nurses in this situation may be asked to divide their time between drug preparation and treating patients, splitting focus in a way that is conducive to errors in both areas. Because nurses learn mixing technique in the physician office setting, rather than in nursing school or other formal mechanisms, there is a high degree of variability in training, knowledge, and experience.

The quality of a nurse's aseptic technique in cancer therapy preparation is highly dependent on the skills of the nurse who is the trainer. Mixing expertise should not be assumed from years of experience, unless more is known about the nurse trainer, practice, and/or system where the nurse was trained.

The Pharmacy Technician

Although a national certification program exists, the pharmacy technician position does not typically require any formal education past high school. Pharmacy technicians can become certified pharmacy technicians (CPhT) by passing a national exam and maintaining continuing education credits. Many states now require this for employment as a pharmacy technician. A CPhT must demonstrate familiarity with USP 797 along with knowledge of drug names, pharmaceutical calculations, and the healthcare system. However, chemotherapy and hazardous drug preparation competence is not emphasized in the current certification process.[7] Plans are under way to create a specialty certification for pharmacy technicians in the area of sterile products.[21] Before working in the oncology setting, pharmacy technicians usually have hospital experience mixing IV medications and hospital cleanroom processes.

Pharmacy technicians play a critical role in many cancer centers but they are an underutilized resource. Pharmacy technicians often prepare and compound cancer therapy, as described previously, but they can also become experts in cleanroom guidelines and maintenance of cleanrooms; they can manage cancer therapy drug inventory, including wholesaler contracts, special ordering, and drug shortages; and they can help maintain documentation for clinical research. Because of their familiarity with drug names and products, pharmacy technicians are often involved in patient billing, obtaining patient and co-pay assistance, and more recently, completing or maintaining required paperwork for US Food and Drug Administration– (FDA-) required programs (eg, risk evaluation and mitigation strategy [REMS] programs). Pharmacy technicians can safely prepare chemotherapy and can perform other tasks when not engaged in preparation. State regulations may restrict how pharmacy technicians are supervised. In some states, the work of a pharmacy technician can be checked by a nurse, while in others a pharmacist or physician might be required to supervise their work.

Ideal Staffing

The ideal cancer therapy preparation area will use staff from all 3 backgrounds, maximizing the skills of each. Determining the right combination of pharmacists, nurses, and pharmacy technicians to balance the tasks and responsibilities of cancer therapy preparation for any one cancer center will depend on many factors, including patient load, services offered, hours of operation, cancer therapy administration, clinical trials, and supportive care. Creation of multidisciplinary staffing models should consider these factors and be designed to provide the most efficient and effective cancer therapy and related services for the cancer center.

SUMMARY

Any setting where cancer therapy is prepared requires several key components: a clean area for production, aseptic practices to maintain sterility, and a multidisciplinary team to perform these tasks. The clean area can be achieved by controlling the environment in a separate area of the clinic and by following national guidelines, particularly USP Chapter 797. Aseptic practices, also outlined in USP Chapter 797, are intended to protect the patient from contamination and the preparation staff from exposure to hazardous agents. Processes should include written policies and procedures and include staff competency and training. Finally, assembling the cancer therapy preparation team should incorporate consideration of the education, unique skills, and experience of available members. Pharmacists, nurses, and pharmacy technicians typically compose this team. With these 3 elements in place, a cancer center can ensure a safer product for patients and a safer environment for staff.

REFERENCES

1. Jochimsen PR. Handling of cytotoxic drugs by healthcare workers: A review of the risks of exposure. *Drug Safety.* 1992;7:374–380.
2. McDiarmid M, Egan T. Acute occupational exposure to antineoplastic agents. *J Occup Med.* 1988;30:984–987.
3. Sessink PJM, Kroese ED, van Kranen HJ, Bos RP. Cancer risk assessment for health care workers occupationally exposed to cyclophosphamide. *Inter Arch Occup Environ Health.* 1993;67:317–323.
4. Blair A, Zheng T, Linos A, Stewart PA, Zhang YW, Cantor KP. Occupation and leukemia: a population-based case-control study in Iowa and Minnesota. *Am J Ind Med.* 2001;40:3–14.
5. Sessik P, Bos R. Drugs hazardous to healthcare workers. *Drug Safety.* 1999;20:347–359.

6. Ruder A, Smith D, Madsen M, Kass F. Is there a benefit to having a clinical oncology pharmacist on staff at a community oncology clinic? *J Oncol Pharm Pract.* 2011;17:425–432.

7. USP 797. *Guidebook to Pharmaceutical Compounding: Sterile Preparations.* Rockville, MD: United States Pharmacopeia; 2008.

8. OSHA. OSHA technical manual, TED 1-0.15A, Sec VI, Chap II: Prevention of employee exposure; 1999. http://www.osha.gov/dts/osta/otm/otm_vi/otm_vi_2.html#5. Accessed May 24, 2013.

9. Controlled Environmental Testing Association guidelines. http://www.cetainternational.org/. Accessed January 10, 2013.

10. Villarini M, Dominici L, Piccinini R, et al. Assessment of primary, oxidative and excision repaired DNA damage in hospital personnel handling antineoplastic drugs. *Mutagenesis.* 2011;26(3):359–369.

11. Dranitsaris G, Johnston M, Poirier S, Boeckmans E, Gillard J, Favier B. Are health care providers who work with cancer drugs at an increased risk for toxic events? A systematic review and meta-analysis of the literature. *J Oncol Pharm Pract.* 2005;11(2):69–78.

12. Fransman W, Roeleveld N, Peelen S, et al. Nurses with dermal exposure to antineoplastic drugs: reproductive outcomes. *Epidemiology.* 2007;18(1):112–119.

13. DHHS (NIOSH). *NIOSH Alert: Preventing Occupational Exposures to Antineoplastic and Other Hazardous Drugs in Health Care Settings.* DHHS (NIOSH) Pub No. 2004–165. Published September 2004.

14. Connor TH, Sessink PJ, Harrison BR, et al. Surface contamination of chemotherapy drug vials and evaluation of new vial-cleaning techniques: results of three studies. *Am J Health Syst Pharm.* 2005;62(5):475–484.

15. Wallemacq PE, Capron A, Vanbinst R, et al. Permeability of 13 different gloves to 13 cytotoxic agents under controlled dynamic conditions. *Am J Health Syst Pharm.* 2006; 63(6):547–556.

16. McAteer, F. Ensure contamination control with effective cleaning processes. *PP&P.* 2011; 8(9):16. http://www.pppmag.com/article/973/September_2011/Ensure_Contamination_Control_with_Effective_Cleaning_Processes/?saturated wipes. Accessed May 24, 2013.

17. Chaffee BW, Armitstead JA, Benjamin BE, et al. Guidelines for the safe handling of hazardous drugs: consensus recommendations. *Am J Health Syst Pharm.* 2010; 67(18):1545–1546.

18. Wong S. Implementing medical grade refrigerators for reliability. *PP&P.* 2011; 8(6):10. http://www.pppmag.com/article/915/June_2011_Temperature_Monitoring/Implementing_Medical_Grade_Refrigerators_for_Reliability. Accessed May 24, 2013.

19. US Environmental Protection Agency. Wastes—Hazardous waste. http://www.epa.gov/waste/hazard/index.htm. Accessed May 24, 2013.

20. US Environmental Protection Agency. Management of hazardous waste pharmaceuticals. http://www.epa.gov/waste/hazard/generation/pharmaceuticals.htm. Accessed May 24, 2013.

21. Pharmacy Technician Certification Board. CREST Initiative. http://www.ptcb.org/about-ptcb/crest-initiative#.UZ__H7Wcl8E. Accessed May 24, 2013.

Oral Cancer Therapy

Beth Chen
Lisa Holle

LEARNING OBJECTIVES

Upon completion of the chapter, the reader will be able to:

1. Outline key components of patient education that should accompany oral cancer therapy.
2. List types of monitoring that must be performed for a patient receiving oral cancer therapy.
3. Identify barriers to successful treatment with oral cancer therapy and describe ways to mitigate these barriers.
4. Describe how to prescribe, dispense, and/or administer oral cancer therapy safely.

INTRODUCTION

The use of oral agents to treat cancer has increased in recent years. Oral agents used to treat cancer include cytotoxic cancer therapy (eg, temozolomide, cyclophosphamide), targeted or biologic agents (eg, imatinib, lenalidomide), and hormonal agents (eg, tamoxifen, anastrozole). **Table 5-1** lists approved oral drugs used in the treatment of cancer along with their original approval dates.[1] While oral agents have been used to treat cancer since the 1950s, the approval of oral cancer therapy, particularly the targeted or biologic agents, has gained momentum in recent years. This trend will likely continue. It is estimated that about 400 cancer therapy drugs are currently in the pipeline, and roughly a quarter of these are being formulated as oral drugs.[2]

Table 5-1 Oral Agents Currently Available for the Treatment of Cancer With Approval Dates[1]

Cytotoxic Cancer Therapy	Targeted/Biologic Agents	Hormonal Agents
6-Mercaptopurine—1953	Thalidomide—1998	Tamoxifen—1977
Methotrexate—1953	Bexarotene—1999	Flutamide—1989
Busulfan—1954	Imatinib—2001	Anastrozole—1995
Chlorambucil—1957	Erlotinib—2004	Bicalutamide—1995
Cyclophosphamide—1959	Tretinoin—2004	Nilutamide—1996
Melphalan—1964	Lenalidomide—2005	Letrozole—1997
Thioguanine—1966	Sorafenib—2005	Exemestane—1999
Procarbazine—1969	Dasatinib—2006	Abiraterone—2011
Lomustine—1976	Sunitinib—2006	Enzalutamide—2012
Estramustine—1981	Vorinostat—2006	
Etoposide—1986	Lapatinib—2007	
Altretamine—1990	Nilotinib—2007	
Capecitabine—1998	Everolimus—2009	
Temozolomide—1999	Pazopanib—2009	
Topotecan—2007	Crizotinib—2011	
Fludarabine—2008	Ruxolitinib—2011	
	Vandetanib—2011	
	Vemurafenib—2011	
	Axitinib—2012	
	Bosutinib—2012	
	Cabozantinib—2012	
	Ponatinib—2012	
	Regorafenib—2012	
	Vismodegib—2012	
	Afatinib—2013	
	Dabrafenib—2013	
	Trametinib—2013	
	Pomalidomide—2013	

Oral agents are often thought to be more convenient, less toxic, and better tolerated compared with intravenous (IV) cancer therapies. This may be true in some cases, but more commonly patients receiving oral agents are faced with similar issues as patients receiving IV cancer therapies. In addition, the use of oral agents creates new patient care challenges that must be identified and managed in order for treatment to be successful.

In contrast to IV anticancer therapies, where the drug is usually administered in a hospital or clinic, patients receiving oral therapy are the primary party responsible for ensuring their medication is administered properly. Oral agents tend to have unique and often bothersome side effect profiles, and because these drugs are often prescribed for chronic administration, the side effects must be managed over a long period of time. Oral agents also tend to have more drug interactions because they are often metabolized in the liver. Some oral cancer therapies have risk evaluation and mitigation strategy (REMS) requirements for prescribing and/or dispensing. Safe handling of oral therapies is not only important during dispensing, but also when patients are administering their medications at home. Finally, many of these drugs are very expensive and present a new financial burden for patients.

DOSING AND ADMINISTRATION

While it is often thought that dosing and administration for oral therapies will be simpler than IV therapies, this is not always the case. Some oral agents are conveniently dosed once daily on a continuous basis; however, many therapies are prescribed for a certain number of days per cycle. Examples of oral therapies that are often given in cycles include capecitabine, lenalidomide, temozolomide, regorafenib, and sunitinib. The drugs may also be given on a continuous basis depending on the patient's specific disease state and treatment plan. In addition, some drugs, such as nilotinib, capecitabine, and sorafenib, are dosed more than once daily. Pharmacists should confirm appropriateness of all dosages for oral cancer therapies. If the prescribed dose is different than that found in the prescribing information or tertiary references, other sources should be consulted, such as the National Comprehensive Cancer Network (NCCN) Guidelines or primary literature, to confirm dosing is appropriate.

Fixed doses, rather than those based on weight or body surface area (BSA), are typically prescribed for the targeted/biologic agents. The dose may then be adjusted due to patient tolerability, drug interactions, or other patient specific factors. In contrast, oral agents classified as cytotoxic cancer therapy are commonly dosed based on weight or BSA as is done with IV cancer therapy (eg, capecitabine, temozolomide, melphalan, and topotecan) and are often available in multiple strengths (**Box 5-1** and **Clinical Pearl 5-1**).[3]

BOX 5-1
Typical Dosing for Capecitabine[3]

Capecitabine is an oral cancer agent that's prescribed based on the patient's BSA. It is available in 2 strengths: 150 mg and 500 mg. Patients may be required to take both strengths to equal the full dosage. For example, a patient with a BSA of 1.9 m^2 is prescribed 1250 mg/m^2 to be taken by mouth twice daily. The total dosage would be 2375 mg, which may be rounded to 2300 mg twice daily. The patient would take four 500 mg tablets and two 150 mg tablets twice daily.

CLINICAL PEARL 5-1

Temozolomide is available in multiple strengths, including 5 mg, 20 mg, 100 mg, 140 mg, 180 mg, and 250 mg capsules. Therefore, most patients will require multiple strengths of capsules per dose, rounding to the nearest capsule size. A separate prescription must be written for each capsule strength. It is recommended that the total dose be listed on each prescription along with full directions about administration.

Oral cancer therapies may represent only part of a patient's overall treatment plan. The patient may also be receiving concurrent IV cancer therapies. Examples include a myeloma patient receiving IV bortezomib in combination with oral lenalidomide and dexamethasone or a colorectal cancer patient receiving IV oxaliplatin in combination with oral capecitabine. Furthermore, oral cancer agents, such as capecitabine and temozolomide, may also be administered in combination with radiation therapy.

Temozolomide is a drug that highlights each of the aforementioned points. When used for glioblastoma multiforme (GBM), it is given initially as a 42-day course along with radiation therapy.[4] This is then followed by a maintenance phase where the drug is given for 5 days of a 28-day cycle. The dose of temozolomide is based on BSA. See **Box 5-2** for an outline of the typical dosing of temozolomide when used in newly diagnosed GBM.

BOX 5-2
Typical Temozolomide Dosing for Newly Diagnosed Glioblastoma Multiforme[4]

Concomitant Phase

75 mg/m² PO once daily for 42 days continuously in combination with radiotherapy.

Maintenance Phase

150 mg/m² PO once daily for 5 consecutive days of a 28-day cycle for 6 cycles. Dose may be increased to 200 mg/m² for cycles 2 through 5 if hematologic and nonhematologic toxicity requirements are met.

Many oral cancer therapies have specific administration guidelines. Certain agents must be taken on an empty stomach while others should be taken after a meal. Some have very specific food-related directions. For example, regorafenib must be taken with a low-fat (<30% fat) breakfast because the fatty foods can increase plasma concentrations of the drug. Studies evaluating regorafenib's efficacy included administration of the drug with a low-fat meal; thus it is recommended to administer the drug in this manner to achieve similar effects as observed in the studies.[5] **Table 5-2** lists administration recommendations of some common oral cancer agents with regard to food.[6] In addition, some agents are best taken at a certain time of day. For example, thalidomide is best taken at bedtime because it may cause somnolence. **Case 5-1** demonstrates the potential complexity with regard to oral cancer therapy dosing and administration.

Table 5-2 Administration of Common Oral Cancer Agents With Regards to Food[6]

Take With Food	Take on an Empty Stomach	Take With or Without Food
Altretamine	Abiraterone	Anastrozole
Bexarotene[a]	Afatinib	Axitinib[a]
Bosutinib[a]	Cabozantinib	Bicalutamide[a]
Capecitabine	Chlorambucil[d]	Busulfan[a,h]
Cyclophosphamide[a]	Dabrafenib	Crizotinib[a]
Exemestane[a,b]	Erlotinib	Dasatinib[a]
Imatinib[a]	Estramustine	Enzalutamide[a]
Regorafenib[a,c]	Etoposide	Everolimus[a]
Tretinoin	Lapatinib	Fludarabine
Vorinostat	Lomustine[e]	Flutamide[a]
	Mercaptopurine	Lenalidomide
	Melphalan	Letrozole
	Methotrexate[f]	Nilutamide
	Nilotinib	Ponatinib[a]
	Pazopanib	Procarbazine[i]
	Pomalidomide	Ruxolitinib[a]
	Sorafenib	Sunitinib[a]
	Thalidomide	Tamoxifen[a]
	Temozolomide[g]	Thioguanine[h]
	Trametinib	Topotecan
		Vandetanib[a]
		Vemurafenib[a]
		Vismodegib

[a] Avoid grapefruit juice.
[b] Recommend to take after a meal; note that fatty meals can increase plasma levels by 40%.
[c] Take with a low-fat (< 30% fat) breakfast.
[d] Absorption is decreased when taken after food.
[e] Take with fluids; no food or drink for 2 hours after administration to decrease nausea.
[f] Food may delay absorption and reduce peak concentrations.
[g] Incidence of nausea/vomiting lower when taken on an empty stomach. Take capsules consistently either with or without food; food affects absorption.
[h] No clear data on food effects.
[i] Avoid tyramine-containing foods (aged or matured cheese, air-dried or cured meats including sausages and salamis; fava or broad bean pods, tap/draft beers, yeast extract concentrate, sauerkraut, soy sauce, and other soybean condiments) because of potential of hypertensive crisis or serotonin syndrome. Improperly stored or spoiled food can also increase tyramine concentrations.

CASE 5-1
Capecitabine and Lapatinib for Metastatic Breast Cancer

KS is a 62-year-old female who comes to the clinic for treatment of her breast cancer. She was initially diagnosed with stage III disease several years ago and was treated with a combination of surgery, radiation therapy, and IV cancer therapy. Her cancer therapy included cyclophosphamide, doxorubicin, and paclitaxel. She is HER2+ and also received trastuzumab. Now she is presenting with metastatic disease, and her oncologist decides to treat her with a combination of capecitabine and lapatinib.

  Her cancer therapy orders are as follows:
  Capecitabine 1500 mg PO BID for 14 days of a 21-day cycle
  Lapatinib 1250 mg PO once daily continuously

1. What should KS be told about proper administration of her regimen?
2. Please list possible side effects that KS may experience.
3. Both of these drugs are metabolized by cytochrome P450. Describe the potential cytochrome P450-related drug interactions that can occur with capecitabine and lapatinib.

SIDE EFFECTS

Oral cancer treatments can cause a wide variety of side effects. Oral cytotoxic cancer therapy will cause similar side effects as their IV counterparts including myelosuppression, mucositis, and nausea and vomiting. The emergence of the newer targeted or biologic therapies has brought about a new spectrum of side effects that must be anticipated and managed. Hormonal agents used for the treatment of breast and prostate cancers also have unique side effects. In addition, targeted and hormonal agents are often prescribed for chronic administration causing the need for these side effects to be managed over a prolonged period of time. **Table 5-3** outlines common side effects associated with selected oral cancer therapies.[6] For a complete list of side effects, please refer to the product labeling for each drug.

Table 5-3 Common Side Effects Associated With Oral Cancer Agents[a,6]

Dermatologic Side Effects

Hand-foot syndrome: Afatinib, axitinib, capecitabine, cabozantinib, dabrafenib, regorafenib, sorafenib, sunitinib, trametinib

Papulopustular conditions/EGFR rash: afatinib, erlotinib, lapatinib, trametinib, vandetanib

Cardiovascular Side Effects

Hypertension: Abiraterone acetate, anastrozole, axitinib, cabozantinib, enzalutamide, everolimus, exemestane, pazopanib, ponatinib, regorafenib, sorafenib, sunitinib, tamoxifen, trametinib, tretinoin, vandetanib

Thrombosis: Anastrozole, cabozantinib, everolimus, lenalidomide, letrozole, pomalidomide, ponatinib, tamoxifen, thalidomide, vorinostat

Left ventricular dysfunction: Dasatinib, imatinib, lapatinib, ponatinib, sunitinib, trametinib

QTc prolongation: Bosutinib, crizotinib, dasatinib, lapatinib, nilotinib, pazopanib, sunitinib, vandetanib, vemurafenib

Edema/fluid retention: Abiraterone acetate, bicalutamide, bosutinib, crizotinib, dasatinib, enzalutamide, estramustine, everolimus, fludarabine, imatinib, letrozole, pomalidomide, ruxolitinib, tamoxifen, temozolomide, tretinoin

Gastrointestinal Side Effects

Diarrhea: Afatinib, axitinib, bicalutamide, bosutinib, capecitabine, cabozantinib, crizotinib, dasatinib, erlotinib, enzalutamide, etoposide, everolimus, fludarabine, imatinib, lapatinib, melphalan, pazopanib, pomalidomide, ponatinib, procarbazine, regorafenib, ruxolitinib, sorafenib, sunitinib, topotecan, trametinib, vandetanib, vismodegib, vorinostat

Constipation: Cabozantinib, crizotinib, dabrafenib, everolimus, pomalidomide, ruxolitinib, temozolomide, thalidomide, topotecan, vismodegib

Fatigue

Virtually all

Somnolence: Thalidomide

[a] For a complete list of side effects with each drug, please refer to the product labeling.
EGFR, epidermal growth factor receptor.

Skin Toxicity

A variety of cutaneous reactions can be caused by oral cancer therapies. Hand-foot syndrome (HFS), also known as *palmar-plantar erythrodysesthesia* or *acral erythema*, is a common, non–life-threatening side effect that results in tingling, dysesthesia with or without erythema on the plantar surface of hands and/or feet. The symptoms can progress to pain, dryness, cracking, blisters, ulcerations, and edema. Left unmanaged, it can impair a patient's ability to carry on his or her daily activities (eg, writing, holding objects, walking). Oral cancer agents that cause HFS include afatinib, axitinib, capecitabine, cabozantinib, dabrafenib, regorafenib, sunitinib, and sorafenib; trametinib less commonly causes HFS (<2%). Patients should be encouraged to protect their hands and feet with a good moisturizer and report any symptoms to their health care provider. Management is aimed at prevention and supportive care when it occurs; tips for managing HFS are provided in **Box 5-3**. In some cases, dose adjustment or breaks in therapy are required.[7]

Many types of rashes can develop as a result of oral cancer therapy. These rashes can range from mild redness to severe reactions, such as Stevens-Johnson syndrome. Agents that target the epidermal growth factor receptor (EGFR), such

BOX 5-3

Tips for Managing Hand-Foot Syndrome[7]

- Avoid the sun and intense heat
- Elevate the hands and feet
- Limit the use of hot water on the hands and feet
- Pat skin dry as opposed to rubbing
- Cool hands and feet with ice packs or cool wet towels for 15–20 minutes; avoid ice directly on skin
- Gently apply (avoid rubbing or massaging) a mild moisturizer on the hands and feet several times a day
- Wear clothes and shoes that are loose and comfortable
- Avoid contact with harsh chemicals
- Avoid contact with tools or household items that require pressing hand against hard surface
- Avoid activities that cause unnecessary friction on hands or feet during the first 6 weeks of treatment

as erlotinib, commonly cause a papulopustular skin eruption. This rash usually appears on the face, scalp, neck, and upper trunk and can appear within 2 weeks after the start of therapy in greater than 50% of patients. Development of the rash may indicate clinical efficacy of the EGFR inhibitor; therefore, the rash should be managed while a patient continues therapy when possible.[8] Patients should notify their oncologist if they experience a rash and keep their skin moisturized with an alcohol-free moisturizer, avoid the sun, or use sunscreen as proactive measures to help minimize the severity of the rash. Treatment depends on severity and particular symptoms but may include topical corticosteroids and topical or systemic antibiotics.[9]

Cardiovascular Toxicity

A range of cardiovascular toxicities has emerged with the newer oral antineoplastics. Drugs which inhibit vascular endothelial grown factor (VEGF) receptor such as axitinib, cabozantinib, pazopanib, ponatinib, regorafenib, sorafenib, sunitinib, and vandetanib may cause hypertension.[6] Other drugs may also cause hypertension (Table 5-3). Patients with preexisting hypertension should have their blood pressure under good control before starting a VEGF receptor inhibitor or other drugs that may increase hypertension, and blood pressure should be monitored throughout therapy. Hypertension should be aggressively managed to avoid complications, which may develop with excessive or prolonged blood pressure elevations.[10]

Thalidomide and the related compounds, lenalidomide and pomalidomide, are known to increase a patient's risk of thrombosis, particularly when given in combination with dexamethasone or chemotherapy. The American Society of Clinical Oncology (ASCO) and NCCN recommend that patients receiving any of these agents, in combination with dexamethasone or chemotherapy, receive venous thromboembolism prophylaxis with warfarin or a low molecular weight heparin. Some data suggest that aspirin may also be effective.[11,12] Patients receiving thalidomide or lenalidomide as a single agent do not require prophylaxis in the absence of other risk factors for thrombosis. Other drugs that are known to increase risk of thrombosis are shown in Table 5-3. Venous thromboembolism prophylaxis is only recommended with these other agents if additional thrombosis risk factors are present.

Many of the oral cancer therapies in the class known as tyrosine kinase inhibitors can cause cardiotoxicity. Dasatinib, imatinib, lapatinib, ponatinib, and sunitinib can cause varying degrees of left ventricular dysfunction.[6] Patients should report any swelling, shortness of breath, or dizziness to their health care provider. Sorafenib and sunitinib have caused cases of myocardial infarction.[13] The package inserts for nilotinib and vandetanib both contain black box warnings for the risk of QTc prolongation and sudden death.[14,15] In addition, several other drugs may prolong the QTc interval as well (Table 5-3).[6] Particular attention should be given to the patient's medication list for other drugs that cause QTc prolongation or may increase concentrations of the oral cancer therapy. Clinicians must be aware of these potentially serious side effects and monitor patients appropriately.

Gastrointestinal Toxicity

Gastrointestinal side effects, particularly nausea and vomiting, have long been recognized as a toxicity of cancer therapy warranting aggressive prophylaxis and treatment. Oral antineoplastics that are considered to have a moderate to high emetogenic potential are listed in **Table 5-4**.[16] However, most oral cancer therapies, particularly the targeted or biologic agents, are considered to have a low or minimal emetogenic potential.[16] It must be kept in mind that these agents are often given chronically and even a small amount of nausea can cause prolonged discomfort for patients and must be addressed when present.

In contrast to nausea and vomiting, diarrhea occurs frequently with oral cancer therapies and has the potential to result in serious complications for patients.

Table 5-4 Oral Cancer Agents With Moderate to High Emetogenic Potential[16]

Altretamine

Busulfan (> 4 mg/day)

Crizotinib

Cyclophosphamide (≥ 100 mg/m^2/day)

Estramustine

Etoposide

Lomustine

Procarbazine

Temozolomide (> 75 mg/m^2/day)

Vismodegib

Diarrhea can be a dose-limiting toxicity, can substantially impact quality of life, and may even require hospitalization in severe cases due to inadequate hydration and nutrition issues. Table 5-3 provides a list of agents that are known to commonly cause diarrhea. Management of diarrhea often consists of modifying dietary habits and/or using oral antidiarrheal products (**Box 5-4**).[17]

Thalidomide is an oral agent that does not cause diarrhea but instead commonly causes constipation, which can be particularly problematic in the elderly myeloma population where this drug is often used. Constipation may occur with other oral agents as well (Table 5-3). Constipation can be managed with stool softeners and stimulants, similar to constipation prophylaxis associated with opioid therapy.

Fatigue

The NCCN defines cancer-related fatigue as "a distressing, persistent, subjective sense of physical, emotional and/or cognitive tiredness or exhaustion related to cancer or cancer treatment that is not proportional to recent activity and interferes with usual functioning."[18] Fatigue is one of the most challenging and difficult-to-manage concerns for cancer patients. Patients often have multiple causes for fatigue and virtually all cancer therapies can cause some degree of fatigue, including oral cancer anticancer therapy. Fatigue may occur as a result of hypothyroidism, which can be observed with several of the targeted agents, such as axitinib, pazopanib, sorafenib, sunitinib, and vandetanib. When a patient presents with

BOX 5-4

Patient Tips for Managing Diarrhea[17]

- Drink plenty of water and other clear liquids.
- Avoid caffeine, alcohol, dairy, orange juice, and prune juice.
- Eat small, frequent meals throughout the day.
- Eat foods that are easy to digest such as rice, bananas, toast, and applesauce.
- Avoid fiber and greasy or spicy foods.
- Avoid laxatives or stool softeners and metoclopramide.
- Call your healthcare provider if you have more than 4 bowel movements a day or have diarrhea at night.

fatigue, all reversible causes, such as pain, sleep disturbances, and anemia, should be identified and treated. Patients receiving active treatment should be counseled about methods to cope with fatigue, such as energy conservation and distraction. Encouraging patients to engage in moderate physical activity while undergoing and following cancer therapy is also recommended.[18]

Toxicities of Hormonal Agents

Hormonal agents are commonly used in the treatment of breast and prostate cancer. While these drugs may be considered better tolerated than other oral drugs used in cancer treatment, clinicians must be aware of their side effects and how to appropriately prevent and/or manage them.

Hormonal therapies used in the treatment of early-stage and metastatic breast cancer include tamoxifen and the aromatase inhibitors (anastrozole, letrozole, and exemestane). When these drugs are used in the adjuvant setting, they are usually administered for a minimum of 5 years. Because patients taking hormonal therapies for breast cancer are often curable, clinicians must be aware of the long-term side effects of these agents. Many of the side effects of hormonal therapies are due to estrogenic blockade. Hot flashes and mood disturbances can be seen with both tamoxifen and the aromatase inhibitors. Tamoxifen is a selective estrogen receptor modulator and acts as an estrogen receptor antagonist on breast cancer cells. However, tamoxifen also has estrogen receptor agonist activity in some tissues, which can have beneficial or detrimental effects depending on the specific target tissue. Beneficial effects are observed in the bone, the cardiovascular system, and in lipid metabolism. On the other hand, serious or life-threatening adverse events, such as endometrial cancer and thromboembolic disease, can also occur. The aromatase inhibitors do not have estrogenic activity, but, due to the depletion of estrogen, lack the protective effects of estrogen. Musculoskeletal side effects, such as myalgias, arthralgias, and bone loss are common with the aromatase inhibitors. Patients receiving aromatase inhibitors should be screened for bone loss using a history, physical examination, bone mineral density (BMD) testing, and FRAX analysis; make lifestyle modifications (exercise, fall avoidance, avoidance of alcohol and tobacco); ensure an adequate dietary and/or supplement intake of calcium and vitamin D; and receive prophylactic pharmacologic therapy if low BMD or high fracture risk exists.[19] Evidence suggests that the aromatase inhibitors may increase a patient's risk of developing hypercholesterolemia and cardiovascular disease, but further studies are required to confirm this effect.[20]

The antiandrogens (flutamide, bicalutamide, and nilutamide) are sometimes used in combination with a luteinizing hormone-releasing hormone (LHRH) agonist as part of androgen deprivation therapy (ADT) in the treatment of prostate cancer. Antiandrogens are sometimes given temporarily at the initiation of an LHRH agonist to prevent symptoms associated with the flare of testosterone that can occur. They are rarely given as single agents; therefore, the most notable toxicities are a result of complete androgen blockade. Patients undergoing ADT are at risk of osteoporosis, clinical fractures, obesity, insulin resistance, lipid abnormalities, diabetes, and cardiovascular disease.[21] Patients may also experience hot flashes, vasomotor instability, painful gynecomastia, and sexual dysfunction.

Two newer oral hormonal therapies for prostate cancer are abiraterone and enzalutamide. Abiraterone, a CYP17 biosynthesis inhibitor, can cause hypertension, hypokalemia, and fluid retention as a result of increased mineralocorticoid levels from CPY inhibition.[22] Monthly measurements of blood pressure, serum potassium, and fluid retention are recommended. Patients in New York Heart Association class II, III, or IV should not receive this drug as its safety has not been evaluated in these patients. Because abiraterone acetate is administered in combination with prednisone, monitoring for adrenocortical insufficiency is recommended if an interruption of daily prednisone and/or concurrent infection or stress occurs. Laboratory abnormalities are common, including hepatic transaminases elevation, hypophosphatemia, anemia, elevated alkaline phosphatase, hyperglycemia, and hypertriglyceridemia.

Enzalutamide, an androgen receptor inhibitor, is commonly associated with fatigue, musculoskeletal pain/arthralgia, diarrhea, hot flashes, headache, and peripheral edema.[23] It, too, is associated with elevations in hepatic enzymes; therefore, routine monitoring is suggested, particularly in early therapy. One rare side effect is the development of seizures. It is recommended to educate patients about the risk of seizures and falls.

DRUG AND FOOD INTERACTIONS

Clinicians must be aware of the large number of potential drug and food interactions that can occur with oral cancer therapies. Patients with cancer are often on multiple medications and care needs to be taken to minimize potential problems that can occur as a result of drug interactions. Certain foods can affect how some oral cancer therapies are absorbed and/or metabolized. As mentioned before, patients may be on these drugs chronically, causing the management of these interactions to be even more important.

One of the most common types of drug interactions involves the cytochrome P450 (CYP450) family of enzymes. Many drugs, including oral cancer therapies, are metabolized by the CYP450 enzymes. Drugs may either inhibit or induce the activity of one or more CYP450 enzymes. If a drug's metabolism is inhibited by another drug, this may result in increased and potentially toxic blood concentrations. Warfarin, a common anticoagulant used in cancer patients, is metabolized by CYP2C9. If a drug that inhibits the activity of CYP2C9 is initiated, such as capecitabine, a patient may experience increased warfarin exposure and potential bleeding.[3] On the other hand, if a drug's metabolism is induced, a subtherapeutic concentration may result, leading to treatment failure. St. John's wort is an inducer of CYP3A4 and may decrease the concentrations of anticancer therapies metabolized by CYP3A4, such as sunitinib.[24] **Table 5-5** lists oral cancer therapies that are metabolized by the CYP450 system and have potential drug interactions.[6] When a cancer therapy is listed as a substrate, other medications that are inhibitors or inducers of that particular enzyme can affect the cancer agent's blood concentration. When a cancer therapy is listed as an inhibitor or inducer, medications that are metabolized by that particular enzyme may have their blood concentrations affected by the cancer therapy agent.

One specific interaction that is worth mentioning is the interaction between tamoxifen and certain selective serotonin reuptake inhibitors (SSRIs). SSRIs are commonly used to treat depression and, not surprisingly, may be prescribed for women who are receiving tamoxifen for breast cancer. In addition, patients taking tamoxifen may experience hot flashes as a side effect, and the SSRIs are one therapeutic option that may be used to help manage hot flashes. Tamoxifen is a prodrug and is metabolized by CYP2D6 to the active metabolite endoxifen. Some of the SSRIs are strong inhibitors of CYP2D6, and when given with tamoxifen, can decrease the activity of tamoxifen and lead to inferior patient outcomes.[25] SSRIs that are considered strong inhibitors of CYP2D6 include paroxetine and fluoxetine, and should be avoided in patients taking tamoxifen. SSRIs, which are more likely to be safe in patients taking tamoxifen, include citalopram, escitalopram, and venlafaxine because they have little or no effect on CYP2D6.

The solubility of some oral cancer agents is pH dependent and requires the acidic environment of the stomach to be absorbed completely. Some examples are bosutinib, dasatinib, erlotinib, and ponatinib.[9,26–28] When these medications are given to a patient who is also taking a proton pump inhibitor or H2 antagonist, the blood concentrations may be significantly reduced. Increasing the dose is unlikely to overcome the interaction. The concomitant use of proton pump

Table 5-5 Oral Agents With Known or Potential Cytochrome P450 Interactions[a6]

Drug	Substrate of	Inhibits (Unless Otherwise Noted)
Abiraterone	**3A4 (major)**	**1A2, 2D6 (strong)** 2C19, 2C9, 3A4 (moderate)
Anastrozole		1A2, 2C8, 2C9, 3A4 (weak)
Axitinib	**3A4 (major)** 1A2, 2C19 (minor)	
Bexarotene	3A4 (minor)	3A4 (weak/moderate)
Bicalutamide	3A4 (moderate)	
Bosutinib	**3A4 (major)**	
Busulfan	**3A4 (major)**	
Cabozantinib	**3A4 (major)** 2C9 (minor)	
Capecitabine		**2C9 (strong)**
Crizotinib	**3A4 (major)**	3A4 (moderate)
Cyclophosphamide	**2B6 (major)** 2A6, 2C9, 2C19, 3A4 (minor)	3A4 (weak) 2B6, 2C8, 2C9 (weak)
Dabrafenib	**2C8, 3A4 (major)**	Induces: 2B6, 2C19, 3A4 (weak/moderate)
Dasatinib	**3A4 (major)**	3A4 (weak)
Enzalutamide	**2C8 and 3A4 (major)**	**Induces 3A4 (strong)**, 2C9, 2C19 (moderate)
Erlotinib	**3A4 (major)** 1A2 (minor)	
Etoposide	**3A4 (major)** 1A2, 2E1 (minor)	2C9, 3A4 (weak)
Everolimus	**3A4 (major)**	
Exemestane	**3A4 (major)**	
Flutamide	**1A2, 3A4 (major)**	1A2 (weak)
Imatinib	**3A4 (major)** 1A2, 2D6, 2C9, 2C19 (minor)	**3A4 (strong)** 2D6 (moderate) 2C9 (weak)
Lapatinib	**3A4 (major)** 2C8 (minor)	2C8, 3A4 (moderate)
Letrozole	2A6, 3A4 (minor)	**2A6 (strong)** 2C19 (weak)

Lomustine	2D6 (minor)	2D6, 3A4 (week)
Nilotinib	3A4 (major)	3A4 (weak); 2C8, 2C9, 2D6 (moderate) Induces 2B6, 2C8, 2C9 (weak/moderate)
Nilutamide	**2C19 (major)**	2C19 (weak)
Pazopanib	**3A4 (major)** 1A2, 2C8 (minor)	3A4, 2C8,2D6 (weak)
Pomalidomide	**1A2, 3A4 (major)** 2C19, 2D6 (minor)	
Ponatinib	2C8, 2D6, 3A4 (minor)	
Regorafenib	**3A4 (major)**	
Ruxolitinib	**3A4 (major)**	
Sorafenib	3A4 (minor)	**2C8 (strong)** 2B6 (moderate) 2C9 (moderate)
Sunitinib	**3A4 (major)**	
Tamoxifen	**2C9, 2D6, 3A4 (major)** 2A6, 2B6, 2E1 (minor),	2C8 (moderate) 2B6, 2C9, 3A4 (weak)
Tretinoin	**2C8 (major)** 2A6, 2B6, 2C9 (minor)	2C9 (minor) Induces: 2E1 (weak/moderate)
Trametinib	**2C8 (weak)**	Induces 3A4 (weak/moderate)
Vandetanib	**3A4 (major)**	
Vemurafenib	3A4 (minor)	1A2 (moderate), 2D6 (weak) Induces 3A4 (weak/moderate)
Vismodegib	2C9, 2A4 (minor)	2C19 , 2C8, 2C9 (weak)

[a]Bold text represents major subtrates or strong inducer/inhibitors, thus most likely to cause a drug interaction.

inhibitors and H_2 antagonists with dasatinib, erlotinib, or ponatinib should be avoided if possible.[9,24–28] Antacids may be used but should be separated from the cancer agent by at least 2 hours.[9,26–28]

Clinicians should also be aware that some oral cancer agents may interact with food (Table 5-3). Grapefruit juice inhibits CYP3A4 and should be avoided if a patient is taking a cancer therapy that is metabolized by CYP3A4.[6] Procarbazine has monoamine oxidase (MAO) inhibitor activity, and in addition to avoiding other drugs with MAO inhibitor activity, many dietary restrictions apply.

Patients taking procarbazine should avoid foods and beverages with a high tyramine content, which include (but are not limited to) wine, ripe cheese, yogurt, and bananas. Procarbazine can also cause a disulfiram-like reaction if a patient drinks alcohol while on therapy.

Transporter-based interactions (eg, p-glycoprotein) can also occur with oral cancer therapy drugs (eg, afatinib, bosutinib, dabrafenib, pomalidomide), as well as other types of drug interactions.[6,27] A thorough review of a patient's medication list is necessary to ensure drug interactions are not present with the addition of an oral cancer therapy agent. Several electronic sources are available for purchase to help clinicians evaluate drug interactions, including Lexicomp, Clinical Pharmacology, and Micromedex. These databases allow the clinician to input a patient's entire medication list and will analyze the list for drug interactions, and they will typically provide a severity level to any interactions found. Difficulty may arise in deciding if a specific interaction is clinically significant, and a pharmacist may be able to help identify those interactions that can pose a potential problem for a patient. Practitioners must often use clinical judgment and weigh risks versus benefits for a particular patient when evaluating and managing food and drug interactions.

COUNSELING AND MONITORING

As illustrated previously, oral cancer therapies can become challenging for patients because of their side effects, administration guidelines, scheduling, and drug interactions. Thorough patient counseling and continuous monitoring must be performed to ensure patients are taking their medications correctly and safely.

When a patient is initiated on an IV cancer therapy, the patient will typically be seated in the infusion center, clinic, or hospital for several hours. This provides ample time for a clinician to provide initial patient education and counseling. Unfortunately, when a patient is prescribed an oral cancer therapy, this same opportunity is not always available. Patients may be obtaining their prescriptions in a variety of settings, including a retail, mail order, specialty, or cancer center pharmacy. Various pharmacy settings have different capabilities or standards of how they address patient education on oral cancer therapies. Oncology practices should establish procedures to ensure their patients receiving oral cancer agents receive the education they need to be successful on therapy. **Box 5-5** lists general recommendations to guide clinicians regarding initial patient counseling.[29,30]

BOX 5-5

Initial Counseling Recommendations for Patients Receiving Oral Cancer Therapies[29,30]

- A dedicated appointment should be scheduled for patient education. If a patient is unable to return to the clinic, education may be done over the phone at a dedicated time.
- Identify specific clinic staff that is responsible for education.
- Create checklists to guide clinicians through the key elements required for patient education (eg, dosing, administration, side effects and their management, safe handling, when to call the clinic).
- The education plan should include the patient, family, caregivers, and/or any individuals who will be assisting the patient with his or her care.
- Patients/caregivers should be provided with written or electronic patient education materials prior to initiation of therapy.
- Patient education materials should be appropriate for a patient's/caregiver's education level and available in the patient's/caregiver's primary language.
- Provide patients with dosing calendars when appropriate and encourage use of reminder systems such as alarms and pill boxes.
- Provide patients with pill images to ensure patient recognizes the correct medication to receive from the pharmacy.

Once a patient is initiated on an oral anticancer agent, it is critical that the patient be continuously monitored throughout therapy. Compared with patients receiving IV cancer agents, patients receiving oral cancer therapies may have less frequent clinic visits. Because patients are primarily managing their drug therapy at home, they are typically responsible for notifying the healthcare provider if problems arise with their therapy. However, patients may wait too long before reporting a problem such as a side effect, or they may not recognize that a problem that warrants an intervention exists. Practices should establish a proactive approach of reaching out to patients who are receiving oral cancer therapy to ensure patients are taking their medication correctly, and that side effects are being managed as effectively as possible. The frequency of office visits and follow-up phone calls should be defined in the patient's treatment plan.[29] The treatment plan should be tailored to the specific patient situation taking into account the patient's specific drug therapy, comorbidities, education level, and support system. Patient monitoring should continue for the duration of therapy.

ADHERENCE

When deciding if a patient is a candidate for an oral cancer therapy, the patient's ability to adhere to the regimen must be taken into account. The potential of nonadherence can cause a dilemma in the case where a patient is not responding to therapy. It may be difficult to determine if the lack of response is due to nonadherence, drug resistance, or some other reason. Some factors that influence adherence include the patient's socioeconomic state, complexity and toxicity of the regimen, severity or stage of illness, education level, personal beliefs, and relationship with the healthcare team. **Table 5-6** lists factors that may be associated with poor adherence to oral cancer therapy.[2,31]

In contrast to parenteral therapy where assessing adherence is very straight-forward, assessing adherence to oral therapy presents a much greater challenge.

Table 5-6 Factors Associated With Poor Medication Adherence[2,31]

Complicated regimen

Cost of medication

History of mental illness (ie, depression)

Inadequate social support

Inconvenient clinic appointments

Lack of belief in treatment

Missed appointments / poor follow-up

Poor patient–provider relationship

Side effects

Unfilled prescriptions

A wide range of methods exist to monitor adherence, each method having its own strengths and weaknesses. Direct observation is not practical unless a patient is hospitalized or resides in a nursing home. Pharmacokinetic monitoring can ensure adequate blood concentrations but is typically not logistically possible outside of a clinical trial. Perhaps the easiest way to monitor adherence is to simply ask the patient directly; however, patients may not accurately recall how the medication was actually taken, or report better than actual adherence in order to please the clinician. Other methods include monitoring pill counts and refill records or asking patients to fill out a medication diary. The Micro Electronic Monitoring System (MEMS) records each time a prescription bottle is opened and could potentially be an effective means to monitor adherence. However, MEMS is expensive and at this time is not practical for most patients outside of the clinical trial setting.[2,31] Because no approach to adherence monitoring is without its weaknesses, using a combination of methods is more likely to yield an accurate picture of medication adherence. For instance, in the clinic setting, patients could be asked to complete a medication diary or mark doses on a calendar. Patients could then be asked to bring their medication bottles in to the clinic so a pill count can be performed. In the pharmacy setting, a similar approach can be used, but refill records can also be evaluated to assess adherence.

Several interventions can be made to improve medication adherence. Good patient education, including counseling on proper administration and side effects and their management, can help ensure a patient is taking his or her medication appropriately. A plan that addresses side effects should be in place to avoid medication nonadherence. Educating the patient on his or her disease and its treatment as well as including the patient in the decision-making process can help motivate the patient to be more adherent. Monitoring adherence closely using some of the methods described in this text can encourage a patient to pay closer attention to the medication regimen because the patient knows he or she is being monitored. Additionally, regimens should be simplified as much as possible, and care should be coordinated to optimize patients' time commitment to their health care. Financial and social barriers must also be addressed and mitigated. Finally, dosing aids, such as pill boxes and calendars, may be beneficial for some patients.[31] The following patient case demonstrates the complexity and potential consequences of nonadherence (see **Case 5-2**).[32,33]

CASE 5-2
Imatinib for Chronic Myeloid Leukemia

JM is a 42-year-old male who has been diagnosed with chronic myeloid leukemia (CML). His oncologist prescribes imatinib 400 mg by mouth once daily, and he achieves a complete hematologic response at 3 months. However, at his 6-month evaluation, he did not achieve a complete cytogenetic response. After sitting down with JM to discuss his treatment, you learn that he has not been taking his imatinib every day.

1. Please list possible reasons why JM is not adherent to his imatinib regimen.
2. Assuming JM was adherent to his regimen, what other possible reasons may explain why JM has not achieved an optimal response to therapy?

SAFE PRESCRIBING AND DISPENSING PRACTICES

Certain safety practices have become standard when dealing with the prescribing and dispensing of IV cancer therapy. For instance, most practices use either pre-printed or electronic systems to order cancer therapy. In addition, several practitioners, including the prescribing physician, pharmacists, and nurses, typically verify orders for IV cancer therapy. Likewise, multiple-check systems are also standard in verifying correct compounding of an IV cancer therapy. Unfortunately, these same safety practices are inconsistent for oral cancer treatments, causing a potential for medication errors. In fact, a report by Weingart and colleagues demonstrated that the most commonly made errors associated with oral cancer therapy were during ordering and dispensing.[34] This problem is compounded because prescriptions for oral cancer therapy may be filled in a variety of different settings including retail, specialty, mail-order, or cancer center pharmacies. Each of these pharmacy settings may have pharmacists with differing expertise in oncology filling prescriptions for oral cancer therapy and have different systems in place for dispensing prescriptions and educating patients. Until recently, no specific guidelines had been published to guide clinicians as to safe practices with oral cancer therapy agents. However, in 2013, the American Society of Clinical Oncology (ASCO) and the Oncology Nursing Society (ONS) published cancer therapy administration safety standards, which include practices for safe administration and management of oral cancer therapies. In general, the standards demonstrate that practices for oral agents should reflect those for IV cancer therapy, with special focus ensuring patients fill prescriptions and adhere to their oral therapies as well as patient education including administration schedules, exception procedures, disposal of unused medication, and continuity of care.[29] **Box 5-6** lists several recommendations that pertain to prescribing and dispensing oral cancer therapies. These recommendations can be used by oncology practices in the development of policies and procedures to ensure safe prescribing and dispensing of oral cancer therapies.

BOX 5-6
Cancer Therapy Prescribing and Dispensing Recommendations[29,30]

- Orders should be written and prepared by a clinician who is qualified according to the practice's policies and procedures.
- Verbal orders should not be used except to hold or discontinue treatment.
- New orders and changes in orders should be made in writing.
- Standardized, preprinted or electronic orders should be used for prescribing oral cancer therapy.
- Full generic names should be used, unless a brand name identifies a unique drug formulation.
- Doses may be rounded to nearest tablet/capsule size or specify alternating doses each day to obtain correct overall dose; use a leading zero for all doses < 1 mg (eg, 0.5 mg).
- A prescription for an oral cancer therapy should include:
  - Patient's full name, second patient identifier, date.
  - Drug name.
  - Height, weight, and/or BSA when applicable to calculate dose and methodology used to calculate dose.

- Dosage, quantity to be dispensed, route, frequency of administration, and duration of therapy or number of days to take therapy if not continual.
- Number of refills (should be written with a time limitation to ensure appropriate patient evaluation).
- A second qualified clinician should independently verify each medication order.
- Standardized data entry should be used in the dispensing of oral cancer therapy.
- Barcode technology should be implemented in dispensing.
- Patients should be provided with pill images.
- A multiple-check system should be implemented during the dispensing process.

BSA, body surface area.

Risk Evaluation Mitigation Strategy (REMS) Requirements

Several oral cancer therapies have a REMS program, some of which have requirements that must be met before dispensing the drug. See **Box 5-7** for the REMS requirements for lenalidomide. The number of REMS programs is likely to increase as more oral therapies become approved. Please see the *Drug Safety and Risk Management* chapter of this text for more information regarding REMS. **Table 5-7** outlines the basic components of oral cancer therapies that currently require REMS.[35] The FDA website provides detailed information of each REMS program.[35]

BOX 5-7
Risk Evaluation Mitigation Strategy (REMS) Requirements for Lenalidomide[35]

RevAssist is the REMS program for lenalidomide, which exists because of the drug's side effects and potential for birth defects.

The following are required for RevAssist: A medication guide must be dispensed with each prescription.

- Prescribers, pharmacies, and patients must be enrolled in the RevAssist program to prescribe, dispense, or take lenalidomide
- Patients are assigned a risk category based on their childbearing potential
- Strict pregnancy testing is performed based on the patient's risk category
- A unique number is assigned to each lenalidomide prescription that is prescribed, and a separate number is assigned for each prescription that is dispensed
- Prescriptions must be filled when 7 days or fewer are remaining on existing prescription and 7 days from the last pregnancy test
- No more than a 28-day supply can be prescribed or dispensed, and no refills are permitted
- Patients receive counseling with each dispensed prescription by a healthcare professional certified to perform the counseling
- The manufacturer has an implementation system in place to ensure compliance with the RevAssist program

Table 5-7 Approved REMS for Oral Cancer Agents[35]

Drug	REMS Components
Lenalidomide	ETASU, implementation system
Pomalidomide	ETASU, implementation system
Thalidomide	ETASU, implementation system
Vandetanib	Medication guide, communication plan, ETASU, implementation system

ETASU, elements to assure safe use; REMS, risk evaluation and mitigation strategies.

SAFE HANDLING

Like IV cancer therapy, the use of oral cancer agents presents the risk of exposure to healthcare workers and patients. However, because oral cancer therapies are typically administered in the home, the family and caregivers of patients are also at risk of exposure from these agents. Care must be taken to ensure that unnecessary exposure is minimized to all who may be in contact with these drugs. Safe handling is important in the preparation, dispensing, administration, and disposal of oral cancer therapies.[36] While risk is likely greatest with cytotoxic cancer therapy, safe handling practices should occur for oral cancer therapies including targeted and biologic agents. All anticancer therapies, however, do not carry the same risk of exposure. For example, dexamethasone is a corticosteroid used in the treatment of several hematological malignancies and does not require special handling. Likewise, most hormonal agents do not require special handling.

In order to protect healthcare providers, proper storage and handling practices should be followed.[36] Oral cancer agents should be stored separately from other medications, and separate equipment (eg, counting trays) should be used for drug preparation. Automatic counting machines should not be used. Disposable gloves should be worn when handling the cancer agents, and hands should be washed before and after glove application. Any manipulations such as compounding, crushing, or breaking tablets should be done in a biological safety cabinet, and proper personal protective equipment similar to that used to prepare IV cancer therapy should be used. An updated list of hazardous medications should be available to personnel, and a written emergency plan to handle a spills or accidental exposure should be in place. All disposable equipment and clothing that is used while handling oral cancer agents should be disposed of as cytotoxic waste according to local regulatory guidelines, and nondisposable equipment should be washed and/or decontaminated after use. All personnel who may come in contact with hazardous substances should receive training of proper handling of these substances. Exposure to hazardous substances by personnel who are pregnant or trying to conceive should be minimized or eliminated whenever possible.

Patient counseling should include education and training to ensure that patients and their caregivers understand proper safe handling procedures.[36] If possible, patients and caregivers should wear gloves when handling oral cancer therapy and wash hands before and after gloves are donned. If gloves are not worn, tablets or capsules should be tipped into a disposable medicine cup rather than into the hands. Tablets should not be split or crushed, and capsules should not be opened. Patients should have information readily available in the event of an accidental exposure. Patients who are receiving cytotoxic cancer therapy should have their clothing and bed linens washed separately from others in the household, and the toilet should be flushed twice after use. If patients have unused medications, they should be returned to the pharmacy, hospital, or clinic for proper disposal rather than flushed in the toilet or thrown away in the trash. The number of individuals who come in contact with the oral anticancer agent should be minimized. Oral cancer agents should be stored away from where food is kept or consumed. They should be kept in a dry area, out of direct sunlight, and out of reach of children and pets.

FINANCIAL CONSIDERATIONS

An important aspect of oral cancer therapies that must not be overlooked is the cost. Traditionally, a patient's medical insurance benefit, or Medicare Part B has covered IV cancer therapy. However, oral cancer therapies are now typically billed to a patient's prescription insurance or Medicare Part D. Medicare Part D was created by the Medicare Modernization Act (MMA) and allows coverage for virtually all oral cancer agents. Many different private insurance companies offer Part D plans with different deductibles and co-pays. Information regarding the different Part D plans can be found at https://www.medicare.gov/find-a-plan/questions/home.aspx. Oral chemotherapies that have an IV counterpart are still covered under Part B, and patients are typically responsible for 20% of the cost after paying a deductible. Examples of such agents include capecitabine, temozolomide, and etoposide. The fact that oral agents may be covered by multiple insurance plans, along with the multitude of Part D plans available, can be very confusing for patients and clinicians. In addition, even when a patient has prescription insurance, high co-pays, deductibles, and coinsurance can cause a significant financial burden for patients. It is critical that a patient's financial resources and insurance coverage are evaluated when assessing a patient for an oral cancer therapy. Also, because these therapies are often given chronically, the patient's financial situation must be assessed periodically.[1] Because oral cancer therapies can be very expensive, financial assistance is sometimes available for patients who qualify. Most of the newer agents have manufacturer-sponsored programs for the uninsured or underinsured. Several agencies exist to help patients who have insurance but still have co-pays or coinsurance that cause a financial burden. **Table 5-8** lists some of these agencies with their contact information. Qualification for assistance from these agencies depends on the patient's diagnosis, treatment plan, financial need, and availability of funding.

Table 5-8 Agencies That Provide Financial Assistance for Patients on Oral Cancer Agents

Agency	Website	Phone Number
CancerCare	www.cancercarecopay.org	(866) 552-6729
Chronic Disease Fund (CDF)	www.cdfund.org	(877) 968-7233
HealthWell Foundation	www.healthwellfoundation.org	(800) 675-8416
The Leukemia and Lymphoma Society (LLS)	www.leukemia-lymphoma.org	(800) 955-4572
National Organization for Rare Disorders, Inc. (NORD)	www.rarediseases.org	(800) 999-6673
Patient Access Network (PAN)	www.panfoundation.org	(866) 316-7263
Patient Advocate Foundation (PAF)	www.copays.org	(866) 512-3861
Patient Services Incorporated (PSI)	www.uneedpsi.org	(800) 366-7741

CASE 5-1
Answers

1. Capecitabine should be taken within 30 minutes after a meal with a glass of water. Usually patients take the drug after breakfast and after their evening meal. KS will take three 500-mg tablets twice daily to make her dose. She will take capecitabine for 14 days followed by a 7-day break to make a 21 day cycle. Lapatinib should be taken on an empty stomach, so she should take it at least 1 hour before or 2 hours after a meal with a glass of water. She will take five 250-mg tablets to make her dose. She will take lapatinib once daily continuously with no breaks in dosing.

2. Side effects that KS may experience include diarrhea, hand-foot syndrome, nausea/vomiting, skin rash, and stomatitis.

3. Capecitabine is a strong CYP2C9 inhibitor, and therefore, substrates of CYP2C9, such as warfarin and phenytoin serum levels, can be increased. Lapatinib is a major substrate of CYP3A4 and substrate of CYP2C8. Therefore, strong inhibitors of CYP3A4, such as clarithromycin or itraconazole, can increase the serum concentrations of lapatinib, and strong inducers of CYP3A4, such

as phenytoin, can decrease concentrations of lapatinib. Avoiding strong inhibitors and inducers of CYP3A4 is recommended, or consideration of lapatinib dose reductions or dose increases, respectively. Lapatinib is a moderate inhibitor of CYP2C8 and CYP3A4 and thus may increase serum concentrations of drugs that are substrates of CYP3A4 and CYP2C8.

CASE 5-2
Answers

1. It has been demonstrated in clinical trials that adherence can impact response rates with imatinib therapy.[32,33] A few possible reasons for why JM is not taking his medication every day include:

   - *Side effects causing skipping of doses.* JM states that he is experiencing stomach upset and nausea. Patient interview reveals he usually does not take imatinib with food, which may decrease the incidence of these side effects. However, he notes that when he does take the drug with food, nausea is still present.
   - *Lack of belief in treatment.* He never felt sick when he was initially diagnosed with CML. In fact, he felt better before starting the medication (more energy, no stomach upset) so he doesn't believe he needs the medication.
   - *Cost of medication.* He is unable to afford the monthly co-pay, so he sometimes takes his imatinib every other day to make a prescription last longer. Sometimes he fills his prescription late because he must wait until he has the money to pay for it.
   - *Inadequate social support.* He is currently helping with the care of his mother who recently suffered a stroke. He and his wife both work full-time and are raising 2 children. Sometimes he has trouble remembering to take his own medication with so many other responsibilities.

Many factors contribute to medication adherence. The healthcare team must identify the underlying reason for a patient's nonadherence. In the case of JM, a simple intervention, such as counseling to take with food or prescribing an antiemetic, can make a big impact on his ability to be successful with therapy. JM probably needs further education about his disease and the importance of imatinib therapy. Additionally, he may need the help of a social worker or financial counselor to help mitigate financial or personal barriers to treatment.

2. Many different reasons exist that may influence a patient's response to therapy. While most patients experience a good response to imatinib, mutations can occur that can cause a particular patient's disease to be resistant to the drug. JM may have one of these mutations, causing imatinib to be less effective. Also, imatinib is a major substrate of CYP3A4. Perhaps JM is taking another medication, such as St. John's wort, that is inducing the metabolism of the imatinib resulting in decreased blood concentrations.

SUMMARY

Oral therapies play a key role in the overall treatment of patients with cancer. The use of oral cancer agents is likely to increase as more of these agents become available, and thus clinicians must be prepared to recognize and address the challenges that exist in caring for patients receiving oral cancer therapies. Oral cancer therapies can have complicated dosing schedules, specific administration guidelines, unique side effects, and numerous food and drug interactions. Therefore, healthcare providers should be aware of the unique characteristics of these agents, thoroughly educate patients and caregivers on the side effects, and closely monitor the patients while on therapy. Because oral cancer therapies are hazardous agents like IV cancer therapies, safe practices for prescribing, dispensing, and administering oral therapies should reflect those for IV anticancer therapy. Finally, the financial impact of an oral cancer therapy for a patient should be evaluated prior to initiation of treatment because of the often chronic treatment and lack of full reimbursement for these expensive therapies.

REFERENCES

1. FDA Approved Drug Products. Food and Drug Administration website. http://www.accessdata.fda.gov/scripts/cder/drugsatfda/index.cfm. Accessed May 20, 2013.
2. Weingart SN, Brown E, Bach PB, et al. NCCN task force report: oral chemotherapy. *J Natl Compr Canc Netw.* 2008;6(Suppl 3):S1-S14.
3. Xeloda [package insert]. San Francisco, CA: Genentech, Inc; 2011.
4. Temodar [package insert]. Whitehouse Station, NJ: Merck & Co, Inc; 2013.
5. Stivarga [package insert]. Wayne, NJ: Bayer HealthCare Pharmaceuticals, Inc; 2012.
6. Lexicomp Online website. http://online.lexi.com/crlsql/servlet/crlonline. Accessed May 23, 2013.
7. Cancer.net. Hand-foot syndrome or palmar-plantar erythrodysesthesia. http://www.cancer.net/patient/All+About+Cancer/Treating+Cancer/Managing+Side+Effects/Hand-Foot+Syndrome+or+Palmar-Plantar+Erythrodysesthesia. Accessed May 23, 2013.
8. Wacker B, Nagrani T, Weinberg J, Witt K, Clark G, Cagnoni PJ. Correlation between development of rash and efficacy in patients treated with the epidermal growth factor receptor tyrosine kinase inhibitor erlotinib in two large phase III studies. *Clin Can Res.* 2007;13:3913–3921.
9. Tarceva [package insert]. Melville, NY: OSI Pharmaceuticals, Inc; 2010.
10. Maitland ML, Bakris GL, Black HR, et al. Initial assessment, surveillance, and management of blood pressure in patients receiving vascular endothelial growth factor signaling pathway inhibitors. *J Natl Cancer Inst.* 2010;102:596-604.
11. Lyman GH, Khorana AA, Kuderer NM, et al. Venous thromboembolism prophylaxis and treatment in patients with cancer: American Society of Clinical Oncology Practice guideline update. *J Clin Oncol.* 2013;31:2189-2204.
12. National Comprehensive Cancer Network. Clinical Practice Guidelines in Oncology. Venous thromboembolic disease (version 2.2013). http://www.nccn.org/index.asp. Accessed May 23, 2013.
13. Orphanos GS, Ioannidis GN, Ardavanis AG. Cardiotoxicity induced by tyrosine kinase inhibitors. *Acta Oncol.* 2009;48:964-970.
14. Tasigna [package insert]. East Hanover, NJ: Novartis Pharmaceuticals Corporation; 2011.
15. Vandetanib [package insert]. Wilmington, DE: AstraZeneca Pharmaceuticals; 2011.
16. National Comprehensive Cancer Network. Clinical Practice Guidelines in Oncology. Antiemesis (version 1.2013). http://www.nccn.org/index.asp. Accessed May 23, 2013.
17. Cancer.Net.Diarrhea.http://www.cancer.net/all-about-cancer/treating-cancer/managing-side-effects/diarrhea. Accessed May 23, 2013.
18. National Comprehensive Cancer Network. Clinical practice guidelines in oncology. Cancer-related fatigue (version 1.2013). http://www.nccn.org/index.asp. Accessed May 23, 2013.
19. Grawlow JR, Biermann JS, Farooki A, et al. NCCN task force report: bone health in cancer care. *J Nat Comprehensive Cancer Netw.* 2009;7(suppl 3):S1-S32.
20. Perez EA. Safety profiles of tamoxifen and the aromatase inhibitors in adjuvant therapy of hormone-responsive early breast cancer. *Ann Oncol.* 2007;18(Suppl 8): viii26-viii35.

21. National Comprehensive Cancer Network. Clinical practice guidelines in oncology: prostate cancer (version 2.2013). http://www.nccn.org/index.asp. Accessed May 23, 2013.
22. Abiraterone acetate [package insert]. Horsham, PA: Centocor Ortho Biotech Inc; 2011.
23. Xtandi [package insert]. Northbrook, IL: Astellas Pharma US, Inc; 2012.
24. Sutent [package insert]. New York, NY: Pfizer Inc; 2012.
25. Kelly CM, Juurlink DN, Gomes T, et al. Selective serotonin reuptake inhibitors and breast cancer mortality in women receiving tamoxifen: a population based cohort study. *BMJ*. 2010;340:c693.
26. Sprycel [package insert]. Princeton, NJ: Bristol-Myers Squibb Company; 2012.
27. Bosulif [package insert]. New York, NY: Pfizer; 2012.
28. Iclusig [package insert]. Cambridge, MA: Ariad Pharmaceuticals, Inc; 2012.
29. Neuss MN, Polovich M, McNiff K, et al. 2013 updated American Society of Clinical Oncology/Oncology Nursing Society chemotherapy administration safety standards including standards for safe administration and management of oral chemotherapy. *J Oncol Pract*. 2013;9:1S-13S.
30. Weingart SN, Spencer J, Buia S, et al. Medication safety of five oral chemotherapies: a proactive risk assessment. *J Oncol Pract*. 2011;7:2-6.
31. Ruddy K, Mayer E, Partridge A. Patient adherence and persistence with oral anticancer treatment. *CA Cancer J Clin*. 2009;59:56-66.
32. Noens L, van Lierde M, De Bock R, et al. Prevalence, determinants, and outcomes of nonadherence to imatinib therapy in patients with chronic myeloid leukemia: the ADAGIO study. *Blood*. 2009;113:5401-5411.
33. Marin D, Bazeos A, Mahon F, et al. Adherence is the critical factor for achieving molecular responses in patients with chronic myeloid leukemia who complete cytogenetic responses to imatinib. *J Clin Oncol*. 2010;28:2381-2388.
34. Weingart SN, Toro J, Spencer J, et al. Medication errors involving oral chemotherapy. *Cancer*. 2010;116:2455-2364.
35. US Food and Drug Administration. Approved risk evaluation and mitigation strategies (REMS). http://www.fda.gov/Drugs/DrugSafety/PostmarketDrugSafetyInformation forPatientsandProviders/ucm111350.htm. Accessed May 23, 2013.
36. Goodin S, Griffith N, Chen B, et al. Safe handling of oral chemotherapeutic agents in clinical practice: recommendations from an international pharmacy panel. *J Oncol Pract*. 2011;7:7-12.

CHAPTER 6

Drug Safety and Risk Management

Karen R. Smethers

LEARNING OBJECTIVES

Upon completion of the chapter, the reader will be able to:

1. Describe an example of a chemotherapy occurrence and classify the occurrence node, error type, and potential contributing factors.
2. Identify an error prevention strategy that could be employed to prevent an oncology occurrence in each the following stages of the medication use process: procurement, prescribing, transcribing/documenting, compounding/dispensing, administering, and monitoring.
3. Describe an example of a sentinel event that requires reporting to The Joint Commission and outline the actions that need to be taken following the event.
4. Explain the goal of the risk evaluation and mitigation strategy program.

INTRODUCTION

The 1999 Institute of Medicine (IOM) report, *To Err Is Human: Building a Safer Health Care System,* highlighted the need to increase focus on patient safety, specifically recognizing that medical errors cause 44,000 to 98,000 preventable deaths each year, with an associated cost of 17 to 29 billion dollars.[1] It is projected that a minimum of 380,000 to 450,000 preventable adverse drug events occur annually in the hospital, and an even greater number, 530,000, in the ambulatory care setting.[2-5]

Medication errors associated with chemotherapy drugs are particularly concerning due to the narrow therapeutic index of these agents. In order to prevent medication errors in the oncology setting, it is important to understand what a medication error is, where in the medication use process errors occur, and what types of errors happen.

Medication errors are defined by the National Coordinating Council for Medication Error Reporting and Prevention (NCC MERP) as "any preventable event that may cause or lead to inappropriate medication use or patient harm while the medication is in the control of the health care professional, patient, or consumer."[6] Chemotherapy errors can occur at any point in the medication use process including during the procuring, prescribing, transcribing/documenting, compounding/dispensing, administering, and monitoring nodes. The NCC MERP system provides a comprehensive taxonomy for categorizing medication error types in the medication use process, the causes of error, and contributing factors for errors.[6] A list of key information and suggested categories for medication error reporting is located in **Tables 6-1, 6-2**, and **6-3**.[7,8]

Table 6-1 Patient and Medication Information Used in Medication Error Reporting

Patient name/initials

Patient identifying number or date of birth

Event date

Medication information

>   Name

>   Dosage form, dose

>   Route

>   Rate

>   Schedule, number of doses, days of therapy

Table 6-2 Categories for Medication Error Reporting[7,8]

Node

Procuring, prescribing, transcribing/documenting, dispensing, administering, or monitoring

Types of Errors

- Incorrect patient
- Prescribing error[a] (drug–drug interaction, documented allergy, drug–disease interaction)
- Dose omission
- Incorrect medication
- Incorrect dosage form
- Incorrect dose (overdosage, underdosage, extra dose)
- Incorrect strength/concentration
- Incorrect medication administration technique
- Incorrect route
- Incorrect rate
- Incorrect duration
- Incorrect frequency/time
- Drug therapy monitoring issue
- Deteriorated, expired, or contaminated medication

Contributing Factors

- Patient information not available
- Medication information not available
- Communication issue
- Medication name, label, packaging issue
- Medication storage or delivery issue
- Environment or workflow issue
- Staff education issue
- Patient education issue
- Quality control or independent check systems issue

[a] Some categorize prescribing error types of error as a drug therapy monitoring issue.

Table 6-3 NCC MERP Index for Categorizing Medication Errors[6]

Index		Description
A	No error	Circumstances or events that have the capacity to cause error.
B	Error, no harm	An error occurred but the error did not reach the patient. (An error of omission *does* reach the patient.)
C	Error, no harm	An error that reached the patient but did not cause patient harm occurred.
D	Error, no harm	An error that reached the patient and required monitoring to confirm that it resulted in no harm to the patient and/or required intervention to preclude harm occurred.
E	Error, harm	An error that may have contributed to or resulted in temporary harm to the patient and required intervention occurred.
F	Error, harm	An error that may have contributed to or resulted in temporary harm to the patient and required initial or prolonged hospitalization occurred.
G	Error, harm	An error that may have contributed to or resulted in permanent patient harm occurred.
H	Error, harm	An error that required intervention necessary to sustain life occurred.
I	Error, death	An error that may have contributed to or resulted in the patient's death occurred.

Definitions

Harm: Impairment of the physical, emotional, or psychological function or structure of the body and/or pain resulting therefrom.

Monitoring: To observe or record relevant physiological or psychological signs.

Intervention: May include change in therapy or active medical/surgical treatment.

Intervention necessary to sustain life: Includes cardiovascular and respiratory support (eg, CPR, defibrillation, intubation, etc).

[a] © 2001 National Coordinating Council for Medication Error Reporting and Prevention. All Rights Reserved.

TYPES OF CHEMOTHERAPY ERRORS IN THE MEDICATION USE PROCESS

Procurement

Procurement is the phase in the medication use process where the drug product is acquired. Procurement staff are integral to assuring a consistent supply of medications and are frequently responsible for maintaining the environment where the product is stored. Although the IOM Committee on Identifying and Preventing Medication Errors did not identify the procurement node as specifically resulting in mediation errors, it is understood that product selection and availability can be a contributing factor to an occurrence.[9] To help assure correct medication selection, chemotherapy inventory must be standardized, neatly organized, and clearly labeled. **Case Study 6-1** described a wrong dose error that is associated with procurement history and stock location.

CASE STUDY 6-1
Procurement: Wrong Dose Associated With Stock Location

An unusual number of patients are seen in the inpatient setting for high-dose intravenous interferon alfa-2b therapy. Additional supply is acquired from the outpatient clinic where a higher strength, 50-million international unit vial is used for subcutaneous administration. As a result, 2 similar size (nearly identical) vials, 1 containing 18 million international units, and another, 50 million international units, are stored next to each other in the refrigerator. The 50-million international unit vial is readily accessible and selected for reconstitution rather than the 18-million international unit vial, resulting in a preparation error.

The error is identified when a discrepancy in the lot number and expiration date documentation is noticed. This is an example of a wrong dose error type occurring during the dispensing node. However, contributing factors in this occurrence include the procurement history and the manner in which the medication was stored (**Figure 6-1A**).

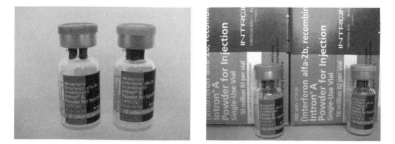

FIGURE 6-1 As seen in the pictures of interferon alfa-2b vials, product labeling by the same company is often similar, both to promote brand recognition and maintain production efficiency.

Medication shortages or contract changes can also lead to errors associated with inventory management. For example, inadvertent ordering of methotrexate containing preservative rather than preservative-free methotrexate or a shortage of methotrexate may necessitate acquisition of a different concentration to maintain adequate supply (eg, 25 mg/mL could be procured in place of a 50 mg/mL product). If pharmacy staff is not familiar with this change or if computer-generated volume calculations are not updated, an incorrect dose error could occur.

Updated procurement contracts can also result in stocking different size and concentration vials. For example, a generic form of DOCEtaxel may replace a brand name product, resulting in stocking 10 mg/mL concentration rather than the previous 20 mg/mL concentration. Effective communication and timely updating of information technology systems are essential to prevent an associated incorrect dose event.

It is also important to have a robust product recall system in order to prevent contaminated or ineffective medications from being dispensed. Recalled medications must be immediately retrieved and sequestered, and an alternative medication must be obtained, as appropriate. Depending on the level of the recall, affected patients may need to be identified and notified with the assistance of the health system legal and/or risk management staff.

Procurement staff that is familiar with the clinical use of products purchased is key to the safe and efficient acquisition of chemotherapy inventory. They can also foster timely communication of product shortages and changes and can facilitate recall activities (**Box 6-1**).

BOX 6-1
Procurement/Stocking Risk-Reduction Strategies

- Maintain an organized, efficient work place free of clutter
- Provide adequate storage space, illumination, and reasonable supply height
- Promote consistent and standard supply of medications
- Reduce the dosage forms and vial sizes stocked
- Procure vial sizes only associated with common medication dose (eg, vinCRIStine 2 mg vs 5 mg)
- Limit stock access depending on location and use
- Limit procurement of vials with similar appearance
- When look-alike vials must be procured, store separately, and label distinctly

- Notify staff when changing medication brand or concentration.
- Notify staff of medication shortages and collaborate in developing action steps/resolution.

Source: Facts About the Sentinel Event Policy. The Joint Commission website. http://www
.jointcommission.org/assets/1/18/Sentinel%20Event%20Policy.pdf. Accessed May 30, 2013.

Prescribing

Prescribing is the phase in the medication use process that involves an action of an authorized prescriber to issue a medication order.[10] The IOM's report, *Preventing Medication Errors: Quality Chasm Series,* recognized prescribing as one of most common nodes involved in medication errors.[9] Depending on the detection method used, 0.61 to 53 errors were identified per 1,000 orders prescribed in health-system settings.[9] The prescribing node involves many error types, including failure to recognize a drug–drug interaction, documented allergy, drug disease interaction, and incorrect medication, frequency, or dose. **Case Study 6-2** described a wrong dose error that is associated with several factors related to prescribing.

CASE STUDY 6-2
Prescribing: Wrong Dose

A 39-year-old breast cancer patient participating in a dose-escalating phase I clinical trial was admitted for high-dose chemotherapy followed by a bone marrow transplant. The dose escalation described in the protocol was misinterpreted by the fellow; cycloPHOSphamide 4000 mg/m² for 4 days was prescribed rather than the intended 1000 mg/m²/day for 4 days.[9] The fourfold overdose was not identified by the hematology/oncology attending physician, the pharmacists compounding and dispensing the medications, or the nurses administering the medications. The patient, Betsey Lehman, a health reporter for the *Boston Globe,* died as a result of the overdose.[9]

This tragic type of incorrect dose error is seen when the total course dose is misinterpreted for the daily dose during the prescribing phase. The factors contributing to the error in this case include the following:

- The protocol was not current and readily accessible
- Descriptions of the protocol dosing was in both total course dose and daily dose formats[11]
- High-dose limits or maximum dose checks were not built into the computer system checking process

Other chemotherapy dosing errors can result from erroneous marks or typos leading to a dose miscalculation or incorrect frequency of medication administration. For example, an incorrect height can be used in a BSA calculation if a stray mark mimics a foot symbol (eg, 5'6" rather than 56"). An incorrect frequency of vinCRIStine was given due to a misprint in a journal article; "Day 1–8" (days 1 through 8) was printed rather than the intended "Day 1, 8" (day 1 and day 8).[12] Missed decimal places can lead to tenfold dosing occurrences, especially when a leading zero is not written and trailing 0s or other insignificant integers are documented. The Joint Commission information management standards require a leading zero (eg, 0.1 mg rather than .1 mg), and prohibit the use of a trailing zero (eg, 1 mg rather than 1.0 mg) in handwritten text, free-text computer entry, and on preprinted forms.[13]

The Institute for Safe Medication Practices-Canada (ISMP-Canada) published a review of medication incidents involving cancer chemotherapy agents reported between 2002 and 2009.[14] Prescribing error themes in this bulletin included incorrect doses due to the complexity of chemotherapy protocols and lack of standard order sets and incorrect frequency due to a reliance on mental determination of dosing schedules. Other errors reported were prescribing a medication to which the patient had a history of a reaction and prescribing incorrect chemotherapy regimens (eg, (folinic acid, fluorouracil, oxaliplatin [FOLFOX] vs. folinic acid, fluorouracil, irinotecan [FOLFIRI]) or phase of a chemotherapy regimen (eg, hyper-CVAD chemotherapy regimen cycle 2 part B vs hyper-CVAD cycle 2 part A).[14]

Transcribing/Documenting

Transcribing/documenting is the phase in the medication use process that involves the act of transcribing a medication order by someone other than the prescriber.[10] The ISMP-Canada identified incorrect medication, incorrect dose, incorrect frequency, and duplicate therapies as the most common chemotherapy related transcription errors.[14]

A list of error-prone abbreviations, symbols, and dose designations is published and regularly updated on the Institute for Safe Medication Practices (ISMP) website.[15] Dangerous abbreviations or symbols used in oncology include *μg*, which is misinterpreted as *mg* (*mcg* is recommended); *cc*, which is misinterpreted as *u* (*mL* is recommended); *IU*, which is misinterpreted as *IV* or *10* (*international units* or *units* is recommended); and *qd* or *QD*, which is misinterpreted as *qid* (daily is recommended).[15] **Case Study 6-3** describes a transcribing/documenting error with use of an abbreviation.

CASE STUDY 6-3

Transcribing/Documenting: Wrong Frequency Associated With Use of Error-Prone Abbreviation

A patient prescribed low dose oral methotrexate 2.5 mg PO three times weekly transitions from an inpatient hospital stay to an outpatient rehabilitation center. During the transition, the patient's medication orders are rewritten and transcribed to a paper medication administration record. The abbreviation TIW, 3 times weekly, is misread for TID, 3 times daily. The rehabilitation center has a consultant pharmacist who reviews medication administration records on site, and fortunately, the error is caught.

This is an example of an incorrect frequency error occurring in the transcribing phase that is caused by the use of an error-prone abbreviation.

Compounding/Dispensing

Compounding/dispensing is the phase in the medication use process that begins with the pharmacist review of the medication order and includes the order entry/processing, preparation, and dispensing.[10] The ISMP-Canada identified the following most common chemotherapy related dispensing occurrences in this phase: incorrect medication due to look-alike medication name (**Figure 6-2**), labeling, and packaging; incorrect dose due to incorrect medication concentration or diluent volume (**Figure 6-3**); and incorrect rate due to elastomeric pump selection.[14] **Case Studies 6-4** and **6-5** describe a compounding/dispensing error with a look-alike, sound-alike product and incorrect dose due to incorrect medication diluent volume, respectively.

CASE STUDY 6-4
Compounding/Dispensing: Wrong Medication Associated With a Look-Alike, Sound-Alike (LASA) Product

A 3-year-old child diagnosed with acute lymphoblastic leukemia is prescribed asparaginase as a part of the treatment regimen.[16] At the time of the occurrence, asparaginase was manufactured in 3 different forms, *Escherichia coli* asparaginase, *Erwinia* asparaginase, and pegylated *E coli* asparaginase. On 8 separate occasions, *E coli* asparaginase was incorrectly used to prepare the lower dose regimen meant for pegylated *E coli* asparaginase.[16] As a result, the patient was undertreated, but fortunately achieved a complete remission.

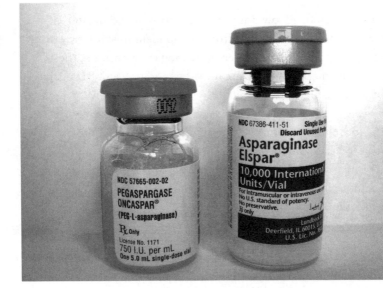

FIGURE 6-2

This description is an example of an incorrect medication type error that occurred in the dispensing node. The similar-sounding medication name was a contributing factor.

CASE STUDY 6-5
Compounding/Dispensing: Wrong Dose

A pharmacy technician unfamiliar with the preparation of temsirolimus was asked to prepare a 25-mg dose. The usual compounding instructions had not been programmed into the computer system; the product was nonformulary. A temsirolimus kit is composed of a medication vial with temsirolimus solution (30 mg in 1.2 mL), which is reconstituted further with 1.8 mL of provided diluent, resulting in a final concentration of 10 mg/mL. The temsirolimus medication vial is labeled 25 mg/mL without a total volume. The pharmacy technician calculated the medication concentration to be 25 mg per 2.8 mL (believing there was 1 mL in the vial along with the 1.8 mL of diluent added), resulting in an 8.9 mg/mL concentration, approximately a 10% difference compared to the actual concentration. The error was caught by the checking pharmacist, when 2.8 mL was drawn up instead of 2.5 mL to provide the 25-mg dose.

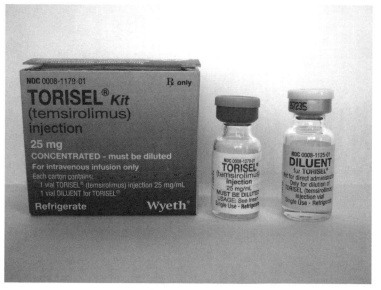

FIGURE 6-3

Contributing factors to this incorrect dose error included an unclear medication label in a setting where reference medication information was not readily available. A systematic process to update medication dilution charts and computer-based volume calculations is important to be sure the information is readily accessible when needed.

Look-alike and sound-alike medications are a well-recognized risk for product selection error. A list of confused drug names and a list of look-alike drug names with recommended tall man letters are available from the ISMP.[15] Chemotherapy products associated with name confusion can be found in **Table 6-4.**

Table 6-4 Examples of Chemotherapy Products With Look-Alike Names[a]

Intended Product	Common Look-Alike Name Product	Additional Look-Alike Name Product
Adriamycin	Aredia	
Afatinib	Axitinib	
Alkeran	Leukeran	Myleran
Escherichia coli asparaginase	Peg-asparaginase	*Erwinia* asparaginase
Anzemet	Avandamet	
AzaCITIDine	AzaTHIOprine	
CISplatin	CARBOplatin	
CycloPHOSphamide	CycloSPORINE	
Cytarabine	Liposomal cytarabine	
DACTINomycin	DAPTOmycin	
DAUNOrubicin	DAUNOrubicin	citrate liposome (DaunoXome)
Darbepoetin alfa	Epoetin alpha	
DOXOrubicin	DAUNOrubicin	IDArubicin
DOXOrubicin	DOXOrubicin liposome (Doxil)	
Epogen	Neupogen	
Femara	Femhrt	
Folic acid	Folinic acid (leucovorin calcium)	
Filgrastim	Pegfilgrastim	
Gemcitabine	Capecitabine	
InFLIXimab	RiTUXimab	
ISOtretinoin	Tretinoin	
Leucovorin calcium	Levoleucovorin	Leukeran
Lomustine	Carmustine	
Lunesta	Neulasta	
Matulane	Materna	
Mitomycin	Mitoxantrone	

Neupogen	Neulasta	Neumega
PEMEtrexed	PRALAtrexate	
PACLitaxel	PACLitaxel protein-bound particles (Abraxane)	
Purinethol	Propylthiouracil	
Taxol	DOCEtaxel	
Taxol	Taxotere	
Trastuzumab (Herceptin)	Ado-trastuzumab emtasine (Kadcyla)	
VinBLAStine	VinCRIStine	VinORELbine
Xeloda	Xenical	
Xtandi	Xgeva	Xofigo
Zytiga	Xgeva	

Administering

Administering is the phase in the medication use process where the medication and the patient interact. It begins with the order being reviewed and the patient being identified, and it continues through the medication administration to the patient.[10] Medication administration involves administering the medication to the right patient at the right time and educating the patient about the medication.[10] The *Preventing Medication Errors: Quality Chasm Series* reported 2.4 to 11.1 administration errors per 100 opportunities or doses.[9] Considering that even one chemotherapy error can be catastrophic, it is important to understand the types of administration errors that occur in this setting. The ISMP-Canada identified incorrect patient, dose omission, incorrect route, and incorrect rate as the most common themes associated with chemotherapy administration errors.[14] **Case Studies 6-6** and **6-7** illustrate administration errors that involve the wrong patient and wrong infusion rate.

CASE STUDY 6-6
Administration: Wrong Patient

Two patients with the same last name are due to be admitted to the outpatient clinic, both with lung cancer. Each is receiving a different regimen, one for small cell lung cancer and the other for non–small cell lung cancer. When the patient with small cell lung cancer arrives first, the nurse mistakenly uses the wrong set of orders and requests the medications from the pharmacy. The pharmacist notices the discrepancy in the regimen and indication, contacts the nurse, and the mix-up is realized.

This wrong patient error is a near miss, or a warning sign that 2 identifiers were not used when reviewing the chemotherapy order, and/or there is another systems issue requiring action. It is important to have a standard process for checking chemotherapy orders to include 2 patient identifiers. (See the chapter called *Basics of Systemic Anticancer Therapy Prescribing and Verification,* elsewhere in this text.)

CASE STUDY 6-7
Administration: Wrong Rate

A patient was being treated in an ambulatory clinic with CISplatin and a 4-day regimen of fluorouracil, administered by an ambulatory intravenous continuous infusion pump.[14] The dose of fluorouracil prescribed was 4000 mg/m² to be infused over 4 days; baseline regimen dose = 1000 mg/m²/day administered by intravenous continuous infusion q24h daily × 4 days = 4000 mg/m² per course. The 4-day medication product was prepared in a 130-mL bag and labeled with both the rate per hour and the rate per 24 hours. The nurse calculated the rate and mistakenly programmed the pump to infuse over 4 hours instead of 4 days. A second nurse did not complete a full independent check, but completed a mental calculation and did not catch the error. When the patient called to report that the bag was empty, the error was discovered. Tragically, the patient developed severe mucositis and neutropenia, followed by multisystem organ failure, and died 22 days later.

The ISMP-Canada published a comprehensive root cause analysis of this wrong-rate event identifying many contributing factors including[17]:

- Unnecessary information on the medication label
- Lack of standard structure for checking functions in nursing
- Lack of smart pump technology to hard stop the incorrect rate

Other events reported during the administration phase include wrong-route errors. One of the most well recognized fatal errors in the treatment of children and adults with leukemia is the inadvertent administration of vinCRIStine by the intrathecal route.[18] Intravenous vinCRIStine is frequently given on the same day as an intrathecal methotrexate and/or cytarabine therapy. Contributing factors associated with wrong-route errors include similar packaging, delivery of both medications at the same time and to the same location, and lack of a systematic checking process for each discipline (**Box 6-2**).[15] See the chapter titled, *Basics of Systemic Anticancer Therapy Prescribing and Verification*, elsewhere in this text, for more information on the steps used in verifying accuracy and appropriateness of cancer therapy orders.

BOX 6-2
Preventing VinCRIStine or Vinca Alkaloids Administration Errors: Error Reduction Strategies[a,15]

- Dilute intravenous vinCRIStine and vinca alkaloids in a minibag rather than a syringe
- Package all intrathecal medications in a distinct manner (eg, sterile packaging)
- Do not unwrap the package until immediately prior to injection.
- Label intravenous vinCRIStine with warning labels stating "For intravenous use only." Include warning on product and outside packaging
- Complete an independent check of intravenous vinCRIStine dose prior to dispensing
- Implement smart pump dose limits for vinca alkaloids
- Establish a setting where intrathecal medications can be safely delivered. Prohibit intravenous medications from being delivered to the same location
- Prohibit intravenous chemotherapy medication in rooms where lumbar punctures are performed
- Consider a handoff directly to the clinician administering the intrathecal medication
- Verify that the intrathecal injection has been administered before dispensing intravenous vinCRIStine

- Require two health professionals independently check IV vinCRIStine doses before administration.
- Educate those who prescribe, prepare, dispense, and administer chemotherapy about published case reports of fatal intrathecal administration of IV vinCRIStine.

ᵃ Adapted from recommendations made through the Institute for Safe Medication Practice.

Monitoring

Monitoring is the phase in the medication use process that involves assessing the patient's physical, emotional, or psychological response to a medication and documenting this response.[10] An example of a monitoring error type includes failure to check or review a methotrexate level and identify the need to increase a leucovorin rescue dose. Another example of a monitoring error is the failure to measure and respond to a change in organ function or specific electrolyte value following therapy. Some health systems include failure to identify a drug–drug interaction, documented allergy, or drug–disease interaction as drug monitoring error. As long as one is consistent with categorizing these medication error types among a health system or group, then the corresponding occurrence rate and associated contributing factors can be effectively addressed.

PREVENTING CHEMOTHERAPY MEDICATION ERRORS

In order to prevent chemotherapy errors, a multidisciplinary team approach must be taken with the understanding that there will always be opportunities to continuously improve the medication use process in each individual setting.

Ready Access to Pertinent Patient Information

Patient information pertinent to processing a chemotherapy order must be readily available.[15] See the chapter titled *Basics of Systemic Anticancer Therapy Prescribing and Verification,* elsewhere in this text, for a checklist of key chemotherapy order and verification elements. Key elements include two patient identifiers, history of the patient's allergies, and previous sensitivities. Patient diagnosis, with ready access to the stage of disease, pathology, and associated therapeutic markers, is also important. A patient's identity should be clarified when the patient is pre-scribed a regimen that is not indicated for the stage or type of disease in order to prevent a potential occurrence. For example, contacting a clinician regarding an order for trastuzumab in a patient with HER-2 negative disease could be the only opportunity to identify a wrong-patient error.

The team must have access to the patient's medication list to verify there are no drug–drug interactions. A patient prescribed a regimen containing irinote-can may begin taking St. John's wort, an over-the-counter antidepressant, which can reduce the effectiveness of the chemotherapy.[19] Other medications may be associated with increased toxicity when taken concurrently with chemotherapy. Itraconazole has been reported to increase neurotoxicity when administered with vinCRIStine.[19] Unless the team is aware that the patient was prescribed this antifungal agent, there will not be an opportunity to prevent or monitor concur-rent administration. The patient's history of previous regimens, including cumu-lative doses of medications, must be available to prevent toxicity associated with exceeding maximum lifetime dose recommendations. Timing of current radiation therapy is important to coordinate with antineoplastic prescribing since patients may be receiving a reduced dose of chemotherapy while receiving radiotherapy.

Not to be overlooked is a careful clinical assessment of the patient and ready access to the patient's most recent laboratory data. Even when an order is written for the right patient and is indicated for the patient's diagnosis, and the dose is calculated correctly, the dose may actually be excessive if the patient's organ function is compromised. For example, if a low absolute neutrophil count value is not available to staff during prescribing, dispensing, or administration, there is a lost opportunity to delay or adjust therapy to prevent a potential admission for febrile neutropenia. It is also beneficial for the team members to be informed of the goal of therapy to understand the basis of treatment decisions, as well as to support and educate the patient.

Ready Access to Medication Information

Team members must have access to medication information when prescribing, compounding, administering, and monitoring chemotherapy.[15] A standardized formulary of drugs and dosage forms that has been evaluated for a medication safety risk, including look-alike sound-alike risk, can help to prevent medication errors. An example of a user-friendly general formulary assessment tool was pub-lished by Pick and colleagues.[20] This tool can be modified to meet the needs of different health systems by individualizing the risk reduction strategy action steps.

Access to primary literature, current investigational protocols, and medication information is also key to be able to prescribe, compound, and administer chemotherapy regimens safely. Pharmacists and pharmacy technicians need to have ready access to standard information on medication reconstitution, dilution, stability, and medication preparation precautions.

Treatment-based algorithms supported by computer physician order entry with clinical decision support can help to standardize care. This type of system guides the clinician to prescribe the appropriate regimens for a specific diagnosis and provides an alert when a dose reduction is recommended. For example, if a patient were prescribed pemetrexed with an estimated creatinine clearance less than 50 mL/min, staff would receive an alert identifying compromised renal function and requiring further assessment. Computer systems should also provide an alert when a dose is prescribed beyond normal dosing range or high dose limit for an individual dose, daily dose, course dose, and cumulative dose. It is ideal if high-dose limits are tailored to the health system's patient population and adjusted for the age and weight of the patient. Order processing systems should also only permit a correct route of administration to be prescribed, processed through pharmacy systems, printed on the product labels, and documented on electronic medication administration records.

Standardized Chemotherapy Order Forms and Checking Process

Physicians and other licensed independent practitioners, pharmacy, and nursing staff need to have a systematic and well-defined procedure for processing chemotherapy orders that supports an independent check of their colleagues. The use of chemotherapy order forms or electronic-based systems with programmed regimens standardizes care and helps prevent errors including those related to illegible handwriting and the use of abbreviations.

The order itself must not appear cluttered but be easy to review. When prompting a calculation of a dose, open boxes are preferred over lines, which could obscure a decimal point. Leading zeros before a decimal place must be used to accentuate the decimal point, (eg, 0.1 mg), and trailing zeros must not be permitted (eg, 1 mg rather than 1.0 mg), to prevent tenfold dose errors. The use of insignificant decimal places must also be discouraged (eg, 30 mg rather than 30.4 mg).

Verbal orders to initiate chemotherapy must be prohibited; however, to reduce risk of continuing toxic therapy, a verbal order to stop chemotherapy may be permitted. Medication names must not be abbreviated; the generic name on the order should match the name on the product label and the name on the medication administration record. In select situations, the use of a trade name may be used in addition to the generic name to reduce the potential for a look-alike or sound-alike error. The use of the trade name Doxil in addition to the generic name DOXOrubicin liposome is an example of a risk reduction strategy to prevent confusion with DOXOrubicin. Symbols and abbreviations, such as *qd*, *U*, and *TIW*, known to result in transcription errors, must be avoided. The patient's height and weight must be documented with consistent units, and a history of height and weight readily accessible. Misinterpretation of a patient's weight (ie, 65 kg for 65 lb), number transcription, or marked weight loss must be readily identified with an automated alert or through a review of the patient's demographic history.

Most importantly, medication doses need to be expressed in a standardized fashion that is clear to each discipline. List the medication name, method of calculation, dose, units (mg preferred), route, rate, frequency, number of doses, and schedule (days). For example, for a patient with a BSA equal to 2 m², the order should read in the following manner: *Cytarabine 100 mg/m²/dose = 200 mg in 500 mL 5% dextrose administered by intravenous continuous infusion over 24 hours daily × 7 days.* Actual dates may be listed if day 1 of therapy is not clear on the ordering form. Calculate a total dose per course only if necessary and only if the daily dose is listed as well. Providing a total course dose in addition to the daily dose is particularly important when dispensing a product that makes up the total course dose of medication, such as an ambulatory continuous infusion fluorouracil pump.

The order-checking process should include verification that the patient understands the purpose of therapy and potential side effects by signing an informed consent. Clinicians involved in the provision of chemotherapy must also assess the patient's medical history and current clinical parameters. This must include a review the last time therapy was administered to verify the appropriate regimen interval (eg, every 14 days vs every 21 days).

Preventing Look-Alike and Sound-Alike Medication Errors

Look-alike and sound-alike (LASA) cancer therapy medication names can result in inadvertent administration of the wrong medication to a patient.[13] Common examples of confused chemotherapy medication names include CISplatin and CARBOplatin (**Figure 6-4**), DOCEtaxel instead of Taxol or PACLitaxel (**Figure 6-5**), and vinCRIStine and vinBLAStine (**Figure 6-6**). See Table 6-4 for other examples of LASA cancer therapies/medications available in a liposome- or albumin-bound formulation in addition to the regular formulation that are at high risk for confusion. The family of anthracyclines including DOXOrubicin,

DOXOrubicin liposome, DAUNOrubicin, and IDArubicin are also at risk for confusion (**Figure 6-7**). To prevent errors associated with LASA medication names, many proactive strategies may be taken. Stock only the medications necessary to meet patient needs, limit the use to a single strength, and purchase products with distinct packaging, including tall man lettering (upper-case lettering).[15] Separate look-alike sound-alike medications in the pharmacy in clearly labeled, individual bins. Use tall man lettering on standard order forms and in computer systems screens to facilitate their appearance on medication labels and medication administration records. Follow published recommendations for clear labeling.[15] Encourage the use of both generic and brand names for confusing medication names. Employ computer-assisted high-dose limits tailored to the health system's population with a hard stop to prevent staff from missing the alert. During the medication preparation process, use a redundant system of checks to include an independent set-up and preparation of the product. Complete a visual and computer-assisted check of the product and volume used during product preparation (eg, pharmacist visual, bar code verification). Lastly, educate staff during about LASA risks during orientation and through ongoing periodic competency assessments.[15] Communicate LASA risks with new formulary products and LASA occurrence as they are identified through reporting systems.

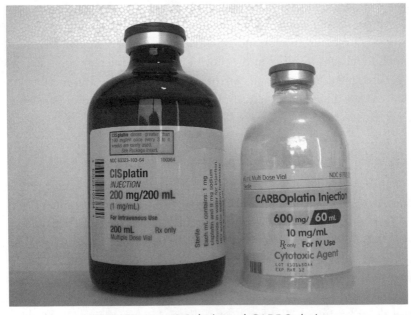

FIGURE 6-4 CISplatin and CARBOplatin

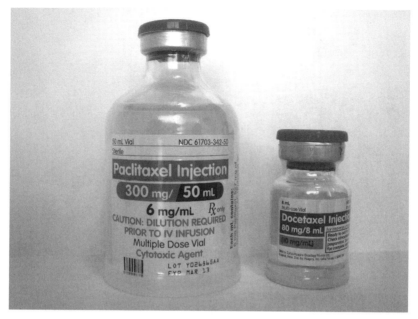

FIGURE 6-5 DOCEtaxel instead of PACLItaxel

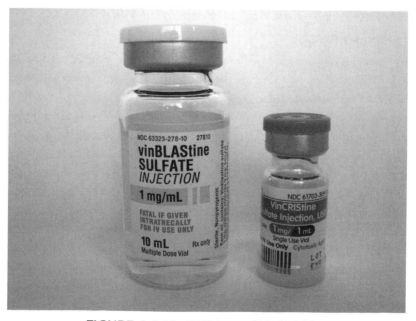

FIGURE 6-6 VinCRIStine and VinBLAStine

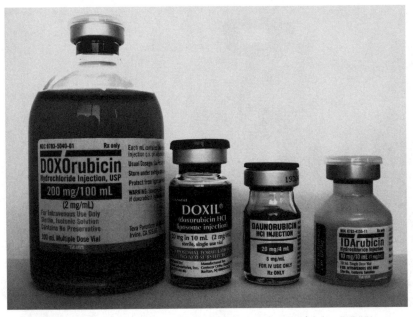

FIGURE 6-7 Family of anthracyclines, DOXOrubicin, DOXIL, DAUNOrubicin, IDArubicin

Preventing Wrong-Route Errors Associated With Intrathecal Therapy

Many strategies may be employed to prevent wrong-route type errors associated with intrathecal therapy.[15] One of the key approaches to prevent inadvertent intrathecal administration is to provide the intrathecal medications in distinct packaging. A large sterile, sealed package can provide a unique visual aid to distinguish an intrathecal dose. Dilute intravenous vinCRIStine or vinca alkaloids in a small fluid bag rather than a syringe. Label vinCRIStine or vinca alkaloids clearly with the identified route of administration on both the product itself and the outer packaging (eg, "For Intravenous Use Only"). Do not label the product with a warning identifying the incorrect route of administration. Establish a systematic process for distributing an intrathecal dose, which should be distinct from doses administered by the intravenous route. Consider handoff directly to the clinician administering the intrathecal medication rather than placing it in a location where other parenteral medications are delivered.[15] Another strategy is to wait until the intrathecal dose has been given before to dispensing the intravenous medication. Include these risk-reduction strategies in employee orientation so new staff members have a clear understanding of the risks of inadvertent intrathecal administration of vincristine and the strategies used to prevent this type of error.

Employ Technology

There are growing opportunities to utilize technology to help prevent medication occurrences. Standardization of order entry through computerized physician order entry (CPOE), when introduced in a structured and planned manner, can immediately prevent illegible handwriting and unclear medication orders. The need to seek and remove old or incorrect order forms is eliminated. CPOE can also allow added levels of safety when combined with clinical decision support to direct medication choices and warn clinicians of potential unsafe medication prescribing.

Other innovations, such as the use of bar coding and/or facial recognition technology to verify the correct medication and diluent are increasingly available and can prevent preparation errors associated with the wrong medication, fluid, or dose.[21,22] Exciting newer technology is using specific gravity to verify the medication volume and is being introduced through robotics and stand-alone scale devices that are integrated with the medication order. This can also help reduce product preparation occurrences.

The use of existing smart pump technology must be employed to prevent free-flow errors and wrong-rate occurrences during the administration process. Smart pumps, which communicate directly with the medication order, will also enhance safety by verifying the patient, medication product, duration, and time of infusion.

Provide a Safe Work Environment

The physical design and organization of the work place needs to support efficient work flow along with appropriate storage space, illumination, supply height, and lack of clutter.[10] Clinicians must be able to work in an area free of distractions when prescribing chemotherapy, when checking chemotherapy orders, and while compounding and verifying medication products. Communication about system issues should be encouraged in a nonpunitive environment. Staff should be encouraged to identify and report errors and be engaged in the solutions to help prevent future occurrences. In addition, staff should be encouraged to continually read and learn about safety risks in their practice area. The ISMP and the ISMP-Canada offers straightforward strategies to prevent errors on their websites and through participation in an oncology medication safety-self assessment program.[14,15]

MEDICATION ERROR REPORTING

MEDMARX is an example of a system originally developed by the US Pharmacopeia that can be used to report, analyze, track, and trend adverse drug events, including oncology medication errors.[10] This system has an established nomenclature based on the NCC MERP taxonomy. The taxonomy helps to systematically define the place (or node) in the system where a medication error occurred as well as the medication error type.[6] Causes of a medication error, contributing factors, and the severity of the medication error are also documented. The NCC MERP Index for categorizing and rating the severity of an event is defined in categories A through I.[6] Category A represents circumstances or events that have the capacity to cause error. Category B indicates that a medication error has occurred but it did not reach the patient (near miss, occurrence; Clinical Pearl 6-5). Categories C and D indicate that a medication error has occurred but did not result in patient harm (Clinical Pearl 6-4). Different levels of harm are reflected in categories E, F, G, and H. Any medication error that resulted in or may have contributed to a patient's death is classified as Category I (Clinical Pearls 6-2 and 6-7). Essential information to collect and suggested categories for medication error documentation and reporting are located in Table 6-1 and Table 6-2.

It is essential to have a supportive culture of safety that encourages error reporting in order to identify opportunities to prevent harm by reducing future occurrences. An emphasis on reporting all occurrences, especially near miss events, must be communicated in each health system. Every member of the healthcare team contributes to patient safety and should participate in the occurrence reporting process. Medication-error and near-miss events may be shared anonymously with the wider community through the ISMP website.[15]

SENTINEL EVENT REPORTING

A sentinel event is an unexpected occurrence involving death, serious physical or psychological injury, or the risk of such an event.[13] Healthcare settings such as hospitals are required to report a subset of sentinel events to The Joint

Commission. These events include an unanticipated death or permanent loss of function, not related to the natural course of the patient's illness or underlying condition, suicide of any patient receiving care or within 72 hours of discharge, hemolytic transfusion reaction involving administration of blood or blood products having major blood group incompatibilities, and/or surgical and nonsurgical invasive procedure on the wrong patient, wrong site, or wrong procedure. For a full description of sentinel events defined by The Joint Commission, go to the website, http://www.jointcommission.org/. Depending on local regulations and health-system policy, medication-related sentinel events may require reporting to the state board of registration in medicine, department of public health, and the National Quality Forum.

Sentinel events signal the need for an immediate response by governing bodies and executive leadership to ensure that everything possible is done to understand what happened and why it happened, and to prevent it from occurring again. This response must include conducting a timely, thorough, and credible root cause analysis.[13] A root cause analysis is a practical problem-solving method that is designed to identify the primary reasons for the event, rather than the more obvious symptoms of the event. A sentinel event root cause analysis must be completed and submitted to The Joint Commission within 45 days of an occurrence for review and acceptance. A basic template to complete a root cause analysis including corresponding action plans is offered by The Joint Commission.[13]

A sentinel event can be the spark that initiates continuous quality improvement to reduce ongoing risk and prevent future occurrences.

ADVERSE EVENT REPORTING

Drug-induced adverse events can range from mild to very severe, such as death.[23] Timely reporting of serious events is important because it assists with communication of such serious adverse effects. In 1993, the Food and Drug Administration created MedWatch, a program designed to educate healthcare professionals about the need to be aware of, monitor for, and report adverse events and to facilitate reporting of adverse events. The FDA considers a serious adverse event to be death, life-threatening event, hospitalization, disability, congenital abnormality, or need for medical/surgical intervention to prevent permanent damage. Healthcare providers can report an adverse event directly to the manufacturer or through the MedWatch program. Refer to the website: http://www.fda.gov/Safety/MedWatch/HowToReport/ucm085568 for more information about reporting adverse events.

RISK EVALUATION AND MITIGATION STRATEGIES

Risk evaluation and mitigation strategies (REMS) were established by the Food and Drug Administration Amendments Act (FDAAA) of 2007 following the publication of a report on drug safety by the IOM in 2006.[24] The IOM recommendations included a clarification of the FDA's role in gathering and communicating additional information on marketed products' risks and benefits as well as an increased role for the FDA's drug safety staff. Title XI of the FDAAA was signed into law on September 27, 2007, and took effect on March 25, 2008.[25]

Section 901 of Title XI granted the FDA new authority to require postmarketing studies for clinical trials of human drugs and to develop a REMS to ensure that the drug's benefits outweigh its risks.[25] Each REMS program has at least one goal—a safety-related health outcome and/or the understanding by the patient or healthcare provider of the serious risk of drug use.

Risk management components of a REMS program may include one or more of the following elements: a medication guide, patient package insert, communication plan, and elements to assure safe use. Medication guides are required when product labeling could help prevent serious adverse effects, the drug product has serious risks relative to its benefits, and/or the drug has important health benefits for which patient adherence is necessary for effectiveness.[25] A communication plan for healthcare providers may include targeted mailings through professional organizations or safety-related notification of healthcare professionals and consumers through the FDA's MedWatch partners program. Elements to assure safe use (ETASUs) are employed when the safe access for patients to the medication with known serious side effects would otherwise be unavailable. These elements may require specific training or certification, patient registration, documentation of safe use conditions such as laboratory tests results, and an implementation system.[26] Some of the most comprehensive REMS programs that affect oncology are listed in **Table 6-5**. Erythropoiesis-stimulating agents (eg, Procrit, [epoetin alfa] Epogen [epoetin alfa], and Aranesp [darbepoetin alfa]) are examples products with REMS programs that require an initial patient acknowledgement form, monthly distribution of a medication guide, health-system and clinician training and registration, and periodic audits to evaluate compliance.

Table 6-5 Examples of Oncology-Focused FDA REMS Programs[26]

Name	Date Approved	REMS Components
Aranesp (darbepoetin alfa) injection	2/16/2010; modified 6/24/2011, 5/31/2012, 3/27/2013	Medication guide, communication plan, elements to assure safe use, implementation system
Caprelsa (vandetanib) tablets	4/6/2011; modified 6/22/2011	Medication guide, communication plan, elements to assure safe use, implementation system
Epogen/Procrit (epoetin alfa) injection	2/16/2010; modified 6/24/2011, 5/31/2012, 3/27/2013	Medication guide, communication plan, elements to assure safe use, implementation system
Nplate (romiplostim) for subcutaneous injection	8/22/2008; modified 8/14/2009, 3/23/2010, 7/29/2011, 12/6/2011	Communication plan
Pomalyst (pomalidomide) capsules	2/8/2013	Elements to assure safe use, implementation system
Promacta (eltrombopag)	11/20/2008; modified 3/5/2010, 2/25/2011, 12/6/2011	Communication plan
Revlimid (lenalidomide) capsules	8/3/2010; modified 5/9/2012, 2/8/2013, 6/5/2013	Elements to assure safe use, implementation system
Soliris (eculizumab) injection	6/4/2010	Medication guide, elements to assure safe use
Thalomid (thalidomide) capsules	8/3/2010; modified 2/8/2013	Elements to assure safe use, implementation system
Yervoy (ipilimumab) injection	3/25/2011; modified 2/16/2012	Communication plan

REMS programs promote safe use of medications, permit approval of medications with serious risks that would not otherwise have been brought to market, and allow others to remain on the market.[24] However, these programs are time consuming for healthcare practitioners, lack reimbursement, and have the potential to disrupt continuity of patient care. All members of the healthcare team need to participate in the future of these programs in order to promote a generation of useful clinical data as well as safety.

SUMMARY

A single medication occurrence related to chemotherapy administration in the cancer patient can be catastrophic to both the patient and the healthcare team. In order to effectively employ risk-reduction strategies and improve the safety of the medication use process, it is important to have a clear understanding of the types of chemotherapy errors that occur, common causes of these errors, and their potential contributing factors. The majority of medical errors are made by good, but fallible people working in imperfect systems.[27] Every member of the healthcare team needs to work collaboratively in order to improve medication safety and reduce risk in the oncology patient. **Box 6-3** provides a summary of strategies that can be used to prevent cancer therapy errors.[28]

BOX 6-3
Chemotherapy Error Prevention Strategies[28]

- Provide ready access to patient information, including pathology, stage, goal of care, allergy history, history of height and weight, comorbid disease state, pregnancy, laboratory values, date of last treatment
- Provide ready access to patient's current medication list
- Provide ready access to resources, including patient protocol, drug information, stability/compatibility, and medication administration record
- Use computerized physician order entry (CPOE) or standardized written chemotherapy preprinted order forms
- Use uncluttered order forms and/or order screens
- Use open boxes rather than lines for dose documentation
- Use high-dose-limit checks in computer systems with hard stops
- Use generic names, add trade names only for look-alike or sound alike risk medications
- Do not use medication abbreviations (eg, CPT-11, 5FU)
- Do not use unit abbreviations (eg, U, use units instead; IU, use international units instead)
- Do not allow verbal orders to prescribe chemotherapy.
- Use a consistent dosage unit (eg, mg)

- Do not use insignificant decimal places (20.4 mg vs 20 mg)
- Use a leading 0, such as 0.1 mg; do not use a trailing 0; use 1 mg
- Use a clear standardized label format
- Take steps to prevent look-alike or sound-alike errors
- Establish a comprehensive chemotherapy order-checking process
- Establish a standardized preparation process
- Establish a standardized chemotherapy administration process
- Establish standard concentrations; standardize chemotherapy reconstitution and dilution
- Take steps to prevent inadvertent intrathecal administration of intravenous medications
- Use smart-pump technology with free-flow protection and high-dose-limit checks
- Provide a physical environment that offers adequate space and lighting, free of distractions
- Engage staff in identifying and reporting errors, and involve staff in determining action plans to prevent future occurrences
- Provide ongoing staff education and competency assessment; encourage board and specialty certification
- Encourage patients to ask questions and communicate concerns

REFERENCES

1. Kohn L, Corrigan J, Donaldson M, eds. *To Err Is Human: Building a Safer Health Care System*. Washington, DC: The National Academies Press; 1999.
2. Classen D, Pestotnik S, Evans R, Lloyd JF, Burke JP. Adverse drug events in hospitalized patients: excess length of stay, extra costs, and attributable mortality. *JAMA*. 1997;277:301–306.
3. Bates D, Cullen D, Laird N, et al. Incidence of adverse drug events and potential adverse drug events: implications for prevention. ADE Prevention Study Group. *JAMA*. 1995;274:29-34.
4. Jha A, Kuperman G, Teich J, et al. Identifying adverse drug events: development of a computer-based monitor and comparison with chart review and stimulated voluntary report. *J Am Med Inform Assoc*. 1998;5:305-314.
5. Gurwitz J, Field T, Harrold L, et al. Incidence and preventability of adverse drug events among older persons in the ambulatory setting. *JAMA*. 2003;289:1107–1116.
6. National Coordinating Council on Medical Error Reduction and Prevention website. http://www.nccmerp.org. Accessed May 30, 2013.

7. National Coordinating Council on Medical Error Reduction and Prevention (NCC MERP). NCC MERP Taxonomy of Medication Errors. Available at: http://www.nccmerp.org/pdf/taxo2001-07-31.pdf. Accessed May 30, 2013.

8. Institute for Safe Medication Practices and Institute for Safe Medication Practices Canada. 2012 ISMP International Medication Safety Self Assessment for Oncology. Available at: https://mssa.ismp-canada.org/oncology. Accessed May 30, 2013.

9. Aspden P, Wolcott J, Bootman L, et al., eds, Committee on Identifying and Preventing Medication Errors. *Preventing Medication Errors: Quality Chasm Series.* Washington, DC: The National Academies Press; 2007.

10. US Pharmacopeial Convention website. http://www.usp.org. Accessed May 30, 2013.

11. Conway J, Weingart S. *Organizational Change in the Face of Highly Public Errors: The Dana-Farber Cancer Institute Experience.* Agency for Healthcare Quality and Research. http://www.webmm.ahrq.gov/perspective.aspx?perspectiveID=3. Accessed May 30, 2013.

12. Cohen M. Misprint in journal articles leads to vincristine overdose. *Hosp Pharm.* 1994;29:294,302.

13. The Joint Commission website. http://www.jointcommission.org. Accessed May 30, 2013.

14. Institute for Safe Medication Practices-Canada website. http://www.ismp-canada.org /index.htm. Accessed May 30, 2013.

15. Institute for Safe Medication Practices. http://www.ismp.org. Accessed May 30, 2013.

16. Cheung, K, van den Bemt P, Torringa M, Tamminga RY, Pieters R, de Smet PA. Erroneous exchange of asparaginase forms in the treatment of acute lymphoblastic leukemia. *J Ped Hematol/Oncol.* 2001;33:e109-e113.

17. *Fluorouracil Incident Root Cause Analysis.* Institute for Safe Medication Practices website. http://www.ismp-canada.org/download/reports/FluorouracilIncidentMay2007 .pdf. Published May 22, 2007. Accessed May 30, 2013.

18. Cohen M. Preventing medication errors in cancer chemotherapy. In: Cohen M, ed. *Medication Errors.* Washington, DC: American Pharmacists Association; 2007:453.

19. *Micromedex Healthcare Series* [intranet database]. Version 2.0. Greenwood Village, CO: Thomson Healthcare.

20. Pick A, Massoomi F, Neff W, Danekas PL, Stoysich AM. A safety assessment tool for formulary candidates. *Am J Health-Syst Pharm.* 2006;63:1269-1272.

21. O'Neal B, Worden J, Couldry R. Telepharmacy and bar-code technology in an iv chemotherapy admixture area. *Am J Health-Syst Pharm.* 2009;66:1211–1217.

22. Poon EG, Cina JL, Churchill W, et al. Medication dispensing errors and potential adverse events before and after implementing bar code technology in the pharmacy. *Ann Intern Med.* 2006;145:426-434.

23. Goldman SA, Kennedy DL, Lieberman R. Clinical therapeutics and the recognition of drug-induced disease. http://www.fda.gov/downloads/Safety/MedWatch /UCM168515.pdf. Published June 1995. Accessed May 30, 2013.

24. Shane R. Risk evaluation and mitigation strategies: impact on patients, health care providers, and health systems. *Am J Health Syst Pharm.* 2009;66(24)(suppl 7):S6–S12.

25. Identification of drug and biological products deemed to have risk evaluation and mitigation strategies for purposes of Food and Drug Administration Amendments Act of 2007. *Federal Register.* 2008;73:16313–16314.

26. Food and Drug Administration. Approved Risk Evaluation and Mitigation Strategies (REMS). http://www.fda.gov/Drugs/DrugSafety/PostmarketDrugSafetyInformation forPatientsandProviders/ucm111350.htm. Updated May 23 2013. Accessed May 30, 2013.

27. Wachter R, Shojania K. *Internal Bleeding: The Truth Behind America's Terrifying Epidemic of Medical Mistakes*. New York, NY: Rugged Land; 2004.

28. Schulmeister L. Preventing chemotherapy errors. *Oncologist.* 2006;11:463–468.

CHAPTER 7

Inventory and Reimbursement

Timothy Tyler
Lisa Holle

LEARNING OBJECTIVES

Upon completion of the chapter, the reader will be able to:

1. Describe the types of accounting methods that can be used to manage hematology/oncology inventory.
2. Explain the methods in which cancer drug therapy can be purchased and the goal of purchasing and maintaining inventory.
3. Discuss the different payer types, including reimbursement of cancer drug therapy.
4. List the four national compendia recognized by Medicare.

INTRODUCTION

Business in the capitalistic model is a very simple concept: items are sold or services provided for clients or customers with a margin of profit. Health care is no different, regardless of the setting. Although the business aspect of cancer care is not always in the forefront of clinicians' minds, it is integral to the overall care of the patient. If business is not managed appropriately, patient care will be impacted. For example, maintaining valuable and skilled staff may be difficult, or attaining and maintaining an inventory of high-cost drugs may not be possible without an appropriate credit line. Therefore, while clinical acumen is essential to cancer care, an aspect that can have no less a devastating impact on patient care is a stable business. A multidisciplinary approach is the best way to ensure that all required resources are available for patients, including inventory and reimbursement.

Inventory is a basic function required of any business, and in oncology, having adequate inventory is essential to providing optimal patient care in a timely manner, despite the expensive nature of many cancer therapies. In addition to inventory, the provision of services and the suitable compensation of those services are probably the most important elements of keeping an oncology practice viable: they are aspects that, if not handled appropriately, will result in the closing of practices and clinics. In the past half-century, several major changes in reimbursement have occurred; however, the key principle remains unchanged: it is imperative to not receive less in payment or remuneration than the cost of providing the service—inclusive of staffing, overhead, and most importantly, the drug inventory.

INVENTORY

Accounting

Inventory control is needed to ensure one of the single largest investments is safe, appropriately managed, and optimized. Two basic models of business accounting exist: cash- and accrual-based transactions. Cash-based accounting, as is implied by the name, means that the income (sales) and outgoes (purchases) are tracked in real time and are logged only once money is collected or actively spent. In this scenario, the transaction is only recorded once the funds are transferred or the check is written. If the credit terms allow purchases to be bought and paid within 30 days, then the payment is not acknowledged until it is paid; that is—only when it actively is paid out of the account would it be recorded. In contrast, accrual-based business accounting is more pragmatic in managing business transactions. Transactions are recorded like keeping a scoreboard. In this scenario, the transaction is recorded immediately. Of course, the party billed might never pay or perhaps the check will not clear, but the transaction is considered valid once the transaction is agreed to and not when it actually transpires. For this reason, when uncertain transactions are recorded, it might be prudent to reserve or not fully count that money until it is in some way validated or collected. Cash-based accounting is difficult to manage in businesses with expanding growth and complex inventories, such as in cancer care; therefore, most oncology-related practices use an accrual-based system.

Inventory seems as if it should be simple, but actually it can be quite complex. Take, for example, a box of syringes. Typically, such a supply would be expensed up front either immediately or over some fixed time period because the supply is needed to run the business and the syringes will be consumed on the premises. Because the syringes are of minimal value, most businesses would consider them an expense when they are purchased rather than an asset to be monitored and tracked. This introduces the concept of materiality threshold in which a dollar value is set and any product that falls below that dollar value would not be inventoried. There can be products that are exempted from the materiality threshold; for example, all drugs are inventoried even if they are below the materiality threshold. This concept forces a business to look at transactions in a very simple light: is the item an asset or an expense? An asset has value and can be recorded on a balance sheet and used in the delivery of a good or service. Conversely, an expense is something that is consumed, and its consumption may be immediate, such as with our box of syringes; thus, we expense them once they are bought rather than subtract their value after each and every use. On the other hand, an expense can be a large item that is used over time, such as an examination table. The table may cost $1,000, but rather than expensing it immediately, a depreciation schedule is created so that the business can remove an appropriate portion off the balance sheet every year it is in service. If the examination table is substituted with 10 vials of a branded cancer therapy agent that is very expensive ($2,400/vial), the method of inventory accounting is likely to differ. Rather than expensing for all 10 vials ($24,000), many practices will only expense the number of vials used (eg, $2,400/vial used). This method allows the assets to not be overstated and not all of the expenses to occur at one time. Several qualities of an inventory item, including materiality (the cost of item), the nature of items for use in the business, their asset value, and the timing or schedule at which the item is used, must be considered when determining the appropriate accounting method.

Pharmacists who are involved in the preparation of the drugs dispensed in a cancer center are poised to assist with managing drug inventory.[1] They can continually monitor drug use and adjust inventory levels accordingly. Additionally, they can track and predict prescribing trends and establish new patient plans of care to anticipate how much of each drug a clinic will need. Finally, minimization of waste of compounded drugs also assists with appropriate inventory levels.

Purchasing

Cancer drug therapies are usually purchased through a wholesaler or distributor, using a purchase order, which is an official agreement to purchase items at specified prices and terms. In the United States, over 50% of the drugs distributed are through the 3 major wholesalers: AmerisourceBergen, Cardinal, and McKesson.[2] See **Clinical Pearl 7-1** about restricted distribution through risk evaluation and mitigation strategy (REMS) programs. Secondary distributors (various) also provide the sourcing of drugs for purchase. Many of the major secondary distributors are divisions of the major wholesalers, but independent distributors also exist. Independent distributors are often regionally based and will compete for purchasing business by offering services because they are smaller and cannot always offer the lowest pricing. Hospitals often use wholesalers for the bulk of their purchases. Wholesalers will typically allow for a daily morning delivery by a courier and will provide added services such as invoicing, credit terms, and label generation to sticker the incoming products. Returns are possible (terms and conditions vary by company and possibly even by product), and other services (eg, inventory management or payment terms), possibly for a fee, are provided at the purchaser's direction. Independent distributors are generally used by physician practices. They provide many of the same services as wholesalers but will typically ship via common carrier such as UPS or FedEx, and shipping across the

CLINICAL PEARL 7-1

Drugs with risk evaluation and mitigation strategy (REMS) programs that have an element to assure safe use (ETASU) have restricted distribution and will require purchase of the drug through a specific distributor, regardless of the practice's usual purchasing mechanisms. In many cases, the provider, pharmacist, and/or patient may also have to register before purchasing can occur. Examples include lenalidomide (Revlimid), pomalidomide (Pomalyst), thalidomide (Thalomid), and ipilimumab (Yervoy). Drugs with REMS programs can be found at http://www.fda.gov/Drugs/DrugSafety /PostmarketDrugSafetyInformationforPatientsandProviders /ucm111350.htm. Click on the drug to find out exact REMS requirements.

country or returns may be restricted or not permitted. Many sites will have one or more of each type of account (wholesalers and independent distributors) to maximize drug availability, combat shortages, and resolve other issues. In general, the majority of purchases are from one entity due to added financial incentives. For example, if business volume is large, a wholesaler will offer attractive terms on financing or even a rebate based on volumes purchased in an attempt to gain the most business. **Clinical Pearls 7-2** and **7-3** illustrate the impact of volume purchasing on the success of wholesalers and the relationship between inventory, respectively. Thus, group purchasing organizations (GPOs) (eg, Premier, Novation, Amerinet) have formed to negotiate contract prices based on the larger volume that can be generated compared with individual institutions.

Few healthcare specialties require such a large capital expenditure as that of hematology/oncology. Because the inventory cost is large, the goal of purchasing and maintaining inventory is to minimize the number of drugs on the shelf and maximize the turnover. See **Case 7-1**. Typically, inventory turnover is desired to be faster (weekly) rather than slower (monthly) because of a concept known as "the time value of money." The amount of capital required to run a business can be dramatically lowered if the business's funds are not tied up needlessly

CLINICAL PEARL 7-2

Because wholesalers' margins are historically extremely small, they must drive their profits from large volume throughput. For example, if they generate 0.01% on every item moved through the organization (whether drop shipped or couriered to a site), the profit will be based on volume. If the amount they move per day totals $1 million vs. $100,000, the difference is an astounding $9000/day with the higher throughput. The success of the wholesaler/distributor is tied closely to the volume moved through the organization.

CLINICAL PEARL 7-3

The 80:20 Rule

Generally, 80% of volume usually comes from only 20% of the drug inventory.

paying off drugs beyond the business's immediate requirements. However, due to drug shipment turnaround times, volume discounts, and shortages or back orders, a larger-than-necessary stock amount is often required. Additionally, price increases, drug shortages, contractual disputes regarding discounts, back charges for drugs that were not billed to the business correctly, recalls and spoilage, and purchasing personnel taking time off for sick and vacation time can impact inventory purchasing practices. The general principle still remains after all of the above factors are considered: excess inventory expense is not desirable because it represents capital that is not available to run the business. To determine the best pattern and process of purchasing for a site, it is best to review the historical purchases, such as a year's worth of invoices or recorded transactions, to determine the usual volume and overall budget for the practice. It is also important to consider that fluctuations with payer mix and volumes of patient types often exist and may influence the inventory maintenance. See **Case 7-2**.

The main reason for purchasing a specific product should be quality (the product is as it is labeled) and reliability in which the drug can be prepared into an appropriate final product for patient consumption. Assuming that all vendors have similar quality products and standards, then price is often the reason for choosing a specific vendor. **Clinical Pearl 7-4** provides suggestions on how to obtain a product that is not routinely stocked by a wholesaler or distributor.

CLINICAL PEARL 7-4

If the primary wholesaler or distributor carries only 3 of the 4 available versions of a particular product, but the fourth product (which is offered at the best contract price) is not stocked on a routine basis, then the purchaser should talk with his or her sales representatives for both the drug and the distribution channel (wholesaler or distributor). Although the wholesaler/distributor sales representative will want to ensure the purchaser's needs are being met, the wholesaler's/distributor's purchaser will want to ensure items that cannot be moved are not stocked. Therefore, the drug manufacturer's sales representative may be of help in getting an item stocked with a particular wholesaler/distributor by collaborating with the manufacturer's public relations personnel.

CASE 7-1
Managing Inventory

A review of the inventory purchases for the past 12-month reporting period reveals a total of $1,345,235 spent, with 47 orders placed with the main distributor, 13 placed with a secondary wholesaler, and 4 exceptional (unusual) orders placed (eg, direct through the manufacturer or through a noncontracted distributor).

1. How often did the inventory turnover in this 12-month period?
2. What was the average purchase amount per order?
3. Can the inventory be managed more effectively?

Bulk purchase may be able to lower the normal cost of inventory; however, it is important to determine if the bulk purchase will in fact be beneficial to the business.

Example: Normally, drug Z costs $2,500 per vial, but if purchased in bulk (minimum of 75 vials), the cost decreases to $2,000 per vial. In this case, purchasing $150,000 worth of drug to save $37,500 in inventory costs makes sense as long as the drug can be used before the expiration date and the price does not naturally drop before inventory is exhausted. In many situations, deals of this sort become available just as a company anticipates losing patent protection on a drug. If it takes the business 6–9 months to use the inventory and the drug becomes generic in 3 months, it may not be worth the bulk purchase.

CASE 7-2
Evaluating Purchase of a Bulk Order of a Patented Drug About to Expire Versus Awaiting a Generic Drug Purchase

To determine whether it is prudent to purchase a bulk order (minimum of 75 vials) of a brand drug about to go off patent or await its generic counterpart to become available, you will need to review your average use of the drug. If the practice or clinic typically uses 25 units per month, and the patent is expected to expire within 3 months, then the anticipated time of the inventory hitting 0 is about the time the patent expires and the bulk purchase would make sense. If, however, usage is less than 10 units per month (on average), the inventory of a large bulk order for the patented drug is likely to remain for 4–5 months after the generic launches. To determine the best purchasing method, a calculation must be made. Often a generic price drops approximately 10% per month.

Assuming the brand price is $2,500/vial discounted unit price is $2,000 / vial and 10% decrease/month once the generic launches, show the calculations needed to determine the best method of purchasing bulk vs awaiting generic release.

Calculation to Determine Best Method: Bulk Versus Awaiting Generic Purchase in an 8-Month Example About "Deals"		
Month No.	No Bulk Purchase	Bulk Purchase
1	$2500 × 10 (brand)	$150,000 (75 × $2000, the discounted unit price)
2	$2500 × 10 (brand)	
3	$2500 × 10 (brand)	
4	$2250 × 10 (generic)	(Note: 10% decrease per month once generic launches in month 4)[a]
5	$2025 × 10 (generic)	
6	$1823 × 10 (generic)	
7	$1640 × 10 (generic)	
8	$1476 × 10 (generic)	
Total	$167,140	$150,000 (difference is $17,140 in favor of bulk buy)

[a] If only one generic manufacturer is on the market, this drop may not be as significant or constant.

Some manufacturers use restricted distribution systems that require the purchase of a drug from a different distributor or wholesaler than the institution's usual source, such as a specialty pharmacy. In these cases, the drug is either sent with the patient to be administered by a provider, a practice called "brown bagging," or the drug is directly shipped to the dispensing pharmacy designated for a specific patient, a practice called "white bagging." In some states (eg, Ohio), white bagging is illegal unless approved by the board of pharmacy and agreed upon by both pharmacies—the specialty pharmacy and the dispensing pharmacy.

Because of the high cost of many cancer therapy agents, counterfeit drug manufacturing or selling is becoming more common.[2] When a lapse in the chain of custody of a drug occurs, several concerns arise including (1) inappropriate drug storage, (2) lower potency of the drugs, (3) incorrect drugs, or (4) no drugs, only inert components. In 2009, a shipment of 110,000 low-dose erythropoietin vials was stolen. The criminals who stole the drug counterfeited labels for the same drug that indicated it was 20 times more potent and sold the misbranded drug at a 20-times higher cost. While this is alarming in the United States, this is a larger problem internationally, where the World Health Organization estimates that 10% of the world drug supply has counterfeit or misbranding issues.[2] Ultimately, having a chain of custody ensures that the drugs purchased are genuine and manufactured in specified conditions that ensure optimum results. A pedigree means that the business can produce proof of contiguous paperwork from the point of manufacture to the point of ultimate consumption. This will minimize the opportunity for inappropriate handling and outright counterfeit or fraud. Several states have chain-of-custody laws or pedigree laws (**Figure 7-1**).[3]

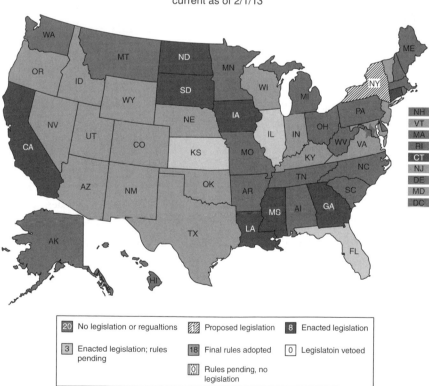

FIGURE 7-1 Reproduced with permission from Healthcare Distribution and Management Association, "Distributor Licensing and Pedigree Requirements by State," http://www.healthcaredistribution.org, 2013. The information included is current as of the publication date.

340B Pricing

Some healthcare clinics, care centers, and hospitals that dispense outpatient drugs qualify for a federal reduced-pricing program, called the 340B program.[4] This program allows the purchase of many drugs at prices far below market price (20%–50% below average price) by institutions that serve indigent or under-served populations. The Affordable Care Act expanded coverage to include freestanding cancer hospitals. In theory, the competitive advantage gained by a nonprofit institution that qualifies for 340B pricing is negated by the fact that it treats a large portion of patients that will not pay for their health care due to poverty. **Clinical Pearl 7-5** describes where information about 340B pricing can be found.

CLINICAL PEARL 7-5

Information about the 340B pricing program, including education tools and resources tools for providers, can be found on the US Department of Health and Human Services Health Resources and Services Administration website at http://www.hrsa.gov/opa/

REIMBURSEMENT

The primary source of income to cover the costs of drugs and supplies, as well as the overhead costs associated with operating a pharmacy business, is the reimbursement received from the patient's insurance company. This section will discuss the various forms of reimbursement.

Payers

Healthcare insurance is currently provided by either private organizations or government agencies. The private insurance includes those policies purchased by an employer or by individual consumers; whereas government agency–provided healthcare insurance includes Medicare, Medicaid, the State Children's Health Insurance Program (SCHIP), military health benefits (including the Department of Defense and Veterans Affairs Health Administration), and the Indian Health Service.

Medicare

The largest payer in the United States is Medicare, the federal government healthcare insurance program administered by the Centers for Medicare & Medicaid Services (CMS). Medicare is available to individuals aged 65 and older, individuals less than 65 years old with certain disabilities, and individuals with end-stage renal disease.[5] Medicare is composed of 4 parts, labeled A through D. Medicare Part A covers inpatient care in hospitals, skilled nursing facilities, hospice, and home care.[5,6] Beneficiaries must meet certain conditions to get these benefits and most do not have to pay a premium for these services because the patient or his or her spouse paid for the service through previous payroll deductions; however, a deductible must be met yearly before full coverage is provided.[5] Medicare Part B covers doctors' services and outpatient care, durable medical equipment, some preventive services, some services such as physical and occupational therapy, and some home health care not covered by Part A.[5,6] These Part B services are only covered when considered medically necessary and the patient usually pays a monthly premium for this service.[5] Additionally, the patient is responsible for a yearly deductible payment and a 20% co-pay on all remaining services, regardless of the price. Medicare Part C (known often as Medicare Advantage) offers healthcare plan options from Medicare-approved insurance companies. These Medicare Advantage plans offer the benefits of services covered under Medicare Part A and B, often Part D coverage as well, and coverage for additional services (eg, eye care and dental care) for a monthly cost.[6] The original Medicare plan does not cover most prescription drugs, although Medicare Part B covers a limited number of outpatient drugs (**Table 7-1**).[7] Therefore, an optional Medicare Part D was created to offer prescription drug coverage through Medicare-approved insurance companies.[5,6] Patients choose to participate in Medicare Part D, select a plan, and pay a monthly premium for coverage.[5] Medicare Part D has a yearly deductible and a 5% co-payment on remaining drug costs until the donut hole amount is reached. The donut hole is the coverage limit of Medicare Part D (in 2013, total drug costs coverage limit is $2,970).[8] Patients who exceed the coverage limit are responsible for the entire cost of prescription drugs until the expense reaches a catastrophic threshold, at which time Medicare coverage begins again (in 2013, the catastrophic limit for total drug costs is $4,750).

For acute care (ie, hospitalizations), the diagnosis-related group (DRG) system calculates reimbursement based on the patient's diagnosis and the average amount of resources that are needed to treat that diagnosis.[9] This reimbursement rate is a fixed, prospectively determined single payment that is to cover all products and services provided, including the drugs administered. If the hospital can provide adequate care during hospitalization and discharge the patient for less that the reimbursement amount, a profit can be made; otherwise a loss may occur.

In the outpatient hospital setting, reimbursement is governed by the Outpatient Prospective Payment Systems (OPPS). Like the DRG, this system uses

Table 7-1 Outpatient Prescription Drugs Covered by Medicare Part B[a,7]

Injectable drugs administered by a licensed medical practitioner

Oral cancer drugs if the drug is available in an injectable form, including the following:

- Busulfan
- Capecitabine
- Cyclophosphamide
- Etoposide
- Melphalan
- Methotrexate
- Temozolomide

Oral antinausea drugs as part of an anticancer regimen if administered within 48 hours and used as full therapeutic replacement for antinausea drugs

Drugs infused through durable medical equipment (eg, infusion pump, nebulizer)

Antigens prepared by a physician and administered under physician supervision

Injectable osteoporosis drugs for qualifying women

Erythropoiesis-stimulating agents for end-stage renal disease or other certain conditions

Blood clotting factors for hemophilia

Immunizations

Immunosuppressive drugs for transplant patients if the transplant is paid for by Medicare in a Medicare-approved facility

Parenteral and enteral feedings

Intravenous immune globulin

[a] Generally covers drugs that usually aren't self-administered and are given as part of a physician service.

a fixed, prospectively determined, bundled payment for hospital-provided outpatient supplies and procedures (including chemotherapy).[10] Services are categorized as ambulatory payment classifications, each corresponding to a specific payment. Some drugs that exceed a specific threshold set annually (eg, $80 for 2013) are paid separately (ie, separately covered outpatient drugs).[10] These drugs are reimbursed at average sales price (ASP) plus a percentage markup (set annually; ASP plus 6% in 2013). The ASP is a US government-derived figure that is published a quarter later by the federal government. The ASP basically seeks to establish the average price (minus all government discounted programs such as the Veterans Administration, Indian Health Services, and 340B drug discounts). Although the Medicare payment rates in the OPPS allow for reimbursement for the administration of intravenous medications, no reimbursement is provided for the drug reconstitution, sterile preparation, and hazardous drug handling by pharmacists and technicians. Instead, the cost for these services is expected to be covered with the amount that is reimbursed for the drug itself.

Physician office practices are reimbursed under Medicare Part B, which for oncology practices will cover both drugs administered in the office and provider services.[11] In Medicare Part B, the drugs are reimbursed through a fee schedule (set annually and published in the *Federal Register* and was ASP plus 6% in 2013). See **Clinical Pearl 7-6**. In addition, the physicians bill for their professional service on a fee-for-service basis. **Table 7-2** compares the differences in hospital OPPS and physician office practice reimbursement.

CLINICAL PEARL 7-6

The proposed and final payment rates for OPPS and Medicare Part B physician's fee schedule are reported in the *Federal Register*, which publishes the proposed rules in August and the final rules in November of the preceding year. See https://www.federalregister.gov/ to search for rules. Average sales price data is updated quarterly and can be found on the Centers for Medicare and Medicaid (CMS) website, Medicare Part B Drug Average Sales Price page at https://www.cms.gov/Medicare/Medicare-Fee-for-Service-Part-B-Drugs/McrPartBDrugAvgSalesPrice/index.html.

Table 7-2 Medicare Part A and B[10,11]

Payment Item	Medicare Part A (Hospital Outpatient)	Medicare Part B (Physician Office)
Payment system	Prospective payment system	Fee schedule
Payment threshold	Yes ($80 in 2013)	No (all paid)
Payment rate	ASP plus 6%[a]	ASP plus 6%[a]
Billing form	UB02 (UB92)	HCFA 1500
340B eligible	Yes (only certain conditions)	No

ASP, average sales price

[a] Sequestration will likely reduce this rate.

Medicaid

Medicaid provides healthcare coverage to children, pregnant women, parents, seniors, and individuals with disabilities, primarily to those with low incomes.[12] The federal government sets minimum standard guidelines for Medicaid eligibility and each state can choose to expand coverage beyond the minimum threshold. State Medicaid agencies pay providers directly for the costs of services or may rely on managed care organizations to arrange payment. Typically, Medicaid covers the same services that Medicare covers and often some additional services. For patients who qualify for and enroll in both Medicare and Medicaid (ie, they are dually eligible), Medicaid also pays for Medicare premiums, deductibles, and co-payments.[13] Each state's Medicaid coverage may vary; therefore, understanding the services and drugs that are reimbursement by a state's Medicaid program is necessary to seek appropriate reimbursement.

Private Insurance

Private or employer-provided insurance can be in the form of a fee-for-service plan or a managed care plan.[14] A fee-for-service plan allows patients to choose a physician and hospital and often requires a deductible to be met before full coverage begins. After the deductible is met, the fee-for-service payer will pay providers for a portion of the total charges billed, with the patient being responsible for the remaining portion or a co-payment. Most private insurers use the Medicare physician fee schedule as the basis for their payment rates.

Managed care plans, such as health maintenance organizations (HMOs), point-of-service (POS), or preferred physician provider organizations (PPOs), usually have lower premiums and co-payments than fee-for-service plans, and they have cost-control programs in place, such as prior authorization for covered services or restrictions on providers within a certain network.[14] HMOs usually cover most expenses but limit providers through an approved network. POS plans are a type of HMO that will allow an outside-of-network provider to provide service, sometimes at a higher coinsurance. PPOs are a hybrid fee-for-service and HMO plan, where coverage is available through a network of providers and facilities included in the PPO, but coverage may be obtained outside of the network for an additional fee. Most managed care companies will require prior authorization or documentation of medical necessity before services are rendered.

Prescription drug coverage under private insurance plans varies based on the type of plan. Many plans have a co-pay associated with each prescription. Oncology-related drugs are often covered in these plans but may require prior authorization or distribution through a specialty pharmacy because of the expense of many of these products.

Coverage

Most Medicare coverage is determined at the local contractor's level with input from healthcare providers. This type of coverage determination is termed local coverage determination. In some instances, Medicare deems it appropriate to offer a national coverage determination. Most private insurers follow the coverage deemed appropriate by Medicare; however, some differences may exist. See **Clinical Pearl 7-7**.

In oncology, therapies are often prescribed for indications that are not Food and Drug Administration–approved, but that have been evaluated in clinical trials. Coverage decisions for the treatment of patients with cancer, thus, are often based on indications listed in 1 or more of the 4 national compendia recognized

CLINICAL PEARL 7-7

The Centers for Medicare and Medicaid Services (CMS) has a searchable database for local coverage determinations and national coverage determinations. To use the database, go to http://www.cms.gov/medicare-coverage-database/search/advanced-search.aspx.

by Medicare, which include (1) Thomson's Micromedex DrugDex, (2) Elsevier's Gold Standard Clinical Pharmacology, (3) the National Comprehensive Cancer Network (NCCN) Drug Information & Biologics Compendium, and (4) the American Hospital Formulary Service Drug Information (AHFS-DI).[15] If at least one of the compendia recommends a treatment, Medicare will provide coverage, as long as another compendium does not advise against the off-label use and Medicare deems the treatment medically necessary. In the absence of compendia-supported off-label indication, peer-reviewed medical literature may be used to justify the prescribing of certain medications. Medicare recognizes 26 peer-reviewed journals to support off-label indications (**Table 7-3**).[15,16]

To avoid payment denials for off-label indications after a medication has been administered, most institutions will employ the process of precertification. Precertification involves submitting a request to an insurer for authorization to treat the patient with the therapy. Preauthorization requirements include: (1) patient-specific information (eg, name, date of birth, insurance number), (2) diagnosis, (3) name, dose, and duration of medications. This process is not exactly the same as verifying insurance benefits. Typically, the physician will dictate a therapy plan. The support staff will then submit the plan for preauthorization and communicate the coverage back to the provider and clinic staff. Authorization requests may be submitted electronically or manually, dependent on the insurer's requirements. When preauthorization occurs, it is not a guarantee of payment but is only a general guidance as to what is and is not acceptable by the insurer.

When insurers pay a claim, typically, a lump sum is paid on a range of items submitted. Therefore, the clinic or practice will need to review the explanation of benefits (EOB) to ensure that all billed items were paid for and that the payment was at the appropriate contracted rate. Mistakes in coding or submitting claims may result in less-than-full payment. Most clinics will have billing personnel responsible for processing precertification, reviewing claims before submission to ensure proper coding, reviewing EOB for appropriate payment, and coordinating appeals for denials. It is a complex process and is best undertaken by personnel with adequate training and expertise.

Patient Assistance Programs

For patients who do not have insurance, are underinsured, or who simply cannot afford their drug therapy or co-pays/deductibles, financial assistance may be available.[17] Pharmaceutical companies and not-for-profit agencies often have programs in which patients can apply to receive free drug or assistance with

Table 7-3 Peer-Reviewed Journals Recognized by Medicare for Off-Label Coverage of Anticancer Therapies[16]

American Journal of Medicine

Annals of Internal Medicine

Annals of Oncology

Annals of Surgical Oncology

Biology of Blood and Marrow Transplantation

Blood

Bone Marrow Transplantation

British Journal of Cancer

British Journal of Hematology

British Medical Journal

Cancer

Clinical Cancer Research

Drugs

European Journal of Cancer

Gynecologic Oncology

International Journal of Radiation, Oncology, Biology, and Physics

The Journal of the American Medical Association

Journal of Clinical Oncology

Journal of National Cancer Institute

Journal of National Comprehensive Cancer Network

Journal of Urology

Lancet

Lancet Oncology

Leukemia

The New England Journal of Medicine

Radiation Oncology

co-payments or deductibles. (See the *Oral Cancer Therapy* chapter for a table listing not-for-profit agencies offering financial assistance.) Each company and organization will have different criteria for eligibility. In some clinics, dedicated pharmacists, technicians, or social workers are involved in identifying candidates, assisting with the application processes, and obtaining a drug supply for eligible patients.[1] This can be a very time consuming process but is very helpful to patients.

CASE 7-1
Answers

1. The inventory turned over 64 times (47 main distributor + 13 secondary wholesaler + 4 unusual orders)
2. The average purchase amount per order was $21,019 ($1,345,235 divided by 64).
3. Reviewing each purchase order is important to determine if the amount of each invoice is near the average of $21,019. If many of the purchase orders deviate greatly from the average of $21,019, then managing the inventory more effectively is warranted to avoid a large portion of the money locked into inventory.

CASE 7-2
Answers

Assuming the brand price is $2,500/vial, discounted unit price is $2,000/vial and 10% decrease/month once the generic launches, show the calculations needed to determine the best method of purchasing bulk vs awaiting generic release.

SUMMARY

To best provide patient care, it is important for all healthcare professionals working in the setting of hematology/oncology to understand the role of inventory and reimbursement. Accrual-based accounting methods are most often used in hematology/oncology because of the complex inventories. The goal of purchasing and maintaining inventory includes minimizing the number of drugs and supplies at any one time and maximizing the turnover of these drugs and supplies. The reimbursement process is complex and is determined by the patient's type of insurance. Understanding the patient's insurance coverage before administering treatment is essential to avoid payment denials.

REFERENCES

1. Ostriker S. The growing value of a pharmacist in community oncology practice. *Oncol Issues*. 2010;38–40. http://accc-cancer.org/oncology_issues/articles/janfeb10/JF10 -Ostriker.pdf. Accessed May 25, 2013.
2. The American Council on Science and Health. *Counterfeit Drugs: Coming to a Pharmacy Near You With an Update for 2009*. http://www.acsh.org/wp-content/uploads /2012/04/20090202_counterfeitdrug09.pdf. Accessed May 25, 2013.
3. Distributor licensing and pedigree requirements by state. Healthcare Distribution Management Association website. http://www.healthcaredistribution.org/gov_affairs /.state/state_legis-static.asp. Accessed May 25, 2013.
4. 340B drug pricing program & pharmacy affairs. US Department of Health and Human Services. Health Resources and Services Administration website. http://www .hrsa.gov/opa/. Accessed May 25, 2013.
5. Medicare program—general information. Centers for Medicare & Medicaid Services website. http://www.cms.gov/Medicare/Medicare-General-Information/MedicareGen Info/index.html. Accessed May 25, 2013.
6. Your Medicare costs. Medicare.gov website. http://www.medicare.gov/your-medicare -costs/index.html. Accessed May 25, 2013.
7. Centers for Medicare & Medicaid Services. *Information Partners Can Use On: Medicare Drug Coverage Under Medicare Part A, Part B, and Part D*. http://www.cms.gov /Outreach-and-Education/Outreach/Partnerships/Downloads/11315-P.pdf. Accessed May 25, 2013.
8. Part D/prescription drug benefits. Center for Medicare Advocacy, Inc website. http://www.medicareadvocacy.org/medicare-info/medicare-part-d/#standard benefit. Accessed May 25, 2013.
9. Acute inpatient PPS. Centers for Medicare & Medicaid Services website. https://www .cms.gov/Medicare/Medicare-Fee-for-Service-Payment/AcuteInpatientPPS/index .html?redirect=/AcuteInpatientPPS/. Accessed May 25, 2013.
10. Medicare and Medicaid programs: hospital outpatient prospective payment and ambulatory surgical center payment systems and quality reporting programs; electronic reporting pilot; inpatient rehabilitation facilities quality reporting program; revision to quality improvement organization regulations; final rule. *Federal Register*. 2012;77(221):68210–68565.
11. Medicare program; revisions to payment policies under the physician fee schedule, DME face-to-face encounters, elimination of requirement for termination of nonrandom prepayment complex medical review and other revisions to Part B for CY 2013; final rule. *Federal Register*. 2012;77(222):68891–69380.
12. Medicaid & CHIP program information. Medicaid website. http://www.medicaid .gov. Accessed May 25, 2013.

13. Centers for Medicare & Medicaid Services. *Medicaid Coverage—Dual Eligibles at a Glance.* http://www.cms.gov/Outreach-and-Education/Medicare-Learning-Network -MLN/MLNProducts/downloads/Medicare_Beneficiaries_Dual_Eligibles_At_a _Glance.pdf. Published March 2013. Accessed May 25, 2013.
14. Health insurance and financial assistance for the cancer patient. The American Cancer Society website. http://www.cancer.org/Treatment/FindingandPayingforTreatment /ManagingInsuranceIssues/HealthInsuranceandFinancialAssistancefortheCancer Patient/health-insurance-and-financial-assistance-priv-plan-types. Revised October 10, 2012. Accessed May 25, 2013.
15. Recent developments in Medicare coverage of off-label cancer therapies. *J Oncol Pract.* 2009;5(1):18–20.
16. Centers for Medicaid and Medicare Services. *Compendia as Authoritative Sources for Use in the Determination of a "Medically Accepted Indication" of Drugs and Biologics Used Off-Label in an Anticancer Chemotherapeutic Regimen.* http://www.cms.gov /Regulations-and-Guidance/Guidance/Transmittals/downloads/r96bp.pdf. Published October 24, 2008. Accessed May 25, 2013.
17. American Cancer Society. *Prescription Drug Assistance Programs.* http://www.cancer.org /acs/groups/cid/documents/webcontent/002570-pdf.pdf. Published 2012. Revised February 1, 2013. Accessed May 25, 2013.

CHAPTER 8

High-Dose Cancer Therapy

Laura E. Wiggins
Ashley Richards

LEARNING OBJECTIVES

Upon completion of the chapter, the reader will be able to:

1. Explain the rationale for the use of high-dose therapy in the treatment of patients with cancer
2. Describe which patients may be at risk for the development of graft-versus-host disease (GVHD) after allogeneic hematopoietic stem cell transplant (HSCT)
3. State potential complications observed after HSCT and recommend management approaches for each complication
4. List common posttransplant infections and discuss the standard prophylaxis and treatment of each

OVERVIEW OF HEMATOPOIETIC STEM CELL TRANSPLANTATION

The bone marrow is the source of hematopoietic stem cells (HSCs), which are capable of self-proliferation and differentiation and are responsible for the production of red and white blood cells and platelets. Hematopoietic stem cell transplantation (HSCT), previously referred to as bone marrow transplantation

(BMT), may be used to treat a number of malignant diseases (eg, acute and chronic leukemia and lymphomas) as well as nonmalignant diseases (eg, aplastic anemia).[1,2] Definitions of terms that may be used frequently throughout this chapter are provided in **Table 8-1**. HSCs can come from several sources, and the type of transplant is classified by the cell source (**Table 8-2**).

Table 8-1 Terminology and Definitions

Term	Definition
Allogeneic	HSCs collected from someone other than the patient
Autologous	HSCs collected from the patient
Conditioning regimen	Chemotherapy regimen administered to patients prior to HSCT; may include radiation therapy or immunotherapy in addition to chemotherapy
Engraftment	The donor's stem cells have been taken up by the patient's bone marrow ("have engrafted") and the patient has evidence of hematopoiesis with "recovery" of peripheral blood counts. The day of neutrophil engraftment is typically defined as the first of 3 consecutive days with an absolute neutrophil count (ANC) > 500/μL. The day of platelet engraftment is typically defined as the first of 3 consecutive days of a platelet count > 20 × 1000/ μL without transfusion.
Graft-versus-host disease (GVHD)	A reaction of the donor cells' immune system against the patient. Common yet serious complication that occurs after an allogeneic HSCT.
Haploidentical	Sharing one haplotype. A haploidentical donor can be a sibling, a parent, or a child of the patient, in which one set of chromosomes (and therefore HLA antigens) are identical, and one set is not.
Hematopoiesis	Generation of blood and blood cells (including red cells, white cells, and platelets)
Hematopoietic stem cells	Cells capable of reestablishing hematopoiesis. These may be collected from the bone marrow, peripheral blood, or umbilical cord.
Human leukocyte antigen (HLA)	Part of the major histocompatibility complex. The HLA system is used to evaluate tissue compatibility, and antigens are genetically determined.

Matched related donor	HSCs are collected from a relative (sibling, parent, or child), usually a sibling, and are a complete (100%) HLA match to the patient.
Matched unrelated donor (MUD)	HSCs are collected from a nonrelative and are a complete (100%) HLA match to the patient
Minitransplant	Nonmyeloablative stem cell transplant
Mismatched related donor	HSCs are collected from a relative (sibling, parent, or child), and are less than a complete HLA match to the patient. A haploidentical donor is one type of mismatched related donor.
Mismatched unrelated donor	HSCs are collected from a nonrelative and are less than a complete HLA match to the patient
Mobilization regimen	Regimen used to mobilize stem cells from the bone marrow to the periphery for collection through apheresis process
Myeloablative conditioning	Conditioning regimen that is designed to ablate the bone marrow that will not allow hematologic recovery. These regimens typically consist of very high doses of alkylating agents, sometimes combined with total body irradiation (TBI).
Nonmyeloablative conditioning	Conditioning regimen that is unlikely to produce significant marrow suppression; drugs and doses are intended to optimize immune suppression. Sometimes referred to as a minitransplant.
Reduced intensity conditioning (RIC)	Drugs and doses may result in varying degrees of marrow suppression, but are usually not fully ablative
Reduced toxicity conditioning	Myeloablative regimen that is designed to produce less severe organ toxicity compared to conventional myeloablative regimens
Tandem transplant	Two sequential courses of high-dose chemotherapy and HSCT. May consist of tandem autologous transplants or an autologous transplant followed by an allogeneic transplant.
Umbilical cord blood (UCB)	HSCs are collected from the umbilical cord blood at the time of delivery. UCB cells are stored in banks and may be donated.

HSC, hematopoietic stem cell; HSCT, hematopoietic stem cell transplant.

Table 8-2 Stem Cell Source and Type of Transplant

Type of Transplant	Stem Cell Donor	Stem Cell Source
Autologous	Patient	Bone marrow Peripheral blood
Allogeneic	Sibling or other family member Unrelated person	Bone marrow Peripheral blood Umbilical cord
Syngeneic	Identical twin	Bone marrow Peripheral blood

Types of HSCT

For many cancer patients, chemotherapy is a critical component of anti-cancer therapy. For chemotherapy-sensitive tumors, it has long been known that increases in chemotherapy dose intensity may result in a proportionate increase in antitumor response. Myelosuppression is the dose-limiting toxicity (DLT) for most chemotherapeutic agents and is a major limitation in the ability to maximize the dose-response relationship of chemotherapy.[1-5] Autologous HSCT is mostly used to reestablish hematopoiesis or rescue patients with tumor types that exhibit steep dose–response relationships after high-dose chemotherapy, thus, bypassing the DLT. Common autologous conditioning regimens include high-dose melphalan, BEAM (carmustine, etoposide, cytarabine, melphalan), BEAC (carmustine, etoposide, cytarabine, cyclophosphamide), and busulfan with cyclophosphamide.[3-5] Allogeneic HSCT is used mostly in those tumor types that will benefit from the immune reconstitution whereby the donor's immune cells destroy the patient's residual tumor cells following high-dose chemotherapy and stem cell infusion.[4,5] As will be discussed later in this chapter, these immune interactions are also largely responsible for a number of the complications that can be observed in a patient undergoing allogeneic HSCT. Historically, conditioning regimens for allogeneic HSCT involved fully myeloablative chemotherapy to ablate the marrow and eradicate residual tumor. Certain therapies at high doses are considered ablative and include busulfan, melphalan, and total body irradiation (TBI). This intensive therapy is typically used in younger patients with good performance status who can be expected to tolerate such rigorous treatment. Two commonly used myeloablative regimens are the combinations of busulfan with cyclophosphamide, and cyclophosphamide with TBI. **Table 8-3** lists the common conditioning regimens.[3,4,6–10] Recently, however, it has become evident that a major benefit of allogeneic HSCT may depend less on intensive conditioning and more on immune reactivity of the donor cells against the patient's underlying malignancy (often referred to as the graft-versus-tumor [GVT] effect). This has led to gentler approaches employing less intensive conditioning therapy without decreasing allogeneic HSCT effectiveness and increases the population of patients who may undergo HSCT.[4,11,12] These gentler approaches may consist of fully myeloablative regimens that are designed to produce less organ toxicity (reduced toxicity or reduced intensity regimens) or of nonablative regimens (sometimes referred to as minitransplants) that do not ablate the marrow and are designed to maximize the GVT effect. The use of reduced intensity or reduced toxicity conditioning regimens has allowed the offering of allogeneic HSCT to a wider population of patients, including older patients and/or patients with medical comorbidities that may have previously made them ineligible for transplantation.[4,11,12] Many nonmyeloablative transplant regimens include a purine analog (fludarabine), antithymocyte globulin, cyclophosphamide, and/or low-dose TBI (Table 8-3).[4] Refer to **Clinical Pearl 8-1** for naming of transplant days. Early after transplant, common chemotherapy toxicities include nausea, vomiting, diarrhea, mucositis, and infections. For certain agents, some toxicities are usually seen soon after the drug is given, such as pericarditis or hemorrhagic cystitis with cyclophosphamide, or seizures and sinusoidal obstruction syndrome with busulfan. Other complications of chemotherapy can occur later, such as secondary malignancies due to alkylating agents or pulmonary fibrosis with busulfan. **Table 8-4** lists the common toxicities of various chemotherapy agents used in HSCT.

CLINICAL PEARL 8-1

The day of hematopoietic stem cell transplant is referred to as day 0. The day the conditioning regimen starts is referred to as day $-x$ and counts down to day 0 (eg, the conditioning regimen starts 4 days before transplant, day -4). The days after transplant are referred to as day $+1$, day $+2$, etc.

Table 8-3 Example Conditioning Regimens for HSCT[3,4,6–10]

Regimen	Drugs	Total Doses[a]	Type of HSCT	Intensity
BEAC	Carmustine	300 mg/m^2/dose IV × 1 day (day -7)	Auto	MA
	Etoposide	100 mg/m^2/dose IV q 12 h × 8 doses (days -6, -5, -4, -3)		
	Cytarabine	100 mg/m^2/dose IV q 12 h × 8 doses (days -6, -5, -4, -3)		
	Cyclophosphamide	35 mg/kg/dose IV daily × 4 days (days -6, -5, -4, -3)		
BEAM	Carmustine	300 mg/m^2/dose IV × 1 day (day -6)	Auto	MA
	Etoposide	200 mg/m^2/dose IV q 12 hr × 4 days (days -5, -4, -3, -2)		
	Cytarabine	200 mg/m^2/dose IV daily × 4 days (days -5, -4, -3, -2)		
	Melphalan	140 mg/m^2/dose IV × 1 day (day -1)		
Bu/Cy (BuCy 2)	Busulfan	1 mg/kg/dose PO q 6 h × 4 days (days -7, -6, -5, -4) or 0.8 mg/kg/dose IV q 6 h × 4 days (days -7, -6, -5, -4)	Allo > auto	MA
	Cyclophosphamide	60 mg/kg/dose IV daily × 2 days (days -3, -2)		
Bu/Flu	Busulfan	130 mg/m^2/dose IV daily × 4 days (days -6, -5, -4, -3)	Allo	MA
	Fludarabine	40 mg/m^2/dose IV daily × 4 days (days -6, -5, -4, -3) ATG may be added based on institution.		
Cy/TBI	Cyclophosphamide	60 mg/kg/dose IV × 2 days (days -5, -4)	Allo	MA
	TBI	200–220 cGy BID × 3 days (days -3, -2, -1)		
Flu/Bu	Fludarabine	30 mg/m^2/dose IV daily × 6 days (days -10, -9, -8, -7, -6, -5)	Allo	NMA
	Busulfan	1 mg/kg/dose PO q 6 h × 8 doses (days -6, -5)		
	ATG (equine)	10 mg/kg/dose IV daily × 4 days (days -4, -3, -2, -1)		

Flu/Cy/ TBI	Fludarabine	40 mg/m^2/dose IV daily × 5 days (days -6, -5, -4, -3, -2)	Allo	NMA
	Cyclophosphamide	50 mg/kg/dose IV daily × 1 day (day -6)		
	TBI	220 cGy × 1 day (days -1)		
Flu/Mel	Fludarabine	25–30 mg/m^2/dose IV daily × 4–5 days (days -6 or -5, -4, -3, -2)	Allo	NMA
	Melphalan	100–180 mg/m^2/dose IV daily × 1 day (day 2)		
Mel	Melphalan	140–200 mg/m^2/dose IV × 1 dose (day -2 or -1)	Auto	MA

[a] Represents 1 dosing scheme; other variations may exist. Clinicians should confirm the dosing and schedule with the primary literature, high-dose chemotherapy reference source, or request the reference from the prescriber in the verification process.
Allo, allogeneic; ATG, antithymocyte globulin; Auto, autologous; MA, myeloablative; NMA, nonmyeloablative; TBI, total body irradiation

Collection of Hematopoietic Stem Cells

Initially, HSCT was performed using bone marrow as a source of stem cells and required a bone marrow harvest, a surgical procedure performed in the operating room (OR) under general anesthesia.[1,4] Marrow harvests are performed before the patient begins high-dose chemotherapy. Marrow cells are collected from multiple aspirations of the posterior iliac crest and the marrow cells must be processed and frozen.

Over the last 20 years, the use of HSCs collected from the peripheral blood (peripheral blood stem cells [PBSCs]) has largely replaced the use of bone marrow because it offers the advantage of collecting large numbers of HSCs via leukapheresis and eliminates the need for general anesthesia and an OR procedure.[13,14] Because the number of circulating HSCs in peripheral blood is relatively low, mobilization strategies are often employed to increase these numbers. Mobilization strategies include (1) administration of chemotherapy in autologous patients only (eg, cyclophosphamide 2–4 grams/m^2 with or without etoposide) with granulocyte colony-stimulating factor (G-CSF; eg, filgrastim 5 mcg/ kg subcutaneously [SC] daily); (2) salvage regimens in autologous patients only (eg, ICE [ifosfamide, carboplatin, etoposide] or ESHAP [etoposide, methylprednisolone, cytarabine, cisplatin]) with collection of cells at the time of marrow

Table 8-4 Common Toxicities in HSCT[a,4]

Drug	Dose-Limiting Toxicities and Other Significant Toxicities[b]	Additional Comments
Busulfan	SOS/VOD (E), seizures (E), pulmonary fibrosis (L), mucositis (E), secondary malignancies (L)	Antiseizure prophylaxis (commonly phenytoin, lorazepam, or levetiracetam) given to all patients during busulfan administration
Carboplatin	Nephrotoxicity (E), elevated liver function tests (E)	
Carmustine	Pulmonary fibrosis (L), SOS/VOD (E), secondary malignancies (L)	
Cyclophosphamide	Hemorrhagic cystitis (E), pericarditis and other cardiac abnormalities (E), secondary malignancies (L)	Mesna often used since very high doses given; aggressive hydration can be given
Cytarabine	Neurotoxicity (E)	
Etoposide	Mucositis (E), neuropathy (E), hypotension during infusion (E), secondary malignancies (L)	Given with IVFs as a high-infusion rate
Fludarabine	Neurotoxicity (E), prolonged immunosuppression (E/L)	Monitor renal function during administration
Melphalan	Mucositis (E), secondary malignancies (L)	Ice chips can reduce mucositis
Total body irradiation	Pulmonary toxicity (E/L), SOS/VOD (E), mucositis (E), neurologic sequelae (L), endocrine dysfunction (L), growth impairment (L), cardiotoxicity (E/L), cataracts (L), secondary malignancies (L)	

[a] In addition to bone marrow suppression.
[b] E indicates early toxicity; L indicates late toxicity.
IVF, intravenous fluids; SOS/VOD, sinusoidal obstruction syndrome/veno-occlusive disease.

recovery; or (3) administration of filgrastim, either alone (typical doses of 10–16 mcg/kg twice daily for autologous patients and 10 mcg/kg/day for healthy allogeneic donors) or combined with the chemokine receptor 4 antagonist plerixafor.[15] Filgrastim is usually started 4 days before apheresis and continued until apheresis is complete. Filgrastim acts by increasing marrow production of HSCs and is universally used in the mobilization of HSCs from both autologous patients and allogeneic donors.[13–15] Inclusion of plerixafor in the mobilization regimen is a newer approach for autologous patients; plerixafor acts by enhancing the release of HSCs from the marrow space (refer to **Clinical Pearl 8-2**). Plerixafor is mainly used with filgrastim, and emerging evidence suggests that it may be safe and effective following chemotherapy mobilization as well.[15,16] Plerixafor is indicated for use in patients with multiple myeloma and non-Hodgkin's lymphoma.[17] It is administered subcutaneously the evening before apheresis and is continued daily until the target number of cells is collected for a maximum of 4 doses.[18] Plerixafor is usually well tolerated. Some adverse effects include injection site pain, erythema, nausea, and diarrhea. The manufacturer recommends administering plerixafor approximately 11 hours before apheresis, which means patients may need to return to the clinic at approximately 10:00 pm each evening for plerixafor. In an effort to improve patient convenience, alternative dosing schedules are being investigated, including 6:00 pm administration times or intravenous (IV) administration in the morning prior to beginning apheresis.[4,19]

CLINICAL PEARL 8-2

Due to the high cost of plerixafor, many transplant centers try to target its use for patients who are most likely to benefit from it. This includes patients who have failed a prior mobilization attempt or patients who may be expected to be a poor mobilizer. Risk factors for poor mobilization include: older age, non-Hodgkin's lymphoma diagnosis (vs multiple myeloma), prior lenalidomide therapy, multiple cycles of chemotherapy (ie, 3 or more prior regimens; 12 or more cycles), and prior radiation to the spine or pelvis.[12]

Infusion of HSCs

HSCs are administered via an IV infusion. Infusion of fresh HSC product (ie, an allogeneic product), is similar to administration of a red blood cell transfusion.[4]

If the donor and recipient (patient) are ABO blood type compatible, premedications are generally not required. If the donor and patient are ABO-incompatible the HSC product should be manipulated to remove as many red cells as possible, and the patient may be given premedications to minimize the risk of an infusion reaction. Infusion of allogeneic/fresh HSCs is generally well tolerated. Side effects are similar to those observed with blood transfusions and may include fevers, mild allergic reactions, or more seriously, hemolysis, pulmonary toxicity (transfusion-related acute lung injury), or severe allergic reactions.[4,20]

If a frozen HSC product is to be administered (usually autologous or umbilical cord blood [UCB] products), then prehydration and administration of premedications is indicated. These products contain dimethyl sulfoxide (DMSO), which is added to stabilize the cells during cryopreservation and will be infused into the patient as part of the HSC infusion (refer to **Clinical Pearl 8-3**). Typical premedications may include diphenhydramine, mannitol, and hydrocortisone (**Table 8-5**). In addition to transfusion reactions that can be seen with

CLINICAL PEARL 8-3

DMSO has a strong, foul-smelling odor that is noticeable immediately after starting the hematopoietic stem cell infusion and can linger for a few days. Some patients complain of nausea or a bad taste in their mouth. Approaches to minimize these adverse effects include the use of peppermint oil in the patient's room to mask the odor or having the patient suck on peppermint candies to improve the taste. Antiemetics may be used for nausea associated with DMSO.

Table 8-5 Hematopoietic Stem Cell Infusion Guidelines–Shands Hospital/University of Florida

Hydration	0.9% NaCl[a] @ 2 mL/kg/hour, beginning 12 hours prior to HSC infusion and continuing for 12 hours following HSC infusion.
Premedication	Diphenhydramine 25-50 mg IV Hydrocortisone 250 mg IV Mannitol 25% 50 mL IV

[a] Electrolytes may be added.

fresh HSC products, infusion of cryopreserved HSCs may be associated with DMSO-associated side effects, which can include itching, rash, flushing, fever, and anaphylactoid reactions.[4,20] The patient is closely monitored during the HSC infusion. The nurse stays with the patient throughout the entire procedure, frequently monitoring vital signs and any adverse effects. Emergency medications such as hydrocortisone, epinephrine, and diphenhydramine should be readily available in the event an anaphylactic reaction occurs.

SUPPORTIVE CARE AND TRANSPLANT-RELATED COMPLICATIONS

Chemotherapy-Induced Nausea and Vomiting

The approach to the prevention and management of nausea and vomiting is similar to that used for patients receiving standard doses of chemotherapy. Because the doses used in the HSCT setting can be significantly higher, most myeloablative conditioning regimens are considered highly emetogenic, and patients are at risk for more severe and/or more prolonged chemotherapy-induced nausea and vomiting (CINV).[4] Guidelines, such as those produced by the National Comprehensive Cancer Network (NCCN), American Society of Clinical Oncology (ASCO), and Multinational Association of Supportive Care in Cancer (MASCC), have extensive recommendations for prophylaxis and treatment of CINV in patients receiving standard-dose therapy. Little guidance exists, however, for prevention of CINV due to high-dose chemotherapy. Due to either practical concerns or a lack of data, agents that are recommended for highly emetogenic standard-dose chemotherapy regimens may not be appropriate in transplant patients, particularly for allogeneic HSCT recipients (refer to **Clinical Pearl 8-4** and **Case 8-1**).

In the HSCT setting, a 5-HT$_3$ antagonist generally should be used for CINV prophylaxis during the conditioning therapy because most myeloablative regimens used are moderately to highly emetogenic. Corticosteroids may be used especially for agents that cause delayed nausea and vomiting; however, some concern exists about using corticosteroids in allogeneic transplant recipients because of their lympholytic actions. While many centers may administer corticosteroids during chemotherapy administration for prevention of nausea and vomiting before the stem cell infusion, these agents should generally be avoided for treatment of delayed or breakthrough CINV early in the posttransplant setting to preserve the potential graft-versus-tumor effects of the donor cells.[4] Because of potential drug–drug interactions, neurokinin-1 (NK-1) antagonists (eg, aprepitant, fosaprepitant) should be used with caution in the HSCT setting. Aprepitant is a substrate for various cytochrome P450 (CYP) enzymes and is a moderate inhibitor of CYP3A4. Medications used during HSCT may potentially interact with aprepitant, including cyclophosphamide, busulfan, etoposide, thiotepa, azole antifungals, tacrolimus, and dexamethasone.[4] A few small trials have demonstrated the safety of aprepitant in various HSCT patient populations; however, more evidence is needed before aprepitant can be widely used in this setting.[21]

CLINICAL PEARL 8-4

There is no consensus currently concerning with which conditioning regimens or patients to use aprepitant or fosaprepitant. Several centers are using aprepitant or fosaprepitant with melphalan-containing regimens for autologous transplant patients (some centers routinely do so while others only use it in patients with history of poor nausea/vomiting control). Use of aprepitant/fosaprepitant with other high-dose chemotherapy regimens is institution-specific or is used on a case-by-case basis.

The American Society of Clinical Oncology (ASCO) specifically addresses high-dose chemotherapy with stem cell transplant in its guidelines and recommends use of a 5-HT3 antagonist with dexamethasone; aprepitant should be considered, although evidence to support its use is lacking in this patient population.

CASE 8-1
Chemotherapy-Induced Nausea and Vomiting

SN is a 67-year-old female diagnosed with multiple myeloma. She is admitted for melphalan 200 mg/m^2 IV on day -2 followed by autologous stem cell rescue. With prior chemotherapy and prior pregnancies, she did experience significant nausea. She tells you she is anxious about receiving chemotherapy because she remembered how miserable she was with her prior therapies.

1. What risk factors does this patient have for chemotherapy-induced nausea and vomiting?
2. What would you recommend for antiemetic prophylaxis for this patient?
3. What is the concern with using aprepitant concomitantly with high-dose chemotherapy, such as that used in hematopoietic stem cell transplant (HSCT)?

SN has some nausea acutely after receiving melphalan, which is mild and self-limiting. However; about 4 days after completing melphalan therapy, she begins to complain of dry heaves and persistent nausea. She has been getting promethazine as needed with some relief.

4. What would you recommend at this time for treating SN's nausea and vomiting?

Cytopenias

The depth and duration of cytopenias depend on the intensity of the conditioning regimen and the agents used, as well as the type of HSCT and graft source.[4] Patients who receive PBSCs will generally have earlier engrafment of stem cells than patients who receive stem cells obtained from the bone marrow. After receiving a myeloablative regimen, the patient is at significant risk for various hematologic deficiencies. Red blood cell and platelet transfusions may be needed until engraftment (the recovery of hematopoiesis) occurs.

Neutrophils recover before platelets in most patients and myeloid engraftment can take between 2 and 4 weeks to occur. Patients undergoing a UCB transplant may have delayed neutrophil engraftment (often longer than 21 days) due to the small amount of stem cells available in the cord.[5] Lymphoid repopulation occurs more slowly; even after lymphocytes recover, these cells have impaired function for more than a year after transplant, especially if the patient has received agents such as fludarabine, antithymocyte globulin, alemtuzumab, a T-cell depleted graft, or if the patient develops graft-versus-host disease (GVHD). Patients are at significant risk of infections during this time. To reduce the risk of infection, most patients will receive antimicrobial prophylaxis at some point during the transplant procedure (further discussed in the *Infection in HSCT Patients* section in this chapter).[4] G-CSFs, such as filgrastim, are often used after transplantation to shorten the time to engraftment, particularly in autologous HSCT patients.

G-CSFs are also often used in many patients undergoing haploidentical (half-matched related donor) and UCB stem cell transplant to reduce the incidence of graft failure.[4] Filgrastim is usually administered at standard doses beginning around 5 to 7 days after HSCT infusion and continued until engraftment of stem cells has occurred. While filgrastim is the most widely used growth factor post-transplantation, sargramostim (GM-CSF) and pegfilgrastim have also been used.

Graft-Versus-Host Disease

Immunocompetent donor T-cells recognize the host (HSC recipient) as foreign, which triggers a complex immune response, referred to as graft-versus-host disease (GVHD).[4,22] GVHD is one of the most serious complications of allogeneic transplant and accounts for a significant proportion of transplant-related morbidity and mortality. GVHD is typically classified as either acute or chronic. Historically, symptoms occurring in the first 100 days posttransplantation were classified as acute GVHD, and symptoms occurring after day +100 were classified as chronic GVHD. However, recently, it has become apparent that it is more accurate to classify GVHD based on presenting signs and symptoms.[22,23]

Acute GVHD results from a complex immune reaction between donor T-cells and host tissues that develops in 3 phases.[4,22–24] First, the conditioning regimen can cause tissue damage to the host/recipient, and these damaged tissues then secrete proinflammatory cytokines, such as interleukin-1 and tumor necrosis factor alpha (TNF-α). Second, donor T-cells recognize the host tissue as foreign, resulting in T-cell activation and proliferation. In the third phase, these activated T-cells produce various inflammatory cytokines (particularly TNF-α) that can interact synergistically with cytotoxic T-lymphocytes involving a complex inflammatory cascade, resulting in amplification of local tissue injury and target organ dysfunction of the host.

Acute GVHD primarily involves the following 3 organ systems: skin, liver, and gastrointestinal (GI) tract. GVHD is often a clinical diagnosis, although biopsy of the affected organ(s) can aid in the diagnosis.[4,5] Skin is the most common organ affected by GVHD and is often the first clinical manifestation. Skin GVHD often coincides with donor cell engraftment and usually presents as an erythematous maculopapular rash. The GI tract is the second most common organ involved in acute GVHD. Signs and symptoms of gut GVHD, such as nausea/vomiting, abdominal cramps, and profuse diarrhea may be difficult to distinguish from those of chemotherapy or radiation toxicity, although GVHD manifestations often occur later. GVHD of the liver is less common; it often manifests as hyperbilirubinemia and/or cholestatic jaundice and elevated alkaline phosphatase. It is often difficult to differentiate liver GVHD from other causes of liver dysfunction.

Acute GVHD is staged according to a clinical grading scale in which each organ system is staged based on the severity of organ involvement.[4,5,22] These stages are combined to determine the overall grade of GVHD. Grade I GVHD is considered mild disease, and grade IV GVHD is life threatening (**Tables 8-6 and 8-7**).

Table 8-6 Clinical Staging of Acute GVHD[45]

Stage	Skin	Liver (Serum Bilirubin Level)	GI Tract (Diarrhea)
1	Rash < 25% of BSA	2–2.9 mg/dL	500–1000 mL/day
2	Rash 25%–50% of BSA	3–6 mg/dL	1000–1500 mL/day
3	Rash > 50% of BSA	6.1–15 mg/dL	1500–2000 mL/day
4	Generalized erythroderma with bullae formation	> 15 mg/dL	> 2000 mL/day or severe abdominal pain ± ileus

Table 8-7 Clinical Grading of Acute GVHD[22]

Grade	Stage
0 (none)	No skin, liver, or gut involvement No functional impairment
I (mild)	Stage 1–2 skin involvement No liver or gut involvement No functional impairment
II (moderate)	Stage 1–3 skin involvement Stage 1 liver and/or stage 1 gut involvement Mild functional impairment
III (severe)	Stage 2–3 skin involvement Stage 2–3 liver and/or gut involvement Moderate functional impairment
IV (life-threatening)	Stage 1–4 skin involvement Stage 2–4 liver and/or gut involvement Severe functional impairment

Prevention of Acute GVHD

For allogeneic stem cell transplant, GVHD prophylaxis is given to all patients (except for syngeneic transplant patients) at the time of transplantation. Despite advances in GHVD prophylaxis, grade II to IV acute GVHD still occurs in approximately 35%-50% of transplant recipients. Since donor T-cell activation is central to the pathophysiology of GVHD, most of the therapies used for prophylaxis are directed at inhibiting T-cell activation and proliferation. T-cell depletion and pharmacologic prophylaxis are the 2 main approaches for GVHD prophylaxis.[4,5,24]

Pharmacologic Prophylaxis of Acute GVHD

Low-dose methotrexate was the first agent used for GVHD prophylaxis. Methotrexate is an antimetabolite cytotoxic agent that inhibits purine synthesis (by inhibiting the enzyme dihydrofolate reductase) in T-cells and subsequently prevents donor T-cell expansion. Cyclosporine is a calcineurin inhibitor (CNI) that inhibits interleukin-2 (IL-2) mediated T-cell expansion. The combination of methotrexate and cyclosporine was shown to be more effective than either cyclosporine or methotrexate alone, and this combination has been considered the standard GVHD prophylaxis regimen for many years.[4,22]

Tacrolimus is a newer CNI that has largely replaced cyclosporine as a mainstay of GVHD prophylaxis, primarily due to its favorable toxicity profile. Newer immunosuppressive agents, such as sirolimus and mycophenolate mofetil, appear to have activity in the treatment of acute GVHD and are being incorporated into prophylaxis regimens in many centers.[24–26] Sirolimus inhibits T-cell activation and proliferation by binding to FK binding proteins, inhibiting mammalian target of rapamycin (mTOR), and may inhibit dendritic cells important in mediating GVHD. Mycophenolate mofetil is a prodrug of mycophenolic acid, which is a selective reversible inhibitor of inosine monophosphate dehydrogenase. Inhibition of this enzyme results in inhibition of de novo synthesis of guanosine nucleotide synthesis and ultimately blocks T-cell proliferation. For myeloablative regimens, the standard is to use more than one agent for GVHD prophylaxis. Some common combinations for GVHD prophylaxis include CNI/methotrexate, mycophenolate mofetil/CNI, and sirolimus/tacrolimus +/- methotrexate, although many combinations are being evaluated. While methotrexate is administered following HSC infusion, other immunosuppressive agents (CNIs, mycophenolate, sirolimus) are usually started 1–3 days before HSC infusion.

Corticosteroids, which are the mainstay for treatment of GVHD, have little role in GHVD prophylaxis, although they may sometimes be used at approximately 1 mg/kg/day of methylprednisolone or its equivalent when the standard GVHD prophylactic agents need to be held (eg, toxicity). As mentioned previously, corticosteroids should be discouraged or used sparingly due to their lymphotoxic effects to the donor graft.

Haploidentical transplantation presents some unique challenges compared with other types of transplantation. Historically, the incidence of severe, fatal acute GVHD has been very high due to the presence of alloreactive T-cells. Recent approaches to GVHD prophylaxis in this patient population differ from what was described previously. Administration of high-dose cyclophosphamide in the early posttransplant period followed by tacrolimus and mycophenolate mofetil has enabled successful haploidentical transplantation with rates of acute GVHD that are comparable to those seen in patients undergoing transplant from a matched sibling donor.[27]

Despite recent additions to the immunosuppression arsenal, acute GVHD remains a major clinical problem in patients undergoing allogeneic HSCT, and clinical trials are ongoing in an attempt to find the optimal GVHD prophylaxis regimen. **Tables 8-8** and **8-9** list common dosing recommendations, monitoring parameters, toxicity profiles, and clinical pearls for agents that are commonly used to prevent GVHD.

Following engraftment, and in the absence of active GVHD, the goal is to wean GVHD prophylaxis agents until patients are off all immunosuppressive agents. For example, tacrolimus can begin to be tapered at approximately 3 months posttransplant with a goal of tapering off tacrolimus by 6 months posttransplant. Unfortunately, it is common for GVHD symptoms to flare during the immunosuppression taper, necessitating continued GVHD therapy.

GVHD Treatment

Once acute GVHD is diagnosed, it should be treated aggressively in most cases. For mild grade I GVHD involving only the skin, no systemic therapy may be required, as this frequently resolves on its own. Development of mild GVHD is often desirable in patients undergoing HSCT for a malignancy (ie, leukemia), because patients who develop GVHD tend to have lower relapse rates compared with patients who do not develop GVHD. This is thought to be due to the antitumor effects of the graft, known as GVT effect. Progression of GVHD beyond grade I or mild disease, however, requires immediate treatment.[4,22,28]

Table 8-8 Common Drugs Used for Acute GVHD Prophylaxis[4,25,26]

Drug	Common Adult Dosage	Metabolism and Excretion	Common Therapeutic Range	Toxicity
Cyclosporine (Gengraf, Neoral, Sandimmune)	• IV: 1.5–2.5 mg/kg every 12 hours • Oral: **Caution**—different preparations with different dosages and conversions. For example: 1:4 for Sandimmune IV: PO, and 1:1–3 for Neoral/micronized or modified IV: PO • Usually starts day -3 to day -1 and is continued at therapeutic levels until ~ day +100 and tapered off by day +180 in the absence of GVHD	• CYP3A4 metabolism in liver and gut wall • Biliary excretion	Trough: 200–400 ng/mL by immunoassay (may be lower if LC-MS assay used, since it does not measure metabolites; for example 150–350 ng/mL)	• Common: hypertension, tremors, nephrotoxicity, hypomagnesemia, hyperkalemia, hirsutism, hyperlipidemia • Uncommon: flushing and painful paresthesias with IV, gingival hyperplasia, seizures, blindness, posterior leukoencephalopathy, thrombotic microangiopathy
Tacrolimus (Prograf)	• IV: 0.02–0.05 mg/kg/day by continuous infusion • PO: 2–4 times IV dose (divided every 12 hours) • Initiation and duration same as for cyclosporine	Same as for cyclosporine	Trough: 5–15 ng/mL	Same as for cyclosporine, but often milder, without hirsutism or gingival hyperplasia
Methotrexate	• Full: 15 mg/m² IV day +1, then 10 mg/m² on days +3, +6, +11 • Mini: 5 mg/m² IV days +1, +3, +6, +11.	• Hepatic and intracellular metabolism • Renal excretion	N/A	• Mucositis • Engraftment delay • Hepatic SOS/VOD

Drug	Dosing/Administration	Metabolism	Therapeutic Level	Toxicities
Sirolimus (Rapamune)	• 6–12 mg PO × 1 loading dose, then 2–4 mg PO once daily • Initiation usually on day -3 • Duration similar to cyclosporine/tacrolimus	CYP450 hepatic metabolism	Trough: 3–12 ng/mL	• Significant hyperlipidemia • ↑ risk of SOS/VOD with myeloablative regimens • Thrombotic microangiopathy • Interstitial lung disease • Possible renal toxicity
Mycophenolate mofetil (CellCept, Myfortic [delayed release])	• 15 mg/kg (actual weight) up to 1000 mg BID to TID (IV and PO dose same for CellCept) • Initiation usually on day -3 • Duration varies with combination/type of HSCT • Myfortic is the delayed-release formulation of mycophenolate. It has FDA approval for allogeneic renal transplant and is not commonly prescribed for allogeneic HSCT.	• Hepatic activation and metabolism • Renal excretion (doses may need to be adjusted for renal impairment)	Limited data to monitor MPA concentrations in HSCT	• GI (nausea, vomiting, diarrhea) symptoms may be indistinguishable from GVHD symptoms • Mild bone marrow suppression

BID, two times daily; CYP, cytochrome; GI, gastrointestinal; FDA, Food and Drug Administration; GVHD, graft-versus-host-disease; HSCT, hematopoietic stem cell transplantation; IV, intravenous; MPA, mycophenolate acid; N/A, not applicable; PO, oral; SOS, sinusoidal obstruction syndrome; TID, three times daily; VOD, venoocclusive disease.

Table 8-9 Clinical Pearls for Immunosuppressive Therapy in HSCT[4,25,26]

Drug	Clinical Pearls	Drug Interactions
Cyclosporine	• Higher and more predictable oral bioavailability with modified oral suspension products (ie, Gengraf or Neoral vs Sandimmune) • Oral suspension should not be administered in polystyrene foam or paper cups • Keep oral capsules in unit-dose foil until ready to take • Hypertension often responds well to dihydropyridine calcium channel blockers, such as amlodipine • May need dose adjustments in hepatic dysfunction • Although not renally cleared, commonly can produce nephrotoxicity • Troughs should not be drawn from same lumen into which drug is infusing; if line contamination occurs, draw samples from peripheral vein • Check troughs every 3–4 days until stable serum concentrations	• CYP 3A4 inducers and inhibitors • May need to adjust dose Examples: • Azoles: decrease dose by 50% when starting voriconazole or by 25%–30% when starting posaconazole • Sirolimus: Administer 4 hours after cyclosporine and keep cyclosporine levels ≤ 200 ng/mL to avoid risk of sirolimus toxicity • Drugs with additive nephrotoxicity
Tacrolimus (Prograf)	• Hypertension often responds well to dihydropyridine calcium channel blockers, such as amlodipine • May need dose adjustments in hepatic dysfunction • Although not renally cleared, commonly can produce nephrotoxicity • If patient on IV, levels can be drawn anytime; do not draw from same lumen into which drug is infusing; if line contamination occurs, draw samples from peripheral vein • Check troughs every 2–3 days until stable	• Similar to cyclosporine • Note: decrease dose of tacrolimus by 50%–67% when starting voriconazole or posaconazole • Keep tacrolimus concentrations ≤ 10 ng/mL when using sirolimus to avoid additive toxicity

Methotrexate	• Start methotrexate approximately 24 hours after stem cell infusion complete • Folinic acid (leucovorin) rescue should be given to patients with severe mucositis or patients with pleural effusions/third spacing to prevent excess toxicity (some centers may give low doses of folinic acid to all patients) • Day +11 methotrexate may be held if severe toxicity occurs; omitting this dose, however, may increase the risk for GVHD	Drugs with additive renal toxicity
Sirolimus (Rapamune)	• Oral suspension should not be administered in polystyrene foam or paper cups • Long half-life (62 hours)—wait 3–4 days to check troughs after loading dose, and check weekly after dosing adjustments	• CYP3A4 inducers/inhibitors • Manufacturer states sirolimus contraindicated with voriconazole or posaconazole • Voriconazole can be used if sirolimus dose is decrease by 90% (ie, weekly dosing) • Target lower tacrolimus or cyclosporine levels due to increased risk of thrombotic microangiopathy
Mycophenolate mofetil	• IV formulation may decrease GI side effects but will not eliminate them • Manufacturer recommendations are to take on empty stomach; may give with light snack to mitigate GI side effects—educate patients on need for consistency	• Cholestyramine • Magnesium and aluminum salts—separate administration

CYP, cytochrome P450; GI, gastrointestinal; GVHD, graft-versus-host-disease; IV, intravenous.

Topical or local corticosteroid therapies may be considered alone in low-grade GVHD of the skin and/or GI tract, or in addition to systemic corticosteroids in moderate to severe GVHD disease. Triamcinolone 0.1% cream/ointment or other intermediate-high potency topical corticosteroid cream can be applied to the affected areas 3 times daily. Hydrocortisone 0.1% cream/ointment or other low-potency topical corticosteroid is applied to more sensitive facial or groin lesions. Topical CNIs (eg, tacrolimus and pimecrolimus) are often used for the treatment of cutaneous GVHD. Oral nonabsorbed steroids such as budesonide (3 mg orally twice or 3 times daily) for lower GI symptoms and beclomethasone (1 mg orally 4 times daily) for upper GI symptoms have efficacy in mild to moderate gut GVHD. These agents may be continued long-term, but sometimes can be held or tapered as GVHD signs and symptoms resolve and may be reinstituted if necessary.[4,22,28]

Systemic corticosteroids are the first-line treatment for significant (grade II or higher) GVHD.[4,22,24,28–30] Corticosteroids inhibit donor lymphocytes and rapidly block the inflammatory cytokine cascade involved in GHVD. The usual starting dose is methylprednisolone 1–2 mg/kg/day IV or an equivalent corticosteroid (eg, prednisone) if the patient is able to take oral medications, (see **Clinical Pearl 8-5**). Higher doses of corticosteroids have failed to show any additional benefit and can lead to added toxicity. For patients who develop GVHD while receiving GVHD prophylaxis, corticosteroids should be added to the current regimen. If the patient develops clinically significant GVHD after immunosuppression has been tapered off, a CNI may be added in addition to corticosteroids. Systemic corticosteroids should be continued for at least 7 days after a complete response followed by a progressive taper. The pace of the corticosteroid taper should be dictated by the patient's clinical response and by the toxicity of the regimen; a typical taper rate may consist of a 10%–25% reduction in the corticosteroid dose per week. If the patient's GVHD symptoms flare after a taper, the taper should be interrupted until the symptoms abate; the dose of the corticosteroid may stay the same or be increased, depending on the severity of

CLINICAL PEARL 8-5

The dose of prednisone is 1.25 times the dose of methylprednisolone and the differences in potency need to be taken into account when prescribing corticosteroids for the treatment of GVHD.

symptoms. However, in patients who develop an opportunistic infection, a more rapid taper should be considered.

Corticosteroids can produce a number of serious side effects, especially when used for long periods of time. Some immediate effects of corticosteroids include insomnia, emotional lability, hypertension, and hyperglycemia. Effects of long-term corticosteroid use include cushingoid effects, myopathies, osteoporosis, avascular necrosis of the hip, and increased susceptibility to various infections. For patients who cannot tolerate steroids, an alternative steroid-sparing immuno-suppressive agent can be initiated to allow for a more rapid corticosteroid withdrawal. For patients in whom steroids are contraindicated, alternative immuno-suppressive therapy such as those used in the treatment of steroid-refractory GVHD may be given.

Steroid Refractory GVHD

While up to half of patients will respond to single-agent corticosteroids, fewer than half of these will have a durable remission. The pace of response varies depending on the organs involved; cutaneous GVHD typically responds more quickly than liver or GI GVHD. No established consensus exists on the defini-tion of steroid-refractory GVHD. It has commonly been defined as progression of GVHD after 3 days of systemic therapy, no change after 7 days of systemic therapy, or an incomplete response after 2 weeks of high-dose corticosteroids.[29,30]

Steroid-refractory GVHD has a very poor outcome, and no clear standard or consensus exists for second-line or salvage treatment. Many agents used as sec-ond-line therapy are the same as those used for GVHD prophylaxis, such as siro-limus or mycophenolate mofetil. A recent clinical trial comparing mycophenolate mofetil to placebo in the treatment of acute GVHD was closed early when the interim analysis showed no benefit from the addition of mycophenolate mofetil. Sirolimus shows promise and is currently under investigation as primary therapy of steroid-refractory acute GVHD. Antithymocyte globulin is commonly used; although its use is limited by the risk of severe opportunistic infections. A variety of doses and schedules are used for antithymocyte globulin. One common regi-men is equine/horse antithymocyte globulin 20 mg/kg IV daily for 5 days. Infu-sion-related reactions are common, and premedications with diphenhydramine, acetaminophen, and hydrocortisone or methylprednisolone are required. While a number of biologically active therapies targeting T-cells and TNF-α have been evaluated for the treatment of steroid-refractory acute GVHD, none have been demonstrated to be clearly effective, and none are considered first-line therapy.

Phototherapy with extracorporeal photopheresis or psoralen and ultraviolet A irradiation (PUVA), while typically used as a treatment for chronic GVHD, has been used in some centers as an adjunctive steroid-sparing treatment for acute GVHD. These techniques expose peripheral blood mononuclear cells to ultraviolet light *ex vivo* through apheresis and appear to have benefit, especially in skin GVHD. Steroid-refractory GVHD remains a significant clinical problem for allogeneic HSCT recipients, and investigation continues in an effort to identify consistently effective therapies.[29–31]

Supportive Care for Acute GVHD

In addition to immunosuppressive therapy, supportive care measures are a critical component of treatment of GVHD.[4,22,24,30] Organ-specific measures include topical therapy and wound care for patients with severe skin involvement. Bowel rest and intravenous hyperalimentation may be needed for patients with severe gut GVHD. Antimotility agents, such as loperamide and/or diphenoxylate with atropine can be used, and octreotide or other somatostatin analogs may be of some benefit when antimotility drugs are ineffective. Octreotide, when used, may be continued until GI symptoms resolve or should be stopped if an ileus forms. Doses are variable and often start at 50 mcg to 100 mcg IV or SC every 8 hours and titrated upwards until response is seen, often up to 500 mcg every 8 hours. It has also been given as a continuous IV infusion. For patients with hepatic GVHD, ursodiol has been used as a supportive care measure, and it is important to avoid hepatotoxins if possible in these patients. The dose and duration of ursodiol varies and it is continued until liver function tests normalize. Other general supportive care measures include pain control, judiciously monitoring for infections, and providing infection prophylaxis.

Chronic GVHD

Chronic GVHD is a major cause of nonrelapse morbidity and mortality after allogeneic HSCT. It is associated with impaired organ function, increased susceptibility to infection, and decreased quality of life.[4,5,32] On the other hand, chronic GVHD is also associated with beneficial GVT effects. Patients who develop chronic GVHD have lower rates of disease relapse than patients without GVHD.

The pathogenesis of chronic GVHD is less well understood compared to acute GVHD. Chronic GVHD seems to be a complex multisystem alloimmune and autoimmune disorder characterized by immune dysregulation, immunodeficiency, and impaired organ function.[4,5,32] As in acute GVHD, alloreactive donor

T-cells have an important role in the pathogenesis. In chronic GVHD; however, the donor T-cells fail to become tolerant to the host. In addition, it is thought that disruption of thymic function can lead to immune dysregulation. Peripheral tissue damage due to previous acute GVHD or inflammation may also lead to auto-antigen development.

Any organ can be affected in chronic GVHD; however, the most common sites of involvement include skin, liver, mouth, and eyes.[4,32,33] Chronic GVHD may manifest in only one organ system, but most often multiple organ sites are involved. Signs and symptoms may range from inflammatory and acute-type manifestations to more fibrotic and chronic manifestations. **Table 8-10** provides a listing of organs involved in chronic GVHD and options for intervention.

The diagnosis of chronic GVHD is based on specific signs, the degree of organ involvement, and additional laboratory or histopathologic confirmation rather than the time of onset after transplant. Historically, the classification of GVHD was simply either limited or extensive. Consensus criteria for the diagnosis and staging of chronic GVHD proposed by the National Institutes of Health (NIH) are available and are widely used in practice.[32] (**Case 8-2**)

Treatment of Chronic GVHD

Multiple approaches have been tried to prevent chronic GVHD with little success. Since acute GVHD is a significant risk factor for chronic GVHD, the most effective prevention of chronic GVHD may be to minimize acute GVHD. Agents used to treat chronic GVHD are similar to those used in acute GVHD treatment. The prior use of prophylactic and treatment agents for acute GVHD in each patient will dictate the choice of treatment for chronic GVHD, as will patient characteristics and the institution's or physicians' preferences. Systemic therapy is indicated in patients with moderate to severe chronic GVHD. Mild GHVD may be monitored without pharmacologic therapy or may be treated with supportive care measures, as necessary.

Corticosteroids are generally considered first-line therapy for chronic GVHD, often at a dose of 1 mg/kg/day of prednisone (or its equivalent).[32–36] Inclusion of CNIs may allow for more rapid tapering of the corticosteroid dose, thus minimizing the long-term effects associated with chronic corticosteroid therapy. Often, patients with chronic GVHD do not tolerate the same doses or serum concentrations that are used in patients with acute GVHD, and the serum concentrations of CNIs may be maintained at the lower end of the therapeutic range. If a patient's clinical manifestations improve with therapy, prednisone can start to be tapered after 1-2 weeks. Prednisone doses for chronic GVHD are generally

Table 8-10 Clinical Manifestations of Chronic Graft-Versus-Host-Disease, Ancillary and Supportive Care Interventions[4,32,33]

Organ	Examples of Clinical Manifestations	Examples of Organ-Specific Interventions
Skin and appendages	Erythematous papular rash (lichenoid) or thick, tight, fragile skin (sclerodermatous), photosensitivity	Photoprotection (sunscreen SPF ≥ 20, avoidance of sun, and protective clothing), monitor for malignancy, range-of-motion exercises For intact skin: topical emollients (ointments or creams), corticosteroids (triamcinolone 0.1% or hydrocortisone 1% for face, groin, axilla), antipruritic agents, topical calcineurin inhibitors (tacrolimus, pimecrolimus), PUVA, treatment of local infections For erosions/ulcerations: topical antimicrobials and monitoring cultures with treatment as necessary, protective films/dressings, wound care consultation, debridement, hyperbaric oxygen
Mouth/oral cavity	Dryness, sensitivity, white plaques (lichenoid planus), ulcerations, mucosal scleroderma	Maintain good oral hygiene with routine cleanings and endocarditis prophylaxis; surveillance of infections and malignancy Topical corticosteroids (fluocinonide gel 0.05%, triamcinolone 0.1%, dexamethasone 0.05 mg/5 mL) and analgesics (lidocaine-based rinses) Fluoride, saliva substitutes, pilocarpine, sugar-free gum for dry mouth
Eyes	Dryness, burning, photophobia, corneal abrasion/ulceration, conjunctivitis, uveitis	Photoprotection, regular ophthalmologic exams Preservative-free artificial tears and ocular ointments, topical steroids or cyclosporine drops, occlusive eye wear, humidified environment, moisture chamber glasses, pilocarpine, surgical (punctual occlusion, tarsorrhaphy), and rarely, gas-permeable scleral contacts and autologous serum eye drops
Vulva and vagina	Lichen planus-like features, vaginal stenosis, dryness, vulvar irritation	Monitor for estrogen deficiency, infection, and malignancy Water-based lubricants, topical estrogens, topical steroids, topical tacrolimus, dilators for vaginal symptoms

Musculoskeletal system	Fasciitis, polymyositis, osteoporosis, joint stiffness	Monitoring range of motion, bone mineral density, calcium and vitamin D levels Physical therapy, calcium and vitamin D supplementation, bisphosphonates
GI tract and liver	Esophageal webs, esophagitis, stenosis/strictures, abnormal motility, malabsorption, diarrhea, anorexia, cholestasis	Surveillance for infection Dietary modification, gastroesophageal reflux management, esophageal dilation, enzyme supplementation for malabsorption, pancreatic enzyme replacement for insufficiency, ursodiol
Lungs	Bronchiolitis obliterans symptoms: dyspnea, wheezing, cough, respiratory failure	Eliminate other etiologies (ie, infections), monitor pulmonary function tests Inhaled corticosteroids, bronchodilators, azithromycin, montelukast, supplementary oxygen, pulmonary rehabilitation, and consideration of lung transplant in appropriate candidates
Neurologic	Neuropathies and myopathies	Monitor calcineurin drug concentrations along with blood pressure control and electrolyte replacements, and seizure prophylaxis if necessary Occupational and physical therapy and treatment of neuropathies (ie, tricyclic antidepressants or anticonvulsants)
Hematologic	Cytopenias (especially thrombocytopenia), eosinophilia	Eliminate other etiologies Growth factors, immunoglobulins if severe
Immunologic	Profound immunodeficiency Functional asplenia Variable IgG levels High risk for pneumococcal, pneumocystis, and invasive fungal infections	Monitor for bacterial, viral, fungal, and atypical infections Immunizations 6–12 months after transplant in the absence of severe GVHD and prophylaxis against *Pneumocystis jiroveci*, varicella zoster, and encapsulated bacteria Consider immunoglobulin replacement based on levels and recurrent infections

GI, gastrointestinal; IgG, immunoglobulin G; PUVA, psoralen and ultraviolet A irradiation; SPF, sun protection factor.

CASE 8-2
Graft-Versus-Host Disease

JD is a 34-year-old male (80 kg) with acute lymphocytic leukemia (ALL) in first remission who received a myeloablative (cyclophosphamide/total body irradiation) allogeneic HSCT from a related donor, his sister, who is a 49-year-old female who has 2 children; she is a 5/6 human leukocyte antigen (HLA) match. Peripheral blood was used. He was given tacrolimus and methotrexate for GVHD prophylaxis. The patient engrafted on day +16. On day +19, the patient developed a maculopapular rash on his face, neck, and upper chest. The next day, his rash had spread to cover 70% of his body surface area (BSA), and the patient began to complain of nausea, abdominal cramps and watery diarrhea (1400 mL/24 hours). On morning labs, his liver function tests, including bilirubin, are normal.

1. What are the JD's risk factors for GVHD?
2. What would be the stage and grade of this patient's acute GVHD?
3. What treatment would be started?
4. Calculate the prednisone dose for this patient.
5. Explain the rationale for reinstituting corticosteroid therapy.
6. What is likely the cause of these symptoms?
7. What other supportive care therapies can be given to this patient to alleviate some of his symptoms?
8. Which antimicrobial prophylaxis regimens should be considered?

The patient has progressive signs and symptoms of chronic GVHD. The team would like to start second-line treatment to try to wean the patient's prednisone.

A Few Options

- Sirolimus
- Extracorporeal photopheresis
- Rituximab
- Pentostatin

Extracorporeal photopheresis would be a good option because it is effective in patients with mouth and skin involvement; however, the patient has a hardship with frequent visits to the clinic, thus, the most convenient therapy would be oral therapy for this patient. The team and patient decide to use sirolimus.

9. What things should be considered when prescribing sirolimus? The patient develops a fungal pneumonia. The team wants to initiate voriconazole therapy. The patient is now taking 2 mg PO twice daily of tacrolimus and 2 mg PO daily of sirolimus.

10. What should the team consider before initiating voriconazole?

tapered more slowly than for treatment of acute GVHD. One approach is to reduce the prednisone dose by 25% per week over 4 weeks to a target schedule of every-other-day dosing while the therapeutic dosing of the CNI continues. The patient is monitored periodically, and if the patient's manifestations are resolved, then the patient is instructed to wean the immunosuppressive slowly. A common practice is to institute a Seattle taper in which the prednisone is eventually dosed every other day, then the CNI is tapered by 25% per week until prednisone is given on alternate days, and eventually the patient is tapered off immunosuppression. If the patient has an incomplete response, then the same doses of prednisone are continued. Often, however, the patient's chronic GVHD symptoms will increase as corticosteroid doses are tapered and the dose of prednisone may need to be increased. It may not be feasible to reattempt another corticosteroid taper for several months. Approximately half of patients will fail to respond to first-line corticosteroids and will require salvage treatment.

Currently no standard second-line therapy exists for chronic GVHD.[32–36] Patients should always be encouraged to enroll in clinical trials if eligible. Mycophenolate mofetil, sirolimus, and/or CNI are commonly used in this setting. Extracorporeal photopheresis is commonly used for chronic GVHD treatment. It is generally well tolerated but requires patients to return to the transplant center frequently; this therapy works best in patients with skin, oral, or liver involvement. PUVA can be used for patients with primarily cutaneous involvement. The TNF-α inhibitors, infliximab and etanercept, have been used with some success. Due to the increasing evidence that B-cells are involved in the pathogenesis of chronic GVHD, rituximab, an anti-CD20 monoclonal antibody, has been shown to be safe and effective in some patients. It is commonly given at the standard dose weekly for 4 weeks. Pentostatin, hydroxychloroquine, and thalidomide have been shown to have some activity, although they are rarely used as the initial salvage therapy. Azithromycin 250 mg orally three times weekly and montelukast 10 mg orally nightly, along with fluticasone inhaled twice daily, have been administered to patients with pulmonary GVHD to diminish the inflammatory responses. Many of these therapies are continued until progressive disease and/or intolerable side effects occur. Studies are ongoing to research the optimal treatment of chronic GVHD and to find novel treatments.

The use of topical therapies for treatment of GVHD may occasionally delay the need for systemic therapy or may allow dose reductions for systemic therapy. Supportive care measures are critical to controlling GVHD as well, including infection prophylaxis, physical and occupational therapy, management of complications of treatments (such as osteoporosis management, lipid and glucose management), nutritional management, pain control, psychosocial support, and drug interaction and adverse effects management. Table 8-10 provides recommendations for supportive care measures and ancillary therapies.

SINUSOIDAL OBSTRUCTION SYNDROME

Sinusoidal obstruction syndrome (SOS), formerly known as venoocclusive disease (VOD), is a serious complication of HSCT with an increased risk of mortality early after HSCT. It usually occurs within the first 30 days of HSCT, but it can occur later. The incidence of SOS ranges from 10% to 60%, and the severity ranges from mild and reversible to severe and fatal. Hepatic injury due to SOS can lead to hepatic failure and eventually multiorgan failure in severe cases.

SOS is a clinical diagnosis; patients present with a classic triad of symptoms, including elevated bilirubin (with or without jaundice), liver enlargement and right upper quadrant tenderness, and weight gain and/or ascites. Often, either the Seattle or Baltimore criteria is used to make the clinical diagnosis (**Table 8-11**). Diagnosis of SOS can be difficult because many other factors can cause hepatotoxicity.[37–39]

Risk factors for SOS include patient characteristics, transplant conditioning regimens, and the type of HSCT, with each influencing the incidence and severity of SOS. The primary event leading to SOS seems to be damage to the sinusoidal endothelial cells and hepatocytes by the transplant conditioning regimen.[37–40]

Selection of a particular conditioning regimen should be based on an individual's risk factors for SOS; if a patient is at high risk for SOS, the conditioning regimen should be one that is expected to have a low incidence of hepatotoxicity. If busulfan is used, IV busulfan is preferred over oral busulfan due to less variable exposure, and targeted busulfan dosing should be considered if the center can

Table 8-11 Diagnosis of SOS[4,46,47]

Seattle Criteria	Baltimore Criteria
Diagnosis requires 2 of the following criteria by day +20 posttransplant: • Hyperbilirubinemia (total serum bilirubin > 2 mg/dL) • Hepatomegaly or RUQ pain • Unexplained weight gain (> 2% of baseline body weight) due to fluid retention	Diagnosis requires hyperbilirubinemia (total bilirubin > 2 mg/dL) and 2 of the following criteria before day +21 posttransplant: • Painful/tender hepatomegaly • Ascites • Weight gain > 5% from baseline

RUQ, right upper quadrant pain.

perform the necessary pharmacokinetic assessments. Monitoring weights daily and maintaining a strict intake/output balance are important. Ursodiol (ursodeoxycholic acid), a hydrophilic bile acid, appears to have benefit based on results from several small trials, although one larger trial failed to show a benefit.[4,37–40] Many transplant centers use ursodiol prophylaxis; the dose, duration, and patient groups who receive ursodiol, however, are extremely variable. Common doses for ursodiol include 300 mg orally two to three times daily or 12–15 mg/kg/day in two to three divided doses. Ursodiol is usually begun at the start of conditioning and is continued to engraftment, or day +30 if liver function tests are normal, or continued up to 6 months posttransplant. Some centers give ursodiol prophylaxis to all patients, others to allogeneic recipients only, and others to high-risk autologous and/or allogeneic recipients only. Ursodiol appears to be safe, with no significant side effects. Low molecular weight heparin (eg, enoxaparin 40 mg SC daily) with ursodiol has been used with conflicting results. Defibrotide is a polydeoxyribonucleotide with local antithrombotic, anti-ischemic, and anti-inflammatory properties and in smaller studies has shown promising results as both a prophylactic agent and as treatment for SOS.[40]

Treatment of SOS

Currently, there is no FDA-approved treatment of SOS, and management consists of best supportive care. Mild disease is usually self-limiting and resolves quickly. Moderate disease is usually reversible, requiring only management of fluid overload. Severe SOS requires treatment due to the high risk of mortality. Whenever possible, exposure to hepatotoxins and nephrotoxins should be avoided. The pharmacokinetics of some drugs may be affected due to abnormal liver metabolism;

methotrexate doses, for example, may need to be adjusted in patients with fluid collections (eg, ascites). Diuretics are commonly used to reduce fluid overload.[4,40]

Many of the same agents used in prophylaxis have been used in the treatment for SOS, with varying degrees of success. Tissue-type plasminogen activator with or without anticoagulation has been used for the treatment of SOS; however, the risk of fatal hemorrhage is high, and this approach is not generally recommended. Defibrotide seems to be the most effective therapy for SOS and appears to be a more effective and safer treatment of SOS compared to heparin, antithrombin, and tissue-type plasminogen activator. Defibrotide binds to adenosine receptors, protects sinusoidal endothelium, and has antithrombotic and fibrinolytic activity without enhancing systemic bleeding. The effectiveness of defibrotide in the treatment of severe SOS has been demonstrated in several trials. Unfortunately, defibrotide is not commercially available and is very costly, and its use should be reserved for patients with severe SOS. The drug can be quickly obtained if an institution review board–approved investigational protocol is already in place; if not, it may take several days to receive the drug from the manufacturer, which may limit its effectiveness. To be effective, this drug should be given as soon as possible to those patients with severe SOS. Transjugular intrahepatic portosystemic shunts have been tried in severe SOS but have not been shown to be safe or effective. Liver transplantation in select patients with severe SOS has been used.[4,40]

Infection in HSCT Patients

The risk of infection following HSCT varies depending on the type of transplant the patient undergoes.[41–43] Almost all patients will develop neutropenia that lasts for 10–14 days after HSCT infusion following completion of the conditioning regimen. During the neutropenic period, patients are at risk for the development of (1) bacterial infection with gram-negative and gram-positive organisms, (2) viral reactivation of herpes simplex virus, and (3) fungal infection. Accordingly, patients should receive preventive therapy with agents such as fluoroquinolones, acyclovir or valacyclovir, and an azole antifungal agent such as fluconazole. **Tables 8-12** and **8-13** provide details about infections and prevention in HSCT recipients.

Following engraftment, the infection risk profile changes substantially for recipients of autologous HSCT compared to recipients of allogeneic HSCT.[41–43] Because autologous HSCT patients do not receive immunosuppressive therapy after transplant, they will experience immune reconstitution at approximately 6 months after transplantation. However, until their immune function is restored, they remain at risk for reactivation of varicella zoster virus and for development of *Pneumocystis jiroveci* (PCP) infection. As a result, these patients should

Table 8-12 Infections in Hematopoietic Stem Cell Transplant Recipients

Patient Type	Time of Occurrence	Infection Type	Risk Factors	Prevention
All HSCT patients (autologous and allogeneic)	Preengraftment	Bacterial (gram-negative, gram-positive)	Neutropenia	Fluoroquinolones
		Fungal		Azole antifungal (fluconazole, voriconazole)
		Viral (HSV reactivation)		Acyclovir, valacyclovir
	Postengraftment	Viral (varicella zoster virus (VZV) or herpes simplex virus (HSV) reactivation)	Delayed immune reconstitution	Acyclovir, valacyclovir
		Other—*Pneumocystis jiroveci* (PCP)		Trimethoprim-sulfamethoxazole, dapsone, aerosolized pentamidine, atovaquone for PCP
Allogeneic HSCT patients only	Postengraftment	Bacterial (encapsulated organisms)	Functional asplenia due to immunosuppression	Trimethoprim-sulfamethoxazole penicillian
		Fungal (molds)	Impaired T-cell function, immunosuppression, GVHD	Azole antifungals (voriconazole, posaconazole), amphotericin/lipid amphotericin products, echinocandins
		Viral (cytomegalovirus [CMV] reactivation)	Impaired T-cell function, immunosuppression, GVHD, CMV serologic mismatch with donor	Preemptive therapy preferred over prophylaxis Agents: ganciclovir, valganciclovir, foscarnet

Table 8-13 Vaccination Recommendations for HSCT Recipients[44]

Vaccine	Schedule	Comments
Haemophilus influenzae type b (Hib) vaccine	A 3-dose regimen should be administered beginning 6 months after transplant; at least 1 month should separate the doses	
Inactivated influenza vaccine	Beginning at least 6 months after HSCT and annually thereafter for the life of the patient	A dose of inactivated influenza vaccine can be given as early as 4 months after HSCT, but a second dose should be considered in this situation. A second dose is recommended routinely for all children receiving influenza vaccine for the first time
Measles, mumps, rubella (MMR) vaccine	All children and seronegative adults, MMR vaccine should be administered 24 months after transplant if the HCT recipient is immunocompetent	In children, 2 doses are favored
Pneumococcal vaccine	Sequential administration of 3 doses of pneumococcal conjugate vaccine (PCV) is recommended, beginning 3–6 months after the transplant, followed by a dose of 23-valent pneumococcal polysaccharide vaccine (PPSV23)	For patients with chronic GVHD who are likely to respond poorly to PPSV23, a fourth dose of the PCV should be considered instead of PPSV23
Tetanus, diphtheria, acellular pertussis vaccine	Three doses beginning 6–12 months after transplant	DTaP is preferred, however, if only Tdap is available (eg, because DTaP is not licensed for adults), administer Tdap

CMV, cytomegalovirus; GVHD, graft-versus-host-disease; HSCT, hematopoietic stem cell transplant; HSV, herpes simplex virus; PCP, *Pneumocystis jiroveci*; VZV, varicella zoster virus.

be maintained on a prophylaxis regimen (eg, valacyclovir and trimethoprim-sulfamethoxazole) to protect them until their immune function returns to baseline.

Because of the need for continued immunosuppression in allogeneic HSCT recipients, these patients remain at risk for opportunistic patients for a prolonged period of time.[41–43] Standard infection prophylaxis for patients on immunosuppressive therapy include PCP prophylaxis with sulfamethoxazole-trimethoprim or an equivalent, antiviral prophylaxis with acyclovir or equivalent to prevent herpes reactivation, and antifungal prophylaxis with at least fluconazole. For patients receiving high-dose corticosteroids ($\geq$ 1 mg/kg/day) for a prolonged period of time, antifungal prophylaxis may be broadened to include activity against *Aspergillus* species, and antiviral prophylaxis against cytomegalovirus may be indicated.

Patients with active GVHD have an even greater risk of infection, both during treatment and after completion of immunosuppressive therapy.[41–43] Mortality associated with chronic GVHD is largely due to infections. These patients are at a very high risk for infection with encapsulated organisms and pneumocystis and should be given appropriate prophylaxis; these agents are generally continued until the patient has been off all immunosuppression for at least 6 months.

Because of the very high risk for infection in HSCT recipients, international consensus guidelines for the prevention of infection in HSCT recipients have recently been updated.[44] Patients should be followed closely after transplant and vaccinations (no live viruses for patients or family members) should be given at recommended intervals, typically starting 12 months posttransplant.

CASE 8-1
Answers

1. Melphalan can cause significant delayed chemotherapy-induced nausea and vomiting (CINV). Also, the patient has a history of nausea and vomiting with prior therapies and during prior pregnancies; thus, this increases her risk of developing CINV with this regimen. She is also at high risk for anticipatory nausea and vomiting.

   It is important to find out from the patient before the conditioning regimen begins what antiemetic regimen has worked in the past as well as what has not worked. The key to any antiemetic regimen is prevention.

2. The patient is at high risk for CINV. Melphalan does not interact with aprepitant, and many practitioners would consider using this medication for this patient. It is recommended to give the patient aprepitant 125 mg PO before her first melphalan dose then give

80 mg PO daily × 2 doses (or fosaprepitant 150 mg once IV before melphalan), along with a 5-HT$_3$ antagonist (eg, ondansetron), and dexamethasone. It would likely be helpful to give SN a benzodiazepine, such as lorazepam, before melphalan, because she may experience anticipatory nausea and vomiting based on past nausea and vomiting experiences.

3. Common medications that are metabolized by the cytochrome P450 3A4 pathway include cyclophosphamide, busulfan, etoposide, and thiotepa. While a few small studies have evaluated the safety and efficacy of using aprepitant with these chemotherapy agents, it is not commonly recommended to use aprepitant with these chemotherapy agents.

   Another concern with the use of aprepitant in HSCT patients is the potential for drug–drug interactions with nonchemotherapy medications. Calcineurin inhibitors (CNIs) such as cyclosporine or tacrolimus are routinely used in allogeneic HSCT. Concomitant administration of aprepitant may result in alterations in metabolism of CNIs, leading to elevated CNI concentrations and an increased risk of CNI-associated toxicity early in the HSCT.

4. The patient can be initiated on scheduled promethazine or prochlorperazine and administered another antiemetic (eg, ondansetron) as needed. The patient should be reassessed and may need another scheduled antiemetic to control her nausea, similar to the practice with standard chemotherapy patients. With high-dose melphalan, patients commonly experience diarrhea, and metoclopramide is not commonly used for CINV because of concern for diarrhea. Ondansetron may not be as effective for delayed nausea/vomiting, although it is often used in clinical practice. Lorazepam is not an ideal antiemetic, although it may help with anxiety associated with vomiting or have an amnesic effect. Autologous transplant recipients can often receive dexamethasone to treat delayed CINV. If the patient had undergone an allogeneic HSCT, it would be prudent to avoid corticosteroids after day 0 due to potential antilymphocyte effects. In some patients who have refractory CINV, olanzapine 5 mg PO twice daily has been effective.

CASE 8-2
Answers

1.
- 5/6 HLA match. This is the most important risk factor for GVHD
- Multiparous female donor
- Myeloablative conditioning regimen
- Peripheral blood stem cell product

2.
- Stage 3 skin (> 50% BSA), stage 0 liver, stage 2 GI tract (1000–1500 mL/day stool output)
- Overall clinical grade of GVHD is grade III acute GVHD (stage 2–3 skin involvement, stage 2–3 gastrointestinal [GI] involvement)

After drug toxicity and infection are ruled out, the patient underwent a skin biopsy and upper and lower endoscopy. Pathology from both the skin and GI tract was consistent with acute GVHD.

3.
- Methylprednisolone 80 mg IV twice daily (2 mg/kg/day)
- Tacrolimus would be continued and maintained at a therapeutic level of 5–15 ng/mL

The patient was continued on tacrolimus, and methylprednisolone therapy was initiated. After 5 days, the patient's skin rash had resolved, and his stool output had decreased to 400 mL/day. At day 7, the team decreased his methylprednisolone to 60 mg IV twice daily (25% dose reduction). He continued to do well, and he was switched to prednisone after 3 doses of the 60 mg methylprednisolone in anticipation for discharge.

4.
- The equivalent dose of prednisone would be 75 mg PO twice daily (1.25 × methylprednisolone dose)

The patient was discharged, and his prednisone was tapered after 7 days to 60 mg PO twice daily, then to 40 mg PO twice daily the week after that. Three days after the taper, the patient presented to clinic with a mild skin rash to his upper chest and face.

His prednisone taper was held and his rash remained stable. After 2 weeks, the patient complained of nausea, increased stool output, and a progressive rash. The patient's prednisone was increased to 75 mg PO twice daily due to his GVHD flare.

5.
- This type of taper is common in clinical practice. Frequently, symptoms of acute GVHD will flare after a taper and the corticosteroid dose may be increased to previous dose levels or may be restarted at 2 mg/kg/day, depending on the severity of symptoms. Typically, the corticosteroid dose would be tapered more slowly to avoid another flare; the time of the course may be dictated by the patient's response to therapy. However, if the patient develops complications to steroids, such as myopathy or infection, it would be important to attempt to taper the prednisone more quickly if the patient can tolerate it.

When the patient was at day +80, he returned to the clinic with complaints of dry itchy skin, dry mouth with ulcers, and feeling like he has sand in his eyes. On exam, he was found to have lichenoid changes in his mouth with ulcerations, scleroderma-like plaques on his extremities, and conjunctivitis. The patient's prednisone is 20 mg PO daily; his tacrolimus level is 8 ng/mL.

6.
- These signs and symptoms are classic features of chronic GVHD. Even though the patient has not reached day +100 after HSCT, his signs and symptoms are more indicative of chronic GVHD than of acute GVHD. This is not unexpected, as the patient previously had acute GVHD, which is a major risk factor for chronic GVHD. Chronic GVHD is preceded by acute GVHD in the majority of cases. Likely, the patient's prednisone would be increased to 1 mg/kg/day and then tapered once his symptoms improve or abate (by 25%, for example, from 80 mg PO daily, to 60 mg PO daily, to 40 mg PO daily, then to 80 mg PO every other day [target is 1 mg/kg every other day] after a 4-week taper.) His tacrolimus therapy would continue to be dosed to reach therapeutic levels.

7.

- Skin: topical emollients, such as Eucerin moisturing cream, to dry areas; oral antihistamine such as diphenhydramine or hydroxyzine for itching; triamcinolone cream 0.1% three times a day to the body and hydrocortisone cream 1% to sensitive areas, such as the face.
- Mouth: fluoride and saliva substitutes can be given for dry mouth; corticosteroid and/or analgesic rinses can be given to improve ulcerations.
- Eyes: artificial tears, topical corticosteroid, or cyclosporine eye drops.

8.

- Patients with chronic GVHD are at high risk for infections, particularly with encapsulated organisms. JD should be placed on antibacterial prophylaxis with penicillin VK 500 mg by mouth three times daily or sulfamethoxazole/trimethoprim 400 mg/80 mg PO daily to twice daily. JD should remain on antiviral prophylaxis while on immunosuppression. Most HSCT clinicians would also prescribe antifungal prophylaxis because of the continued corticosteroid therapy. Fluconazole can be used, although many clinicians may broaden prophylaxis to provide better antimold coverage (eg, posaconazole, voriconazole) for patients receiving high-dose corticosteroids. This patient should also continue to receive *Pneumocystis jiroveci* (PCP) prophylaxis. If the patient has recurrent infections, his care providers should consider checking serum IgG levels and replace with IV immunoglobulin (400 to 500 mg/kg) if IgG levels are low. Patients such as JD should be scheduled for posttransplantation vaccination beginning approximately 12 months after HSCT, as long as chronic GVHD is not severe; live vaccines should be avoided.

9.

- The patient is taking tacrolimus. There is a significant risk of thrombocytopenic purpura/hemolytic uremic syndrome with the combination of tacrolimus and sirolimus, so the tacrolimus level should be maintained between 5 and 10 ng/mL. The dose of

sirolimus for chronic GVHD is typically 2 mg PO daily (a load-
ing dose is often not given for chronic GVHD). Sirolimus levels
should be measured and the concentration of sirolimus should
be maintained between 3 and 12 ng/mL.
  • Lipid levels should be checked routinely
10. A significant interaction with voriconazole and the two
    immunosuppressive agents, tacrolimus and sirolimus, exists.
    Voriconazole is expected to decrease the metabolism of these two
    drugs, resulting in increased concentrations of tacrolimus and
    sirolimus. Normally, it is recommended to decrease tacrolimus to
    one-third or half of the previous dose when initiating voriconazole.
    An appropriate dose reduction of tacrolimus would be to
    change to 0.5 to 1 mg PO twice daily. While it is recommended
    to avoid voriconazole in patients receiving sirolimus, this is a
    relative contraindication. If voriconazole administration cannot
    be avoided, a 90% dose reduction of sirolimus is recommended.
    An appropriate dose of sirolimus in this patient would be either
    0.2 mg (liquid) PO daily or 2 mg PO weekly. When starting
    voriconazole, it is prudent to check tacrolimus and sirolimus
    levels more frequently until a stable serum concentration has been
    obtained.

SUMMARY

Patients receiving high-dose chemotherapy and HSCT are at risk for a number of
serious complications, including many that are unique to the transplant patient
population. Healthcare providers involved in the care of patients receiving high
doses of chemotherapy and HSCT should be familiar with the risk factors for
manifestations of and therapy for these complications.

REFERENCES

1. Armitage JO. History of autologous hematopoietic cell transplantation. In: Appelbaum FR, Forman SJ, Negrin RS, et al. *Thomas' Hematopoietic Cell Transplantation.*
   4th ed. Oxford, UK: Wiley-Blackwell; 2009:8–14.

2. Horowitz MM. Uses and growth of hematopoietic cell transplantation. In: Appelbaum FR, Forman SJ, Negrin RS, et al. *Thomas' Hematopoietic Cell Transplantation*. 4th ed. Oxford, UK: Wiley-Blackwell; 2009:15–21.

3. Dershow JH, Synold TW. Pharmacologic basis for high-dose chemotherapy. In: Appelbaum FR, Forman SJ, Negrin RS, et al. *Thomas' Hematopoietic Cell Transplantation*. 4th ed. Oxford, UK: Wiley-Blackwell, 2009:289–315.

4. Wingard JR, Gastineau DA, Leather HL, et al., eds. *Hematopoietic Stem Cell Transplantation: A Handbook for Clinicians*. Bethesda, MD: AABB; 2009.

5. Copelan EA. Hematopoietic stem-cell transplantation. *New Engl J Med*. 2006;354:1813–1826.

6. Bensinger, WI. High-dose preparatory regimens. In: Appelbaum FR, Forman SJ, Negrin RS, et al. *Thomas' Hematopoietic Cell Transplantation*. 4th ed. Oxford, UK: Wiley-Blackwell, 2009:316–332.

7. Sandmaier BM, Storb R. Reduced-intensity conditioning followed by hematopoietic cell transplantation for hematologic malignancies. In: Appelbaum FR, Forman SJ, Negrin RS, et al. *Thomas' Hematopoietic Cell Transplantation*. 4th ed. Oxford, UK: Wiley-Blackwell, 2009:1043–1058.

8. Barker JN, Weisdrof DJ, DeFor TE, Blazar BR, Miller JS, Wagner JE. Rapid and complete donor chimerism in adult recipients of unrelated donor umbilical cord blood transplantation after reduced-intensity conditioning. *Blood*. 2003;102:1915–1919.

9. Andersson BK, Kashyap A, Gian V, et al. Conditioning therapy with intravenous busulfan and cyclophosphamide (IV BuCy2) for hematologic malignancies prior to allogeneic stem cell transplantation: a phase II study. *Biol Blood Marrow Transplant*. 2002; 8:145–154.

10. Blaise D, Maraninchi D, Archimbaud E, et al. Allogeneic bone marrow transplantation for acute myeloid leukemia in first remission: a randomized trial of busulfan-Cytoxan versus Cytoxan-total body irradiation as preparative regimen: a report from the Group d'Etudes de la Greffe de Moelle Osseuse. *Blood*. 1994; 84:941–949.

11. Alyea EP, Kim HT, Ho V, et al. Comparative outcome of nonmyeloablative and myeloablative allogeneic hematopoietic cell transplantation for patients older than 50 years of age. *Blood*. 2005;105:1810–1814.

12. Aoudjhane M, Labopin M, Gorin, NC, et al. Comparative outcome of reduced intensity and myeloablative conditioning in HLA-identical sibling allogeneic hematopoietic stem cell transplantation for patients older than 50 years of age with acute myeloblastic leukemia: a retrospective survey from the Acute Leukemia Working Party (ALWP) of the European group for blood and marrow transplantation (EBMT). *Leukemia*. 2005;19:2304–2312.

13. Gertz MA. Current status of stem cell mobilization. *Br J Haematol*. 2010;150:647–662.

14. Pusic I, Jiang SY, Landua S, et al. Impact of mobilization and remobilization strategies on achieving sufficient stem cell yields for autologous transplantation. *Biol Blood Marrow Transpl*. 2008;14:1045–1056.

15. Giralt S, Stadtmauer EA, Harousseau JL, et al. International myeloma working group (IMWG) consensus statement and guidelines regarding the current status of stem cell collection and high-dose therapy for multiple myeloma and the role of plerixafor (AMD3100). *Leukemia*. 2009;23:1904–1912.

16. Attolico I, Pavone V, Ostuni A, et al. Plerixafor added to chemotherapy plus G-CSF is safe and allows adequate PBSC collection in predicted poor mobilizer patients with multiple myeloma or lymphoma. *Biol Blood Marrow Transpl*. 2012;18:241–249.

17. Stiff PJ. Management strategies for the hard-to-mobilize patient. *Bone Marrow Transpl.* 1999; 23 suppl 2:S29-S33.

18. Mozobil [package insert]. Cambridge, MA: Genzyme Corporation; 2010. http://www.mozobil.com/document/Package_Insert.pdf. Accessed May 28, 2013.

19. Cooper DL, Pratt K, Baker J, et al. Late afternoon dosing of plerixafor for stem cell mobilization: a practical solution. *Clin Lymphoma Myeloma Leuk.* 2011;11:267–272.

20. Alessandrino P, Bernasconi P, Caldera D, et al. Adverse events occurring during bone marrow or peripheral blood progenitor cell infusion: analysis of 126 cases. *Bone Marrow Transpl.* 1999; 23:533–537.

21. Bubalo JS, Cherala G, McCune JS, Munar MY, Tse S, Maziarz R. Aprepitant pharmacokinetics and assessing the impact of aprepitant on cyclophosphamide metabolism in cancer patients undergoing hematopoietic stem cell transplantation. *J Clin Pharmacol.* 2012;52:586–594.

22. Cutler C, Antin JH. Acute Graft-vs-host disease. In: Appelbaum FR, Forman SJ, Negrin RS, et al. *Thomas' Hematopoietic Cell Transplantation.* 4th ed. Oxford, UK: Wiley-Blackwell, 2009:1287–1303.

23. Morris ES, Hill GR. Advances in the understanding of acute graft-versus-host disease. *Br J Haematol.* 2007;137:3–19.

24. Cutler C, Antin JH. Novel drugs for the prevention and treatment of acute GVHD. *Curr Pharm Des.* 2008;14:1962–1973.

25. Lanum SA. Clinical pearls: cyclosporine and mycophenolate. Presented at BMT Pharmacists Meeting; February 2010. Orlando, FL.

26. Gulbis AM. Clinical pearls: sirolimus and tacrolimus. Presented at BMT Pharmacists Meeting; February 2010. Orlando, FL.

27. Bayraktar UD, Champlin RE, Ciurea SO. Progress in haploidentical stem cell transplantation. *Biol Blood Marrow Transpl.* 2012;18:372–380.

28. Bacigalupo A. Management of acute graft-versus-host disease. *Br J Haematol.* 2007;137:87–98.

29. Pidala J, Anasetti C. Glucocorticoid-refractory acute graft-versus-host disease. *Biol Blood Marrow Transpl.* 2010;16:1504–1518.

30. Paczesny S, Choi SW, Ferrara JM. Acute graft-versus-host disease: new treatment strategies. *Curr Opin Hematol.* 2009;16:427–436.

31. Martin PJ, Inamoto Y, Flowers MED, Carpenter PA. Secondary treatment of acute graft-versus-host disease: a critical review. *Biol Blood Marrow Transpl.* 2012;18;982–988.

32. Filipovich AH, Weisdorf D, Pavletic S, et al. National Institutes of Health consensus development project on criteria for clinical trials in chronic graft-versus-host disease: I. Diagnosis and staging working group report. *Biol Blood Marrow Transpl.* 2005;11:945–955.

33. Bolanos-Meade J, Vogelsang GB. Chronic graft-versus-host-disease. *Curr Pharm Des.* 2008;14(20):1974–1986.

34. Wolff D, Schleuning M, von Harsdorf S, et al. Consensus conference on clinical practice in chronic GVHD: second-line treatment of chronic graft-versus-host disease. *Biol Blood Marrow Transpl.* 2011;17:1–17.

35. Couriel D, Carpenter PA, Cutler C, et al. Ancillary therapy and supportive care of chronic graft-versus-host disease: National Institutes of Health consensus development project on criteria for clinical trials in chronic graft-versus-host disease: V. Ancillary therapy and supportive care working group report. *Biol Blood Marrow Transpl.* 2006;12:375–396.

36. Choi SW, Levine JE, Ferrara JLM. Pathogenesis and management of graft-versus-host disease. *Immunol Allergy Clin North Am.* 2010:75–101.

37. McDonald GB, Hinds MS, Fisher LD, et al. Veno-occlusive disease of the liver and multiorgan failure after BMT: a cohort study of 355 patients. *Ann Int Med.* 1993;118:255–267.

38. Jones RL, Lee KSK, Beschorner WE, et al. Veno-occlusive disease of the liver following bone marrow transplantation. *Transplantation.* 1987;44:778–783.

39. McDonald GB. Hepatobiliary complications of hematopoietic cell transplantation, 40 years on. *Hepatology.* 2010:51:1450–1460.

40. Ho VT, Linden E, Revta C, Richardson PG. Hepatic veno-occlusive disease after hematopoietic stem cell transplantation: review and update of the use of defibrotide. *Semin Thromb Hemost.* 2007;33;373–388.

41. Wingard JR, Hsu J, Hiemenz JW. Hematopoietic stem cell transplantation: an overview of infection risks and epidemiology. *Hematol Oncol Clin North Am.* 2011;25:101–116.

42. Leather HL, Wingard JR. Infections following hematopoietic stem cell transplantation. *Inf Dis Clin North Am.* 2001;15:483–520.

43. Hiemenz JW. Management of infections complicating allogeneic hematopoietic stem cell transplantation. *Semin Hematol.* 2009;46:289–312.

44. Tomblyn M, Chiller T, Einsele H, et al. Guidelines for preventing infectious complications among hematopoietic cell transplantation recipients: a global perspective. *Biol Blood Marrow Transpl.* 2009;15:1143–1238.

45. Glucksberg H, Storb R, Fefer A, et al. Clinical manifestations of graft-versus-host disease in human recipients of marrow from HL-A-matched sibling donors. *Transplantation.* 1974; 18:295–304.

46. McDonald GB, Hinds MS, Fisher, LD, et al. Veno-occlusive disease of the liver and multiorgan failure after bone marrow transplantation: A cohort study of 355 patients. *Ann Intern Med.* 1993;118(4):255–267

47. Jones RJ, Lee KS, Beschorner WE, et al. Venoocclusive disease of the liver following bone marrow transplantation. *Transplantation.* 1987 Dec;44(6):778–83.

CHAPTER 9

Pediatric Oncology

Brooke Bernhardt
Susannah E. Koontz

LEARNING OBJECTIVES

Upon completion of the chapter, the reader will be able to:
1. Describe the epidemiology and etiology of childhood cancers
2. Describe the standard approach to treating children with cancer
3. Identify critical supportive care issues when treating children with cancer

INTRODUCTION

Approximately 12,000 children less than 15 years of age are diagnosed with cancer each year in the United States. While this represents less than 1% of all new cancer diagnoses per year, cancer is the second leading cause of death in children. Childhood mortality from cancer has declined substantially over the past several decades. Most investigators attribute this decline to the high participation rate of children in clinical trials, including cooperative group clinical trials. Nearly one-third of children diagnosed with cancer have some form of leukemia, making leukemia of all types as the most common type of cancer in children. Brain tumors and tumors of the central nervous system comprise the next largest group of patients followed by various solid tumors and lymphomas (**Figure 9-1**).[1] Each of the childhood tumor types will be discussed briefly throughout this chapter. The reader should have a general familiarity with hematologic and oncologic malignancies. This chapter will serve to identify specific features of each cancer disease most observed in children and treatment unique to the pediatric patient.

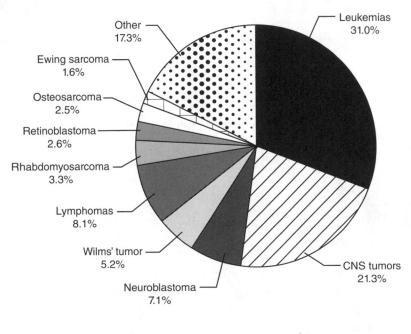

FIGURE 9-1 Childhood Cancers[1]

ROLE OF COOPERATIVE RESEARCH GROUPS

Survival rates from childhood cancers have increased markedly from 10% to almost 80% during the past 50 years. Much of this success can be attributed to the serial efforts and accomplishments of pediatric cancer cooperative group studies formed as early as the mid-1950s.[2] In 2000, four major pediatric oncology cooperative groups, Children's Cancer Group (CCG), Pediatric Oncology Group (POG), Intergroup Rhabdomyosarcoma Study Group (IRSG) and National Wilms' Tumor Study Group (NWTSG), merged to form the Children's Oncology Group (COG). Today, the COG is the largest childhood cancer research organization in the world and is composed of more than 5,000 pediatric health-care specialists at approximately 230 programs located in the United States, Canada, the Netherlands, Switzerland, Australia, and New Zealand. Most member institutions are part of large academic-based medical centers.

Pediatric cancers are rare, and resources to conduct studies, including patients, funding and research infrastructure, are limited. Thus, the work of cooperative groups such as the COG are important because they facilitate enrollment of eligible patients onto studies rather than compete for patients as individual entities. Furthermore, the COG also aggregates data for more expeditious outcome results and establishment of practice standards, shares centralized services (eg, pathology and radiology review centers) to maximize resources, creates and more rapidly refines protocols to harmonize treatment approaches across all patients regardless of treatment center, and provides extensive patient follow-ups to monitor for long-term sequelae resulting from treatments. More than 90% of pediatric patients with a newly diagnosed malignancy in the United States are seen at a COG institution with 50%-60% of these patients enrolled onto a clinical trial. As a result, a majority of pediatric patients are treated with investigational protocols available only to COG member institutions rather than widely available standard of care regimens utilized in adult patients.

INITIAL PRESENTATION AND ONCOLOGIC EMERGENCIES

Initial Presentation

Presenting signs and symptoms of cancer in children are often nonspecific and vary based on the type of malignancy. Some of the general signs and symptoms are similar to those seen in adult patients. Select common signs and symptoms that may indicate a malignancy are presented in **Box 9-1**.[1]

BOX 9-1
Possible Signs and Symptoms of Childhood Cancer[1]

- Swelling, an unusual mass, or a lump
- Unexplained fatigue or pallor
- Easy bruising or bleeding with or without a cause
- Localized pain, including bone or joint pain
- Illness, fever, or weight loss of unknown origin
- Headaches, with or without vomiting
- Ocular or visual changes

Oncologic Emergencies

Children may present with similar types of oncologic emergencies as those seen in adults. Some of the more common oncologic emergencies seen in children are a product of the most common types of malignancies seen in children (eg, leukemias and lymphomas) and include hyperleukocytosis, tumor lysis syndrome, and superior vena cava syndrome.[3]

Hyperleukocytosis

Hyperleukocytosis is an oncologic emergency, which is defined as a peripheral white blood cell (WBC) count greater than 100,000/µL.[3] Hyperleukocytosis is observed in approximately 10% of newly diagnosed children with acute lymphoblastic leukemia (ALL), from 5% to 20% of children with acute myeloid leukemia (AML), and nearly all children in the chronic phase of chronic myeloid leukemia (CML). In some patients, life-threatening complications such as respiratory failure and hemorrhage may occur as a result of increased blood viscosity when the leukocyte volume is greater than 20%-25%. Patients with a WBC count greater than 300,000/µL are at an increased risk of death due to the enhanced risk of hemorrhage, especially in the central nervous system. The management of hyperleukocytosis should include frequent laboratory monitoring (eg, complete blood count, renal function, and serum chemistries every 6-8 hours), aggressive fluid support (often ranging 2-3 times maintenance values—see section called Fluid Management in this chapter), management of actual or anticipated tumor lysis syndrome, cytoreduction with leukapheresis or exchange transfusion, and treatment of the malignancy.

Tumor Lysis Syndrome

Tumor lysis syndrome is defined as a set of metabolic abnormalities commonly seen at initial presentation or at relapse of a hematologic malignancy.[3,4] In some patients with a bulky mediastinal mass, tumor lysis syndrome may occur following the initiation of corticosteroids, regardless of dose.[3] In clinical trials, around 6%-27% of children experience metabolic derangements consistent with tumor lysis syndrome.[4] The most common malignancies associated with tumor lysis syndrome in children include ALL, AML, and non-Hodgkin's lymphoma (NHL); specifically, Burkitt's lymphoma.[3,4]

Of note, the use of rasburicase along with hydration and electrolyte management is clearly defined and should be encouraged in the initial management of pediatric patients at high risk of developing tumor lysis syndrome.[4]

Superior Vena Cava Syndrome

Superior vena cava (SVC) syndrome is an oncologic emergency that may be observed in children with an anterior mediastinal mass, such as that seen with non-Hodgkin's lymphoma.[3] This syndrome is characterized by obstruction or compression of the superior vena cava. As a result, the patient may experience reduced blood flow or airflow. Management includes close respiratory and cardiovascular monitoring along with avoidance of sedatives and general anesthesia until the obstruction or compression can be relieved. Although the use of corticosteroids before obtaining a diagnosis is typically contraindicated, it may be warranted to relieve the pressure induced by an anterior mediastinal mass.

ACUTE LEUKEMIAS

Of children and adolescents less than 19 years of age in the United States, nearly 6,500 are diagnosed with some form of leukemia. About 80% of cases are attributable to ALL, and up to 20% are attributable to AML, with a small percentage presenting as chronic leukemias.[5] Chronic leukemias of childhood will not be discussed in this text; the reader is encouraged to refer to other resources for additional information such as chapters in the pediatric oncology textbooks edited by Pizzo and Poplack and Lanzkowsky.[6,7]

Acute Lymphoblastic Leukemia

ALL is a proliferation of abnormal lymphoblasts of precursor B-cell or T-cell lineage. In childhood ALL, one or more consecutive genetic aberrations contribute to the development of abnormal clones; these abnormalities result in several biologic subtypes of ALL, some of which require specific therapeutic approaches.[8] Over the past several decades, survival for children with ALL has improved dramatically with 5-year event-free survival rate as high as 83% in cooperative groups for all subtypes of childhood ALL.[9] A child's prognosis is based on a variety of features, including age at diagnosis, leukocyte count at diagnosis, the presence of various genetic abnormalities, and the response to induction therapy. Children less than 1 year old or older than 10 years of age have a poorer prognosis. Those with a total leukocyte count greater than 50×10^9/L at diagnosis also have a poorer prognostic outlook.[8,9] Individual genetic aberrations are indicative of prognosis although it is not uncommon for a patient to have more than one abnormality. Additionally, children with a low to absent level of minimal residual disease (MRD) (ie, less than 0.01% blast cell measurement by flow cytometry or polymerase chain reaction analysis) following initiation of induction chemotherapy have an improved prognosis and reduced risk of relapse.[8,10] Together, these risk factors assist in the determination of a patient's overall prognosis and planned risk-based treatment assignment.

In children, typical therapy for the treatment of ALL includes induction, central nervous system (CNS) -directed therapy, consolidation, reinduction (delayed intensification), and maintenance therapy, though various terms have been used by cooperative groups. The role of each of these treatment elements is highlighted in **Table 9-1**.[9] Children with specific genetic abnormalities may benefit from the addition of targeted therapies to a therapeutic backbone. Such is the case in children with the BCR-ABL fusion gene; these children are characterized as having very high-risk ALL and receive more aggressive therapy than other children. Therapy for children with the BCR-ABL fusion gene may include intensive chemotherapy with the addition of a tyrosine kinase inhibitor, such as imatinib.[8-10]

Several questions pertaining to therapy for ALL still remain. Controversy exists regarding the amount, type, and timing of the corticosteroid used throughout therapy. Additionally, the optimal role and timing of allogeneic stem cell

Table 9-1 Treatment Backbone for Childhood Acute Lymphoblastic Leukemia [9]

Component	Goal of Therapy	Agents Employed
Induction	Induce morphologic remission Restore normal hematopoiesis	Glucocorticoid (dexamethasone or prednisone) Vincristine PEG-asparaginase or L-asparaginase Daunorubicin (high-risk patients only)
CNS-directed therapy	Prevent CNS relapse	Intrathecal therapy (given during most phases depending on disease at presentation)
Consolidation/ intensification	Reduce systemic minimal residual disease	High-dose methotrexate (especially for T-cell disease), mercaptopurine, cyclophosphamide, cytarabine
Reinduction	Reduce the risk of relapse	Similar agents as in induction and consolidation
Maintenance	Maintain long-term remission	Mercaptopurine, methotrexate, glucocorticoids, vincristine

CNS, central nervous system; PEG, polyethylene glycol.

transplantation is unclear.[9] Patients with certain high-risk features such as those with a poor response to induction therapy or BCR/ABL+ ALL may be good candidates for an allogeneic transplant; however, the majority of the remaining patients (ie, standard-risk patients with good response to therapy) are typically only eligible for transplant following first relapse.[9]

The ability to minimize toxicities while still maintaining a high level of long-term survival is of utmost importance and concern in children with ALL. Children with ALL are at an elevated risk of late cardiac toxicity (secondary to anthracyclines), potentially permanent neuropathies (vinca alkaloids), avascular necrosis (steroids), and cognitive delay (antimetabolites) as a result of the various agents used throughout therapy. Moreover, patients with genetic polymorphisms affecting the activity of drug metabolism may exhibit widely variable effects and toxicities.[8,9] For example, patients with homozygous or heterozygous deficiencies of thiopurine methyltransferase (TPMT) may experience increased myelosuppression from mercaptopurine compared with patients with no genetic deficiency of this enzyme (see **Clinical Pearl 9-1**). Children with this deficiency may require empiric dosage adjustments (as per cooperative group protocol guidelines or recently published consortium guidelines) prior to initiation of mercaptopurine in the setting of maintenance therapy. In one institution, a pharmacist-managed clinical pharmacogenetics service was developed to interpret TPMT results and provide recommendations for dosing to other clinicians.[11] The refinement of administration techniques of therapeutic agents such as mercaptopurine has also proven to be important. Studies have demonstrated that mercaptopurine should be administered in the evening, as its efficacy is enhanced compared to administration in the morning. Additionally, it should not be administered with milk or milk products containing xanthine oxidase, as the efficacy of mercaptopurine may be compromised.[12,13] As a result, clinicians recommend administering mercaptopurine to children on an empty stomach at night prior to going to bed.

CLINICAL PEARL 9-1

Patients with homozygous or heterozygous deficiencies of thiopurine methyltransferase (TPMT) may experience increased myelosuppression from mercaptopurine and may require an empiric dosage adjustment during maintenance therapy.

Down Syndrome and ALL

Children with Down syndrome are at an increased risk of developing ALL and have poorer outcomes; this is in contrast to the outcomes seen in children with Down syndrome and AML.[14] Poor outcomes may be a result of alterations in chemotherapy pharmacokinetics and variation in chemotherapy sensitivity (eg, children with Down syndrome may be at increased risk of mucositis and infectious complications due to enhanced sensitivity to methotrexate).

Acute Myeloid Leukemia

AML arises from the development and proliferation of abnormal myeloid (granulocytic, erythroid, monocytic, and megakaryocytic) cell precursors.[5] Over the past several decades, complete remission rates as high as 90% have been achieved. Relapse is common, occurring in 30%-40% of patients, with subsequent 5-year event-free and overall survival rates in the range of 30%-60% across cooperative groups using similar therapy. In children, typical therapy for the treatment of AML includes 4 or 5 courses of intense chemotherapy. Regardless of where the patient is treated, each course typically contains cytarabine in a high or intermediate dose with etoposide, an anthracycline, or both. The anthracycline used in induction varies based on the cooperative group; typically daunorubicin is used in the United States, while idarubicin and mitoxantrone may be used in other countries. Cumulative chemotherapy doses and related outcomes from select cooperative groups are depicted in **Table 9-2**[5]. The role and timing of allogeneic stem cell transplantation is still not clear. Most cooperative groups agree that patients with certain cytogenetic high-risk features should receive a transplant following 2 to 3 courses of chemotherapy while in first remission. For other patients, including those with favorable prognoses such as Down syndrome, transplantation should be reserved for salvage therapy.

The predicted prognosis for an individual patient with AML is affected by a variety of clinical features as well as genetic factors. Poorer outcomes have been associated with age greater than 10 years at diagnosis, underweight or overweight body mass index, African American race, and failure to achieve remission after the first course of induction therapy. Disease-related features may also play a role in predicting survival; children with AML of the M0 or M7 subtype (without Down syndrome) may have worse outcomes than other subtypes of AML.

Table 9-2 Cumulative Chemotherapy Doses and Related Outcomes[5]

Study	Cytarabine (g/m^2)	Etoposide (mg/m^2)	Anthracycline DE[a] (mg/m^2)	CR (%)	5-year EFS (%)	5-year OS (%)
AML-BFM93[b]	41.1	950	300-400	83	51	58
CCG2891[c]	14.6	1100	180	78	34	47
POG8821[d]	55.7	2250	360	77	31	42
St Jude-AML91	3.8	1200	270	79	44	57
UK MRC[e] AML10	10.6	500-1500	550	93	49	58
UK MRC AML12	4.6-34.6	1500	300-610	92	56	66

CR, complete response; DE, daunorubicin equivalent; EFS, event-free survival; OS, overall survival.

[a] Anthracycline DE (daunorubicin equivalents) based on the following conversions: doxorubicin:daunorubicin (1:1), idarubicin:daunorubicin (5:1), mitoxantrone:daunorubicin (5:1).
[b] BFM: Berlin-Frankfurt-Munster.
[c] CCG: Children's Cancer Group.
[d] POG: Pediatric Oncology Group.
[e] UK MRC: United Kingdom Medical Research Council.

Down Syndrome and AML

Children with Down syndrome have a 10- to 20-fold increased risk of developing leukemia compared to children without Down syndrome. At least 10% of newborn children with Down syndrome may develop transient myeloproliferative disorder (TMD). Abnormal blasts will spontaneously disappear and the blood count will normalize in the majority of patients with TMD; however, nearly 20% of patients with TMD will develop leukemia between the ages of 0 to 2 years.[14] The majority will develop the M7 subtype of AML, known as acute megakaryocytic leukemia, resulting in a 500-fold higher risk of developing acute megakaryocytic leukemia compared to children without Down syndrome.[14,15] Typically, children with Down syndrome and AML have a greater event-free survival rate and a lower relapse rate than children without Down syndrome. This enhanced response may be a result of the greater sensitivity to cytarabine and other types of chemotherapy. As a result, investigational efforts are aimed at minimizing the toxicities of chemotherapy while maintaining efficacy. In lieu of etoposide, children with Down syndrome and AML may receive thioguanine with standard-dose cytarabine and an anthracycline during induction and consolidation therapy.[14]

Acute Promyelocytic Leukemia

Children with the M3 subtype of AML, known also as acute promyelocytic leukemia (APL), receive therapy with all-*trans*-retinoic acid (ATRA, tretinoin) and have excellent complete remission rates of greater than 95%, 5-year event free survival rate over 70%, and overall survival rate of around 90%.[16-18] A small percentage of patients die during induction; nearly half as a result of APL-related coagulopathy and hemorrhagic complications. Early initiation of treatment with ATRA is recommended to achieve rapid disease control and to minimize hemorrhagic complications.

In more than 90% of all children with AML, at least one known genomic alteration can be detected. The acquisition of multiple genetic mutations or chromosomal rearrangements may result in abnormal hematopoietic precursors, which leads to impaired differentiation, apoptosis, and subsequent development of AML. In some patients, one or more of these and other abnormalities may be present, making prognostic prediction and treatment decisions difficult.[10] One of the more notable abnormalities currently under investigation is internal tandem duplications of *FLT3* (*FLT3* ITD). It is known that *FLT3* ITD portends unfavorable outcomes and is a strong predictor of relapse with event-free survival rates in the range of 7%-29%.[5] Current research efforts are directed toward identification of these mutations and targeted agents that may possess activity against them (eg, sorafenib activity against *FLT3* ITD). The reader is encouraged to seek additional resources for more detailed information.

LYMPHOMAS

After leukemias and CNS tumors, malignant lymphomas are the third most common group of malignancies in children. NHL comprise nearly two-thirds of all lymphomas in children.[1]

Hodgkin's Lymphoma

Hodgkin's lymphoma (HL) is well recognized as having a bimodal distribution; the first peak in adolescents and young adults (15-35 years of age) and the second later in adulthood (over 50 years of age).[19] Patients with HL commonly present with painless supraclavicular or cervical lymphadenopathy. Other signs and symptoms include generalized pruritus, fatigue, anorexia, weight loss, fever, and night sweats; the latter three symptoms are referred to as constitutional B symptoms and carry an unfavorable prognosis.

HL may present as 2 major histologic subtypes: nodular lymphocyte predominant HL and classical HL. Although many subtypes exist, the treatment is not based on the histologic subtype; rather, it is based on the clinical stage at diagnosis and the presence of B symptoms. Children and adolescents with HL are staged with the Ann Arbor staging classification, similar to adult patients with HL. Based on the clinical stage, patients will receive chemotherapy alone or in combination with involved-field radiation. Multiagent chemotherapy used in children varies based on stage but typically incorporates several of the following agents: doxorubicin, bleomycin, vincristine, vinblastine, procarbazine, cyclophosphamide, prednisone, etoposide, and mechlorethamine.

Prognosis following treatment for HL is excellent; at least 80% of children are expected to be cured of their disease. Relapsed disease is not common. Relapse within the first year after completion of initial therapy carries a poor prognosis; a relapse that occurs later is frequently salvageable with additional chemotherapy, radiation, and/or high-dose chemotherapy followed by stem cell transplantation.

HL is associated with a variety of late effects as a result of the chemotherapy and radiation employed in the treatment of the disease. Depending on the agents used, the patient may experience late effects such as pulmonary dysfunction, fertility complications, cardiac dysfunction, and secondary malignancies. Patients cured of their disease should receive long-term follow-up for late toxicities.

Non-Hodgkin's Lymphoma

All malignant lymphomas in children, exclusive of Hodgkin's lymphoma, are categorized as NHLs. Approximately 40% of lymphomas in children are Burkitt's or Burkitt's-like lymphomas while lymphoblastic lymphomas (precursor B-cell and precursor T-cell lymphoma) represent around 35% of NHL in children.[20,21] The most common subtype of the mature T-cell/natural killer-cell lymphoma subgroup is anaplastic large cell lymphoma (ALCL). Although ALCL is a rare tumor, recent investigations into the genetic basis of the disease have sparked interest in the t(2:5)(p23;q35) chromosomal rearrangement, also known as the *NPM-ALK* rearrangement.[20] This rearrangement is of particular interest due to the potential therapeutic role of crizotinib, a tyrosine kinase inhibitor that inhibits anaplastic lymphoma kinase (ALK).

As with adults, staging for NHL is based on the extent of disease spread. In children, the St. Jude Children's Research Hospital staging system is commonly used and categorizes disease in 4 stages based on the extent of spread from a single site of disease to diffuse spread including the CNS and/or bone marrow.[20] Treatment is based upon the subtype, stage, and extent of disease. Treatment may include surgery (eg, Burkitt's lymphoma of the gastrointestinal tract diagnosed during a ruling out of another nonmalignant process).[21] In general, NHLs are chemosensitive, and management with chemotherapy alone is commonplace. Agents with activity in childhood NHLs are similar to those used in adults and include cyclophosphamide, vincristine, corticosteroids (ie, prednisone), doxorubicin, etoposide, rituximab, and methotrexate (specifically, high-dose and intrathecal methotrexate).[20] See **Clinical Pearl 9-2** for specifics about administering rituximab in children. Because many of these tumors are rapidly growing, clinicians should pay close attention to the potential development of tumor lysis syndrome when initiating therapy. The predicted prognosis for all subtypes of NHLs is good; upwards of 80%-85% of children with NHLs will have long-term disease-free survival.[20,21]

CLINICAL PEARL 9-2
Rituximab Administration in Children

Rituximab administration in children is based on a mg/kg/hour rate, capping at the adult hourly rate (400 mg/hour)

- An initial dose may commonly be infused at 0.5 mg/kg/hour (maximum of 50 mg/hour) and titrated at 1 mg/kg/hour up to a maximum of 400 mg/hour
- Subsequent infusions could start at 1 mg/kg/hour with similar maximum hourly rate as in previous bullet point
- More rapid infusions have not been studied in children (unpublished observation, authors)

CENTRAL NERVOUS SYSTEM TUMORS

CNS tumors as a group are the second most common malignancy in children and the most common solid tumor in children. Types of CNS tumors seen in children are identified in **Box 9-2**.[22]

BOX 9-2
Malignant Central Nervous System Tumors of Childhood[22]

Gliomas[a]

Embryonal tumors[b]

Craniopharyngiomas

Choroid plexus tumors

Germ cell tumors

[a] Includes low-grade astrocytomas, malignant/high-grade gliomas (eg, diffuse pontine gliomas), and ependymomas.

[b] Includes medulloblastomas, atypical teratoid rhabdoid tumors, and central nervous system primitive neuroectodermal tumors.

The management of CNS tumors in general will be reviewed; the management of each specific tumor will not be discussed. The reader is encouraged to seek other references for additional details in pediatric oncology, particularly textbooks edited by Pizzo and Poplack and by Lanzkowsky.[6,7]

Children with CNS tumors may present with a variety of signs and symptoms, some of which include vomiting, visual changes, seizures, speech alterations, and endocrine abnormalities. Vomiting may be associated with increased intracranial pressure (ICP); children with increased ICP may require high-dose dexamethasone to reduce the edema surrounding the tumor. If the increased ICP is a result of obstructive hydrocephalus, an external ventricular drain or ventriculoperitoneal shunt may be required. Patients with endocrine abnormalities may require supplemental therapy based on the type and extent of the endocrinopathy.

The management of CNS tumors typically includes surgery, radiation, and chemotherapy. The goal of surgery is to obtain a histologic diagnosis and gross total resection. In some patients, the location and size of the tumor may prevent total resection; in others, the location and size of the tumor may prevent surgery altogether. Radiation therapy is used for a variety of CNS tumors, and it is associated with acute and late toxicities that vary based on the site and extent of the area irradiated. Chemotherapy is useful in some types of CNS tumors of childhood, though the number of effective agents is limited due to the presence and activity of the blood–brain barrier.[22] Agents commonly utilized in brain tumor protocols include carboplatin, cisplatin, lomustine, vincristine, temozolomide, vorinostat, and high-dose methotrexate.[22,23] Attempts have been made to administer chemotherapy using creative approaches to overcome the effect of the blood–brain barrier; examples include intrathecal chemotherapy, intratumoral chemotherapy, high-dose chemotherapy (with stem cell rescue), and combination chemotherapy with or without agents that are known to disrupt the blood–brain barrier (eg, mannitol).[23]

Children with long-term survival following diagnosis with a CNS tumor are at an increased risk of a variety of late effects such as neurocognitive deficits, depression, and endocrine abnormalities. Long-term follow-up recommendations are reviewed later in this chapter.

COMMON SOLID TUMORS OF CHILDHOOD

Neuroblastoma

Neuroblastoma is one of the most common solid tumors of childhood, representing 8%-10% of all childhood cancers and a disproportionate 15% of deaths from childhood cancer. Survival from neuroblastoma varies greatly based on the disease stratification. Patients with low or intermediate risk disease have a much higher chance of long-term survival compared to those with high-risk disease. Historically, overall survival was achievable in less than 40% of patients with high-risk disease, despite aggressive multimodal therapy with induction chemotherapy, surgery, radiation, purged autologous stem cell transplantation, and maintenance therapy with isotretinoin.[24] Several chemotherapeutic agents possess activity in the disease state; these agents are presented in **Table 9-3**.

Recently, results from a multi-institutional phase III clinical trial indicate that survival may be augmented with the addition of targeted immunotherapy to

Table 9-3 Active Chemotherapeutic Agents in the Treatment of Neuroblastoma

Induction Chemotherapy	Transplantation	Salvage
Vincristine	Carboplatin	Topotecan
Doxorubicin	Etoposide	Cyclophosphamide
Cyclophosphamide	Busulfan	Irinotecan
Cisplatin	Melphalan	Temozolomide
Carboplatin		
Etoposide		
Ifosfamide		

isotretinoin in the maintenance phase. Immunotherapy consisted of 5 courses of therapy with the ch14.18 monoclonal antibody against the GD2 receptor located on neuroblastoma cells. Aldesleukin or granulocyte-macrophage colony-stimulating factor (GM-CSF) was added to ch14.18 in an alternating fashion from one course to the next. Although survival was increased in the group receiving additional immunotherapy, this cohort of patients experienced significant toxicities including pain, fever, hypersensitivity reactions, capillary leak syndrome, hypokalemia, hyponatremia, and elevations in liver transaminases.[25] As a result of the positive preliminary data, additional studies are under way to further characterize the toxicity profile of this promising therapy.[26]

Wilms' Tumor

Approximately 500 new cases of Wilms' tumor are diagnosed each year in the United States; the vast majority of which occur in children less than 5 years of age.[27] Cooperative group clinical trials for the treatment of Wilms' tumor date back to 1969 with the creation of the National Wilms' Tumor Study (NWTS). Since that time, successive clinical trials have increased the overall survival for Wilms' tumor of all types from less than 30% to more than 90%. The NWTS group is now part of COG. Historical clinical trials executed by the NWTS group highlight the success of cooperative group clinical trials in the understanding of and treatment of this tumor. Currently, ongoing clinical trials are evaluating a variety of patient- and disease-related factors for treatment outcomes and prognosis; some of the factors include age at diagnosis, tumor size, histology (favorable or unfavorable/anaplastic), initial response to therapy, and chromosome 1p and 16q allelic status.

Rhabdomyosarcoma

Rhabdomyosarcoma is the most common type of soft tissue sarcoma in children less than 15 years old. It accounts for approximately 4%-6% of all childhood cancers and has a peak incidence in children less than 5 years old. The most common sites of presentation include the head or neck, the genitourinary tract, and the extremities.[28]

Contemporary treatment for rhabdomyosarcoma is based on the patient's risk category at diagnosis. Treatment for all patients, regardless of presentation, will include surgery, chemotherapy, and in most cases, radiation therapy. In the United States, the most commonly employed standard treatment regimen is triplet therapy with vincristine, actinomycin D, and cyclophosphamide

(VAC). Approaches under clinical investigation in the United States include doublet therapy with vincristine and actinomycin D (VA) in lower risk patients and vincristine plus irinotecan (VI) doublet therapy as an up-front window treatment in high-risk patients prior to VAC. Other agents under investigation for recurrent disease include oral metronomic cyclophosphamide with intravenous vinorelbine, temsirolimus, and bevacizumab.

Osteosarcoma

Osteosarcoma is the most common malignant bone tumor in children and adolescents. Osteosarcoma has a peak incidence during the second decade of life and occurs slightly more often in males than females. Children in families with the Li-Fraumeni cancer syndrome are at an increased risk of developing osteosarcoma; up to 3% of children with osteosarcoma have a germ line mutation in p53. Patients commonly present with dull, aching pain in the limb; up to 15% of patients may also present with a pathologic fracture. Around 80% of patients present with a primary tumor in the distal extremities (ie, the proximal tibia, proximal humerus, or distal femur). Nearly 80% of patients present with localized disease at diagnosis; these patients have a long-term survival rate of 60%-70%. Of the 20% who present with metastatic disease, the major site of metastases is the lungs; these patients have an overall survival rate of only 20%.[29]

Treatment includes neoadjuvant chemotherapy with high-dose methotrexate and leucovorin rescue alternating with cisplatin and doxorubicin. After up to 3 months of systemic therapy, surgery is performed for local control. The extent of tumor necrosis from neoadjuvant chemotherapy at the time of surgery is an important prognostic indicator; patients with at least 90% tumor necrosis are defined as good responders and will receive several additional months of adjuvant chemotherapy (same agents as given in the neoadjuvant setting) after surgery. For poor responders with less than 90% tumor necrosis, additional agents may be added in an alternating fashion with the agents used in the neoadjuvant setting.

Ewing's Sarcoma

Ewing's sarcoma (ES) is a peripheral primitive neuroectodermal tumor (PNET) in the Ewing's sarcoma family of tumors (ESFT). ES is the second most common bone tumor in children.[30] In the United States, 250-400 patients are diagnosed with ES each year, with close to 80% of cases occurring in children.[31] ES most commonly occurs in the second decade of life with a peak age at initial diagnosis of 15 years.[31] Like osteosarcoma, Ewing's sarcoma has a slightly higher incidence in male compared to female patients.[30] It is also much more common in white, Caucasian children than in other ethnicities. ES typically arises from the bone; however, it may also arise from the soft tissue surrounding the bone.[31] Like osteosarcoma, the most common site of metastasis is the lung followed by metastases in the bone marrow and bone.[30,31]

The treatment of ES includes multiagent, combination chemotherapy regardless of the extent of disease at presentation. Patients with localized disease should also receive local control with radiation, surgery, or both.[30,31] The most commonly used regimen for pediatric patients in the United States is outlined in **Table 9-4**. The prognosis for children with nonmetastatic disease at presentation is much better than the prognosis for children with metastatic disease at presentation. Children with recurrent ES have a dismal prognosis with a 5-year event-free survival rate at merely 10% of patients.[30] Chemotherapy for recurrent disease may include topotecan with cyclophosphamide, irinotecan with temozolomide, and a variety of investigational or targeted agents.[30,31]

Retinoblastoma

Retinoblastoma is the most common primary intraocular malignancy in children in the United States. The majority of cases are diagnosed by 3 or 4 years of age, with the median being diagnosed by 2 years of life. Like many other childhood cancers, survival rates have improved over the past few decades, with current survival estimates as high as 99% in developed countries. In developing countries, survival rates are much lower due to later detection of the tumor and a subsequent reduction in prognosis associated with more advanced disease.[32]

Table 9-4 Chemotherapy for Ewing's Sarcoma[30,31]

Disease at Diagnosis	Regimen	Survival Estimate
Localized	VDC alternating with IE Cycles alternate every 2 weeks with G-CSF support	91%[a]
Metastatic	VDC alternating with IE Cycles alternate every 2 weeks with G-CSF support	
	VDC Cycles given every 2-3 weeks	

VDC: vincristine, doxorubicin, cyclophosphamide; IE: ifosfamide, etoposide
[a] 4-year overall survival time

Leukokoria and strabismus are the 2 most common presenting signs of retino-blastoma.[33] Further work-up for retinoblastoma should occur for patients with either of these conditions.

The treatment of retinoblastoma depends upon the extent of disease at presentation; however, multimodal therapy is used in all patients. Modalities employed include chemotherapy, cryotherapy, brachytherapy, transpupillary thermotherapy, external beam radiation (EBR), and enucleation. Because many patients with retinoblastoma may have an increased risk of second malignancies due to germ line mutations, contemporary protocols have sought to minimize the use of EBR due to its association with secondary malignancies. The triple combination of intravenous carboplatin, etoposide, and vincristine is commonly employed in the management of children with retinoblastoma. More recently, some investigators have added intra-arterial chemotherapy or subtenon carboplatin (periocular administration of carboplatin into the episcleral space beyond the Tenon's capsule and sclera of the eye) to this regimen for more advanced disease.[32]

SUPPORTIVE CARE

As with adult patients, children may experience a variety of toxicities as a result of antineoplastic therapy. The specific areas of supportive care, which will be addressed here, include chemotherapy-induced nausea and vomiting and bone marrow support. Description and management of other supportive care issues encountered in pediatric oncology are detailed elsewhere (see *Handbook of Supportive Care in Pediatric Oncology*).[3]

CHEMOTHERAPY-INDUCED NAUSEA AND VOMITING

Chemotherapy-induced nausea and vomiting (CINV) is a troubling side effect for children with cancer and their caregivers. The emetogenicity of single agents has not been as widely studied or characterized in children as it has been in adults. Little data is available regarding the use of some of the newer agents (eg, palonosetron, aprepitant) in children of all ages with cancer.[34,35] Of the older agents used for CINV, promethazine, prochlorperazine, and metoclopramide have been associated with adverse toxicities in children.[35] Specifically, children less than 2 years of age should not be given promethazine due to the risk of potentially fatal respiratory depression; this adverse event is noted as a black box warning in the package insert.[36] Prochlorperazine and metoclopramide have been associated with extrapyramidal side effects (EPS); these effects have been reported to be more common in children than in adults. An antihistamine, such as diphenhydramine, can be used to mitigate EPS.[37]

BONE MARROW SUPPORT

A child with cancer should receive empiric growth factor support based on the individual treatment or clinical protocol, which frequently mirrors guidelines published for adult patients. Filgrastim, pegfilgrastim, and sargramostim have all been used in children with cancer. Application of topical anesthetics (eg, lidocaine and prilocaine) 30-60 minutes prior to subcutaneous injections of these agents is routine to decrease pain. Of special note, pegfilgrastim is commercially available only as a 6 mg/0.6 mL single-dose prefilled syringe.[38] Older children weighing at least 45 kg may be eligible to receive the full syringe dose, and the most widely studied dose in patients weighing less than 45 kg is 100 mcg/kg (capping at the adult dose).[39] The appropriate dosing volume for children less than 45 kg should be drawn into a syringe using appropriate aseptic technique. For some patients, receiving doses of pegfilgrastim less than 6 mg may present a logistical problem with regards to insurance coverage and reimbursement.

Lastly, cancer- and chemotherapy-induced anemia is managed differently in children compared to adult patients. Erythropoiesis-stimulating agents (ESAs) are not commonly used in the pediatric setting; rather, blood transfusions are more commonly used when indicated.[40] If a provider elects to use an ESA, he or she would be required to follow the steps in the APPRISE (Assisting Providers and Cancer Patients with Risk Information for the Safe use of ESAs) program as would be required for any adult patient, and prescribed doses of these agents in children mirror those for adults.[41] (see Drug Safety and Risk Management chapter more information on ESA risk and evaluation mitigation strategies program).

SURVIVORSHIP AND LONG-TERM TOXICITIES

Cure from cancer is a realization for almost 80% of pediatric patients. Thus, a shift in focus from a patient's primary cancer to late-occurring toxicities and secondary malignancies begins 5-10 years from the end of the therapy for the primary cancer. One of the most serious late-occurring effects is a secondary malignancy, which is most commonly associated with alkylating, anthracycline, and epipodophyllotoxin chemotherapy as well as radiation therapy. Long-term toxicities, those occurring during or shortly after therapy cessation and continuing past the end of cancer treatment, are frequent and can be serious, although many are modifiable with appropriate monitoring and early intervention.[42] The reader is referred to the Children's Oncology Group Long-Term Follow-Up Guidelines for Survivors of Childhood, Adolescent, and Young Adult Cancers (www.survivorshipguidelines.org) for comprehensive information on screening recommendation and toxicity management for late effects, including information specifically written for patients and families.[43]

SPECIAL DOSING CONSIDERATIONS

Some of the features of chemotherapy unique to the pediatric population are discussed in **Table 9-5**.

Table 9-5 Unique Features of Chemotherapy in the Pediatric Population

Agent(s)	Unique Features
Asparaginase products	• Pegylated and *Erwinia asparaginase* products available; *Escherichia coli* asparaginase was discontinued in early 2013
	• Most contemporary ALL protocols use pegaspargase as front-line agent due to superior antitumor efficacy and reduced toxicity compared to L-asparaginase
	• Some protocols use L-asparaginase as part of a Capizzi cytarabine arm
	• Erwinia asparaginase reserved for patients with hypersensitivity reaction to pegaspargase; may be less effective and requires additional injections to achieve an equivalent dose
	• Routine premedication or fibrinogen replacement not included in pediatric protocols
	• Consult protocol for recommendations on when to hold or resume therapy for children with pancreatitis
Carboplatin	• Dosing techniques vary among protocols
	• Options may include the following:
	o Standard dosing by mg/m^2 or mg/kg
	o Alternate dosing by AUC. One of the following formulas may be used, based on experience in the particular tumor type:
	▪ Kushner
	▪ Mann
	▪ Marina
	▪ Newell/modified Calvert
	▪ Pinkerton

Cisplatin	• Brainstem auditory evoked response may be performed in children too young or impaired to participate in an audiogram • Children with variants of the TPMT gene (*TPMT*3B* and *TPMT*3C*) are at an increased risk of cisplatin-induced ototoxicity
Dactinomycin	• May cause sinusoidal obstruction syndrome
Daunorubicin, doxorubicin, idarubicin	• Cooperative group clinical trials are designed to keep cumulative anthracycline dose below the standard threshold • In children, cardiomyopathy typically measured by the SF, whereas EF is more commonly used in adult patients • For doxorubicin: Some protocols include instructions for converting from bolus to continuous infusion anthracycline, or from either of the prior to bolus with dexrazoxane when a patient meets a certain dose level and/or is at a specific level or percent reduction in SF
Dexamethasone, prednisone, prednisolone	• Steroids are a critically important part of therapy for children with leukemia and lymphoma. Ensure the patient has filled his or her prescription or has definitive access to the medication upon discharge to prevent gaps in therapy • Gastric prophylaxis may be used in patients receiving high doses of steroids as anticancer therapy (eg, induction therapy for ALL) • Consult the protocol prior to converting from one agent to the other to ensure that a substitution is appropriate per protocol • Steroids are often avoided in children with brain tumors due to the theoretical risk of reducing the CNS penetration of chemotherapy
Etoposide	• Standard blood pressure norms for children differ from adults and vary among age levels. The age-related norm and the patient-specific baseline should be used when determining whether the patient has become hypotensive as a result of etoposide
Ifosfamide	• Hyperhydration and mesna should be incorporated with all doses • Fanconi-like electrolyte wasting may occur, especially with higher doses and prolonged exposure as seen in sarcoma protocols. Monitor serum sodium, potassium, and phosphorus, and replace as necessary • Neurotoxicity possible due to accumulation of toxic metabolite
Isotretinoin	• Must be obtained through the iPledge program. Most patients will be eligible to obtain the agent through the route for patients of nonchildbearing potential • Counsel caregivers administering the agent to children about the potential adverse reactions and pregnancy considerations associated with the agent

(continues)

Table 9-5 Unique Features of Chemotherapy in the Pediatric Population (*continued*)

Irinotecan	• Oral irinotecan may be administered in some regimens. To achieve this, the injectable product is drawn into oral syringes and mixed with cranberry juice just prior to administration to mask the flavor • Oral cefixime or cefpodoxime is used in many protocols to minimize irinotecan-associated diarrhea and to increase accumulation of the active metabolite • Oral atropine and loperamide are commonly prescribed for diarrhea associated with irinotecan
Mercaptopurine, thioguanine	• Oral doses should be administered at night. Do not give with food or milk • When given in maintenance for ALL, titrate dose to target ANC per protocol • Check TPMT status for children with prolonged or unexpected myelosuppression. Some protocols recommend up-front testing and empiric dose reductions for children with deficiencies in 6-thioguanine and 6-mercaptopurine metabolism • Thioguanine: May cause sinusoidal obstruction syndrome or similar toxicities
Methotrexate	• Leucovorin rescue and alkalinized intravenous fluids should be given with all intermediate and high doses of methotrexate. Leucovorin doses > 25 mg should be given intravenously • Glucarpidase should be considered in the setting of excessively delayed clearance despite leucovorin and fluid rescue • Two doses of oral leucovorin should be given at hours 48 and 60 after methotrexate-containing intrathecal therapy to children with Down syndrome and ALL in all phases of therapy except maintenance • When given orally in maintenance for ALL, titrate the dose to target ANC per protocol
Vincristine	• Neurotoxicity measured and managed based on Balis scale. Jaw pain and foot drop may be some of the first signs of neurotoxicity • Prophylaxis against constipation is generally recommended due to serial dosing of vincristine in most protocols
Rasburicase	• Rasburicase should be used on a risk-based approach as published without using a capped dose[4] • When rasburicase use is needed urgently and G6PD status is unknown, the family history of anemia and food allergies should be assessed to determine if G6PD deficiency is present/possible

Abbreviations: ALL, acute lymphoblastic leukemia; ANC, absolute neutrophil count; AUC, area under the curve; CNS, central nervous system; EF; ejection fraction; G6PD, glucose-6-phosphate dehydrogenase; SF, shortening fraction; TPMT, thiopurine methyltransferase.

FLUID MANAGEMENT

Fluid management is a critical component in the care of children receiving chemotherapy. A stepwise approach may be used for anticipating and providing intravenous (IV) fluids to children receiving chemotherapy, particularly in the inpatient setting. In adult patients, standard IV dosing volumes and premixed bags such as 250 mL, 500 mL, or even 1000 mL can be used to dilute chemotherapy. This practice is not always practical in children; large volumes of chemotherapy over short time periods are unsuitable for younger and smaller children. Refer to the checklist in **Table 9-6** for details on how to estimate maintenance fluid requirements and fluid requirements for chemotherapy dilution.

Table 9-6 Fluid Management Checklist

Step	Questions to Consider
1. Calculate the maintenance IV fluid rate	• Should the fluid requirement be calculated based on the Holliday-Segar[44] or body surface area method? • Does the patient's treatment or research protocol state which method should be used?
2. Determine whether the patient requires fluids less than or in excess of the maintenance fluid rate. Adjust the hourly rate accordingly	• Does the patient have any sensible or insensible losses? • Does the patient have any conditions that may require adjustment of the fluid rate (eg, tumor lysis syndrome, renal failure)? • Will the patient be receiving chemotherapy that could benefit from hyperhydration (eg, high-dose methotrexate)? • Is the patient receiving fluids from any other source?
3. Ensure the hourly fluid rate is maintained, even when chemotherapy is infusing	• Will the nurse stop IV fluids to infuse chemotherapy or will they run concomitantly? • Is chemotherapy diluted to an appropriate volume in an appropriate fluid to ensure the appropriate level of hydration?
4. Check electrolytes	• Is the electrolyte makeup of the IV fluid appropriate for patient age, size, and clinical status? • Do any electrolytes need to be added or removed based on the patient's clinical status? • Do any electrolytes need to be added or removed in anticipation of wasting or sparing caused by the chemotherapy? • Does the patient have appropriate venous access for the prescribed IV fluid with added electrolytes?
5. Follow laboratory parameters	• How frequently should the electrolytes, urine-specific gravity, urine pH, or other parameters for these fluids or for the treatment protocol be checked?

IV, intravenous.

Note that some patients are appropriately able to consume oral fluids; in these situations it may be appropriate to use oral fluid hydration. In all situations, the treatment or research protocol should be consulted for additional information.

CHEMOTHERAPY DOSING IN INFANTS

The approach to dosing anticancer therapy in infants and young children is a unique challenge. Very little is known about anticancer therapy pharmacokinetics in premature, newborn, and infant patients. These patients have developmentally related differences in renal function, hepatic function, gastric acid production, and total body water compared with older children and adults. These differences contribute significantly to drug absorption, metabolism, and excretion. Some of the differences are highlighted in **Table 9-7**.[45] Several clinical trials have revealed an increased risk of chemotherapy-related toxicities in infants when chemotherapy is dosed based on using a body surface area calculation as is used in older children and adults. Some of the toxicities noted include enhanced vincristine-related neurotoxicity, pronounced chemotherapy-related myelosuppression from triplet therapy of vincristine, dactinomycin, and doxorubicin, marked dactinomycin-related hepatotoxicity, and enhanced acute toxicity (eg, electrolyte wasting with cisplatin).

Table 9-7 Developmental Challenges in Infant Dosing[45]

Parameter	Age-Related Differences in Neonates and Infants
Total body water	Increased total body water compared to older children/adults • Infants: 60%-75% of total body weight • Older children/adults: 50%-60% of total body weight Decreased extracellular water compared to older children/adults • Infants: up to 45% of total body weight, decreases to 25%-30% by 12 months of life • Older children/adults: ~ 20% of total body weight *Impact*: variable exposure to chemotherapy based on drug properties

Hepatic function	Decreased bile acid metabolism Variable enzyme activity; pertinent examples include: • CYP2D6: 50% present at 30 days after birth, fully developed by age 3-6 months • CYP3A4: appears during the first week after birth; full activity by age 3 months • NAT2: adult levels by 3-4 years old *Impact*: alterations in hepatic activation or detoxification, potentially leading to variations in efficacy and/or toxicity
Renal function	Decreased renal blood flow Decreased glomerular filtration rate Decreased ability to concentrate/acidify urine Underdeveloped organic ion/active transport *Impact*: decreased renal elimination and increased half-life of certain agents
Gastric absorption	Decreased gastric pH Prolonged gastric emptying time *Impact*: alterations in absorption of oral chemotherapy
Protein binding	Decreased binding capacity due to the following: • Presence of fetal albumin • Decreased plasma albumin and total protein • Competition for binding sites with other protein-bound substances (eg, bilirubin) • Lower blood pH *Impact*: higher volume of distribution
Blood–brain barrier	Increased permeability of blood–brain barrier, possibly as a result of the following: • Incomplete myelination • Decreased CNS p-glycoprotein efflux pump activity *Impact*: Increased presence of chemotherapy in the CNS leading to increased exposure/toxicity
CSF, spinal cord, brain tissue quantity	Increased size and volume compared to older children relative to BSA *Impact*: variable exposure vs other populations if dose based on BSA

BSA, body surface area; CSF, cerebral spinal fluid; CNS, central nervous system; CYP, cytochrome; NAT2, n = -acetyltransferase 2.

In order to reduce severe chemotherapy-related toxicities in the infant population, empiric dose modification strategies have been recommended. The most widely used dose reduction strategy involves a conversion from a body surface area dose (mg/m²) to a dose per body weight (mg/kg) calculation. Investigators have proposed that infants (children less than 12 months of age) receive chemotherapy using a dose based on body weight (mg/kg) (see **Clinical Pearl 9-3**). This dose reduction has also been suggested for body weight less than 6-12 kilograms regardless of age, depending on the protocol and agents employed (unpublished observation, authors). The dose per body weight (mg/kg) is typically derived by dividing the dose based on BSA (mg/m²) by a factor of 30; this factor is extrapolated based on the estimation that an average 1 m² patient would weigh approximately 30 kilograms.[46]

CLINICAL PEARL 9-3
Dosing

The dose per body weight (mg/kg) for infants is derived by dividing the dose based on BSA (mg/m²) by a factor of 30.

Example:
What should be the dose of vincristine for a 9-month-old infant weighing 9 kg who is 27 inches with a BSA = 0.41 m²?
Vincristine is normally dosed at 1.5 mg/m².

Using mg/kg dosing:
Step 1: 1.5 mg/m² divided by 30 = 0.05 mg/kg
Step 2: 0.05 mg × 9 kg = 0.45 mg
Dose = 0.45 mg (correct answer)

Using mg/m² dosing:
1.5 mg × 0.41 = 0.615 mg (round dose to 0.62 mg since 0.615 mg not measurable in a 1-mL syringe)
Dose = 0.62 mg (incorrect answer)

The mg/m² dosing calculation would have resulted in an approximate 1.5 × increase in dose compared to the mg/kg calculation and may attribute to increased toxicity.

OBESE CHILDREN

Very little is known about the pharmacokinetics of anticancer agents in obese children. What is known is that obese children, as well as malnourished children, do not tolerate chemotherapy as well as children of normal weight and as a result have reduced outcomes. Moreover, a recent study with a limited patient population suggested that doxorubicinol, but not doxorubicin, clearance was reduced in obese patients with more than 30% body fat.[47] Additional research is needed in this area before any official recommendations can be made.

CASE 9-1
Pediatric Oncology

RW is a 3-year-old male with newly diagnosed B-cell ALL. He is determined to be standard risk and is scheduled to start induction chemotherapy tomorrow consisting of dexamethasone, vincristine, and PEG-L-asparaginase in addition to intrathecal chemotherapy. RW is 38 inches tall, weighs 35 pounds, and his laboratory analysis is unremarkable except for potassium = 5.2 mEq/L, phosphorus = 6.5 mg/dL, uric acid = 7.2 mg/dL, LDH = 970 units/L, and WBC = $28.2 \times 10^3/mm^3$. He has no known drug or food allergies.

1. Based on the height and weight stated, how will you use these values to calculate RW's chemotherapy doses?
2. Based on RW's diagnosis and laboratory values, he is at greatest risk for which oncologic emergency?
3. What preventive measures should be employed in RW to prevent such an oncologic emergency?
4. What are the goals of induction therapy in RW?
5. Which supportive care medications should RW receive during his induction therapy?

OUTPATIENT PEDIATRIC ONCOLOGY

Medication Errors in the Outpatient Setting

As previously mentioned in this chapter, the most common malignancy in children is ALL. The management of ALL involves extensive outpatient chemotherapy, including the use of oral chemotherapy in the home setting. A published prospective case series of children with ALL treated at a large tertiary care center revealed nearly 10% of all chemotherapeutic agents used in the outpatient setting were associated with either a prescribing or administration-related medication error.[48] Only oral agents used in the home setting as administered by the caregiver for antileukemic effect were evaluated. Compliance was not assessed. This error rate corresponds with at least one chemotherapy-related medication error in nearly 19% of all patients evaluated. Of the medication errors that were identified, more than two-thirds (70%) were categorized by investigators as administration errors. Agents involved in these errors included mercaptopurine, methotrexate, prednisone, and dexamethasone. Of the errors associated with corticosteroid administration, the mean discrepancy between the prescribed dose and the administered dose was approximately 15.4%. The remaining errors were identified as prescribing errors and involved mercaptopurine, methotrexate, and dexamethasone. Each of the prescribing errors was characterized as a miscalculated dose; a mean difference of 22% was discovered between the intended and prescribed dose for this group. No pharmacy dispensing errors were noted in the sample, although the authors note that the majority of prescriptions were filled by pharmacists at the tertiary care center who are familiar with the protocols and doses used in the treatment of the sample patients. Although limitations may be inherent in the study, the results should not be ignored; significant potential exists for administration errors in the outpatient management of children with ALL. Healthcare professionals have a unique opportunity to work with caregivers to ensure that medications used in the home setting are accurately administered. See **Table 9-8** for recommended steps in reviewing inpatient or outpatient intravenous anticancer therapy orders in pediatrics. These steps will help minimize the potential for medication errors.

Oral Chemotherapy Formulations

Medication errors in the outpatient setting may be partially attributed to the limited availability of appropriate ready-to-administer anticancer agents. Pediatric patients vary substantially in size and developmental level across age groups.

Table 9-8 Inpatient or Outpatient IV Anticancer Therapy in Pediatrics—
Chemotherapy Order Checklist

Step	Questions to Consider
1. Check for treatment consent	• Has the patient and/or caregiver given appropriate consent to the prescribed treatment regimen? • If the patient is enrolled on a particular protocol, is the protocol number listed and is access to the protocol and associated treatment plans available?
2. Check patient demographic and vital information	• Is the height and weight listed on the order form current? • Is the height and weight measured and listed in appropriate units (preferably height in cm and weight in kg)? • Is the BSA calculation correct and does it appear appropriate for the patient age? • If the patient is significantly above or below ideal body weight, is an adjusted body weight being used in dosing calculations? If so, are adjusted weight and BSA calculated correctly? • Is the patient an infant (age less than 12 months) or does the patient weigh less than 6-12 kg? If so, dosing should be calculated based on dose per body weight (mg/kg), in most cases
3. Check for necessary and appropriate pretreatment tests, laboratory analysis, and other requirements	• Has the patient received a pregnancy test (if a postmenarcheal female)? Alternately, has the patient received counseling for appropriate contraceptive use? • Does the patient have adequate renal function to receive chemotherapy at the prescribed doses? For some patients, this is specifically measured by a 12- or 24-hour urine collection for creatinine clearance calculation • Does the patient have adequate liver function to receive chemotherapy at the prescribed doses? • Does the patient have adequate blood counts to receive chemotherapy? • Has the patient received or will he or she receive appropriate IV fluids prior to starting chemotherapy? For some patients, a specific urine output, urine-specific gravity and/or urinary pH need to be met before starting chemotherapy • Has the patient had a recent ECHO if he or she is to receive an anthracycline? • If electrolytes need repletion prior to starting chemotherapy, has this been done appropriately?
4. Check fluid, chemotherapy, ancillary medication, and laboratory orders	• Are the treatment phase or cycle as well as day number indicated on the order and does this match the treatment plan in the medical record? • Are pre-, peri-, and posttreatment fluid orders calculated appropriately in relation to the patient's maintenance fluid needs? Are electrolytes included or excluded as appropriate?

- Are chemotherapy doses calculated correctly in relation to the patient's weight and/or BSA?
- If dose rounding occurs, does it align with protocol guidelines or institutional policies?
- If a chemotherapy dose adjustment is made, is it clear as to why it is being done, and is the adjusted dose correctly calculated?
- Are chemotherapy agents prescribed in the correct order, if applicable, in relation to one another and/or radiation therapy?
- Does the patient have the appropriate venous access to receive the chemotherapy as ordered and dispensed?
- If the patient is unable to swallow solid dosage forms, are liquid formulations available?
- Are necessary supportive care medications ordered with the chemotherapy such as antiemetics, mouth care regimen, prophylactic growth factors and prophylactic antibiotics?
- Have orders been checked for drug–drug interactions?
- If medications are contraindicated during chemotherapy, have these medications been appropriately held or discontinued?
- Are necessary laboratory values ordered to adequately monitor the patient for treatment toxicity?
- Are drug levels, if applicable, ordered appropriately along with any necessary interventions or ancillary therapies?

5. Check discharge orders	• Has the patient met the criteria for discharge including completion of posttherapy hydration and laboratory analysis?
	• Is it okay to resume medications that needed to be held during chemotherapy?
	• Does the patient have prescriptions for all prescribed medications that are to be continued at home? Do these prescriptions match what is prescribed in the treatment protocol?

BSA, body surface area; ECHO, echocardiogram; IV, intravenous.

Many anticancer agents are only available in solid dosage forms that are too high in dose per unit, even at the smallest dosage unit, and must be manipulated into a compounded oral suspension. Complicating matters, not all oral agents have a published recipe for a suspension; for those agents that have a recipe available, there is frequently limited stability or bioavailability data.[49] As an example, lomustine is frequently used in the management of various brain tumors in children. These children may either be too young to swallow the necessary number of capsules or may have an impaired ability to swallow. The latter type of patient will frequently require oral medication administration via gastric tube. Unfortunately, lomustine is insoluble in water and is only soluble in absolute alcohol or 10% ethanol, impairing its ability to be prepared as an oral suspension suitable for children. Complicating matters even more, agents with limited or no stability data must be prepared extemporaneously in the home by the caregiver, potentially exposing the caregiver to harmful antineoplastic agents. There is a great need for additional research in the area of extemporaneous preparation and safe handling of anticancer agents, particularly for pediatric patients and their caregivers.

Outpatient Pediatric Oncology

Children who survive following therapy for the treatment of a malignancy should receive long-term follow-up on a regular, predetermined schedule by clinicians familiar with the treatment and pertinent toxicities associated with the therapy received. In the time period immediately following the completion of therapy, patients should receive close follow-up for disease recurrence and any immediate toxicities. For many patients, long-term follow-up may include one or more of the following: cardiac monitoring, renal function assessment, hepatic function assessment, bone scans and evaluation, and psychological assessments.

CASE 9-1
Answers

1. Since RW is not an infant, his chemotherapy doses should be calculated based on his body surface area. Body surface area (BSA) calculations in pediatric patients mirror those for adults, with the Mosteller formula being the most widely used. Height and weight for chemotherapy orders are best expressed in metric measurements (cm and kg, respectively) although the US customary system of inches and pounds can be used to calculate BSA with the corresponding formula. Using the Mosteller formula and metric measurements of 96.5 cm and 15.9 kg, RW's BSA = $(96.5 \times 15.9)^{1/2}/60 = 0.65$ m^2.

2. RW is at the greatest risk for developing tumor lysis syndrome (TLS). He has been diagnosed with ALL and has elevations in WBC, potassium, phosphorus, and LDH. It should be noted that

young children have different normal limits to their laboratory values from adults. Particularly, his phosphorus is only slightly above the upper limit of normal for his age.

3. The following measures are recommended to decrease the likelihood for development of TLS in RW:

   • Infuse IVF at a rate of 1.5 to 2 times maintenance fluid rate with a target urine output of > 3 mL/kg/hour
   • Remove electrolytes from IVF and discontinue oral electrolyte supplements
   • Avoid or limit the use of nephrotoxic medications
   • Administer one dose of rasburicase and monitor the need for additional doses
   • Monitor labs every 6-8 hours as appropriate
   • Urinary alkalinization is not recommended with the use of rasburicase

4. Induction chemotherapy goals are to induce a morphologic remission and restore normal hematopoiesis.

5. In addition to TLS preventative measures, it is suggested RW receive the following:

   • Gastric prophylaxis in conjunction with dexamethasone
   • Prophylaxis against constipation due to vincristine
   • Antiemetics to prevent chemotherapy-induced nausea/vomiting associated with mild emetogenic potential agents (vincristine and intrathecal therapies)
   • Antimicrobial prophylaxis directed against *Pneumocystis jiroveci* (other antimicrobial prophylaxis is not generally recommended)
   • The routine use of growth factors is not generally recommended

SUMMARY

Despite their rarity and heterogeneity, pediatric cancers are treatable with cure being a reasonable expectation and outcome. The accomplishments realized in the field of pediatric oncology are a result of decades of collaborative work by multidisciplinary teams of healthcare practitioners around the world. Efforts are continuing by these practitioners to achieve a cure rate of 100% in all childhood cancers while minimizing short- and long-term effects of cancer treatments.

REFERENCES

1. American Cancer Society. *Cancer Facts & Figures 2012.* Atlanta, GA: American Cancer Society; 2012. Available at http://www.cancer.org/Research/CancerFactsFigures/CancerFactsFigures/cancer-facts-figures-2012. Accessed May 29, 2013.
2. O'Leary M, Krailo M, Anderson JR, Reaman GH, Children's Oncology Group. Progress in childhood cancer: 50 years of research collaboration, a report from the Children's Oncology Group. *Semin Oncol.* 2008;35:484–493.
3. Abla O, ed. *Handbook of Supportive Care in Pediatric Oncology.* Sudbury, MA: Jones & Bartlett, 2010.
4. Coiffier B, Altman A, Pui CH, Younes A, Cairo MS. Guidelines for the management of pediatric and adult tumor lysis syndrome: an evidence-based review. *J Clin Oncol.* 2008;26(16):2767–2778.
5. Rubnitz JE, Gibson B, Smith FO. Acute myeloid leukemia. *Henatol Oncol Clin North Am.* 2010;24:35–63.
6. Pizzo PA, Poplack DG, eds. *Principles and Practice of Pediatric Oncology.* 6th ed. Philadelphia, PA: Lippincott Williams & Wilkins; 2011.
7. Lanzkowsky P, ed. *Manual of Pediatric Hematology and Oncology.* 5th ed. Burlington, MA: Elsevier; 2011.
8. Carroll WL, Raetz EA. Clinical and laboratory biology of childhood acute lymphoblastic leukemia. *J Pediatr.* 2012;160:10–18.
9. Pieters R, Carroll WL. Biology and treatment of acute lymphoblastic leukemia. *Henatol Oncol Clin North Am.* 2010;24:1–18.
10. Pui C-H, Carroll WL, Meshinchi S, Arceci RJ. Biology, risk stratification, and therapy of pediatric acute leukemias: an update. *J Clin Oncol.* 2011;29:551–565.
11. Crews KR, Cross SJ, McCormick JN, et al. Development and implementation of a pharmacist-managed clinical pharmacogenetics service. *Am J Health Syst Pharm.* 2011;68(2):143–150.
12. Schmiegelow K, Glomstein A, Kristinsson J, Salmi T, Schrøder H, Björk O. Impact of morning versus evening schedule for oral methotrexate and 6-mercaptopurine on relapse risk for children with acute lymphoblastic leukemia. Nordic Society for Pediatric Hematology and Oncology (NOPHO). *J Pediatr Henatol Oncol.* 1997;19(2):102–109.
13. De Lemos ML, Hamata L, Jennings S, Leduc T. Interaction between mercaptopurine and milk. *J Oncol Pharm Pract.* 2007;13:237–240.
14. Zwaan CM, Reinhardt D, Hitzler J, Paresh V. Acute leukemias in children with Down syndrome. *Henatol Oncol Clin North Am.* 2010;24:19–34.
15. Massey GV, Zipursky A, Chang MN, et al. A prospective study of the natural history of transient leukemia (TL) in neonates with Down syndrome (DS): Children's Oncology Group (COG) study and POG–9481. *Blood.* 2006;107:4606–4613.
16. de Botton S, Coiteux V, Rayon C, et al. Outcome of childhood acute promyelocytic leukemia with all-trans-retinoic acid and chemotherapy. *J Clin Oncol.* 2004;22:1404–1412.

17. Testi AM, Biondi A, Lo Coco F, et al. GIMEMA-AIEOP AIDA protocol for the treatment of newly diagnosed acute promyelocytic leukemia (APL) in children. *Blood.* 2005;106:447–453.
18. Ortega JJ, Madero L, Martin G, et al. Treatment with all-trans-retinoic acid and anthracyclines monochemotherapy for children with promyelocytic leukemia: a multicenter study by the PETHEMA Group. *J Clin Oncol.* 2005;23:7632–7640.
19. Hochberg J, Waxman IM, Kelly KM, Morris E, Cairo MS. Adolescent non-Hodgkin lymphoma and Hodgkin lymphoma: state of the science. *Br J Haematol.* 2009;144:24–40.
20. Jaglowski SM, Linden E, Termuhlen AM, Flynn JM. Lymphoma in adolescents and young adults. *Semin Oncol.* 2009;36:381–418.
21. Miles RR, Arnold S, Cairo MS. Risk factors and treatment of childhood and adolescent Burkitt lymphoma/leukaemia. *Br J Haematol.* 2012;156:730–743.
22. Fleming AJ, Chi SN. Brain tumors in children. *Curr Probl Pediatr Adolesc Health Care.* 2012;42:80–103.
23. Motl S, Zhuang Y, Waters CM, Stewart CF. Pharmacokinetic considerations in the treatment of CNS tumours. *Clin Pharmacokinet.* 2006;45:871–903.
24. Park JR, Eggert A, Caron H. Neuroblastoma: biology, prognosis, and treatment. *Henatol Oncol Clin North Am.* 2010;24:65–86.
25. Yu AL, Gilman AL, Ozkaynak MF, et al. Anti-GD2 antibody with GM-CSF, interleukin-2, and isotretinoin for neuroblastoma. *N Engl J Med.* 2010;363:1324–1334.
26. Maris JM. Recent advances in neuroblastoma. *New Engl J Med.* 2010;362:2202–2211.
27. Davidoff AM. Wilms' tumor. *Curr Opin Pediatr.* 2009;21:357–364.
28. Walterhouse D, Watson A. Optimal management strategies for rhabdomyosarcoma in children. *Pediatr Drugs.* 2007;9(6)391–400.
29. Heare T, Hensley MA, Dell'Orfano S. Bone tumors: osteosarcoma and Ewing's sarcoma. *Curr Opin Pediatr.* 2009;21:365–372.
30. Balamuth NJ, Womer RB. Ewing's sarcoma. *Lancet Oncol.* 2010;11:184–192.
31. Karosas AO. Ewing's sarcoma. *Am J Health Syst Pharm.* 2010;67:1599–1605.
32. Kim JW, Abramson DH, Dunkel IJ. Current management strategies for intraocular retinoblastoma. *Drugs.* 2007;67(15):2173–2185.
33. Shields CL, Shields JA. Retinoblastoma management: advances in enucleation, intravenous chemoreduction, and intra-arterial chemotherapy. *Curr Opin Ophthalmol.* 2010;21:203–212.
34. Jordan K, Roila F, Molassiotis A, et al. Antiemetics in children receiving chemotherapy. MASCC/ESMO guideline update 2009. *Support Care Cancer.* 2009;19 (Suppl 1):S37–S42.
35. Phillips RS, Gopaul S, Gibson F, et al. Antiemetic medication for prevention and treatment of chemotherapy induced nausea and vomiting in childhood. *Cochrane Database Syst Rev.* 2010;8:CD007786.
36. Promethazine hydrochloride injection, USP [package insert]. Irvine, CA: Teva Parenteral Medicines, Inc; 2009.
37. Vinson DR. Diphenhydramine in the treatment of akathisia induced by prochlorperazine. *J Emerg Med.* 2004;26:265–270.
38. Neulasta [package insert]. Thousand Oaks, CA: Amgen Inc; 2012.

39. Spunt SL, Irving H, Frost J, et al. Phase II, randomized, open-labeled study of pegfilgrastim-supported VDC/IE chemotherapy in pediatric sarcoma patients. *J Clin Oncol.* 2010;28:1329–1336.

40. Shankar AG. The role of recombinant erythropoietin in childhood cancer. *Oncologist.* 2008;13:157–166.

41. Reeves DJ, Quebe AK, Patel R. The ESA APPRISE oncology program. A history of REMS requirements, a review of data, and an approach to compliance in the hospital. *P T.* 2011;36:423–433.

42. Oeffinger KC, Hudson MM, Landier W. Survivorship: childhood cancer survivors. *Prim Care.* 2009;36:743–780.

43. Children's Oncology Group. *Long-term follow-up guidelines for survivors of childhood, adolescent and young adult cancers*, Version 3.0. Arcadia, CA: Children's Oncology Group; 2008. www.survivorshipguidelines.org. Accessed May 29, 2013.

44. Holliday MA, Segar WE. The maintenance need for water in parenteral fluid therapy. *Pediatrics.*1957;19:823–832.

45. Kearns GL, Abdel-Rahman SM, Alander SW, Blowey DL, Leeder JS, Kauffman RE. Developmental pharmacology—drug disposition, action, and therapy in infants and children. *N Engl J Med.* 2003;349(12):1157–1167.

46. Talbot NB, Richie RH. The advantage of surface area of the body as a basis for calculating pediatric dosages. *Pediatrics.* 1959;24:495–498.

47. Thompson PA, Rosner GL, Matthay KK, et al. Impact of body composition on pharmacokinetics of doxorubicin in children: a Glaser Pediatric Research Network study. *Cancer Chemother Pharmacol,* 2009;64:243–251.

48. Taylor JA, Winter L, Geyer LJ, Hawkins DS. Oral outpatient chemotherapy medication errors in children with acute lymphoblastic leukemia. *Cancer.* 2006;107: 1400–1406.

49. Lam MS. Extemporaneous compounding of oral liquid dosage formulations and alternative drug delivery methods for anticancer drugs. *Pharmacother.* 2011;31:164–192.

CHAPTER 10

Investigational Drugs

Theresa A. Mays
Leslie Smetzer

LEARNING OBJECTIVES

Upon completion of the chapter, the reader will be able to:

1. Explain the difference between processing orders for conventional chemotherapy versus investigational chemotherapy
2. Describe the federal regulations governing investigational chemotherapy medications
3. Maintain appropriate records for investigational chemotherapy medications
4. Verify dose modifications based on protocol requirements and the Common Terminology Criteria (CTC) for adverse events
5. Perform appropriate concomitant medication screening for patients on investigational chemotherapy medications

INTRODUCTION

Initially, the process involved in assessing patients and preparing therapy for investigational agents appears very similar to the process for conventional chemotherapy treatments. However, the requirements for investigational agents are more extensive and time consuming. Verification of chemotherapy orders requires review of the patient's height, weight, body surface area (BSA), laboratory values, and assessment of toxicities. Review of investigational chemotherapy orders includes all of the aforementioned parameters, in addition to verifying that the patient has signed the appropriate informed consent documents and meets the protocol-specific requirements for either initial or repeat treatment. Several federal guidelines that specify how clinical research should be conducted in human subjects exist.[1,2] This chapter will discuss the unique aspects of participating in oncology clinical trials, including the management and dispensing of investigational chemotherapy medications.

There are 4 phases of clinical trials performed in the United States.[3]

- **Phase I** clinical trials are conducted to determine a safe dosage range and to identify adverse effects of the investigational agent or combination.
- **Phase II** trials further investigate the dose determined by the phase I study and evaluate if it is effective in addition to further evaluating product(s) safety.
- **Phase III** trials compare the investigational agent or combination to an existing standard treatment to confirm the effectiveness and to further evaluate the product's or products' safety.
- **Phase IV** trials are postmarketing studies that further provide additional information about the agent, including the benefits versus risks of the medication and optimal use.

DOCUMENTATION

Documentation is the backbone of participation in investigational protocols. There is a saying that if it is not documented, it did not happen. Every site participating in clinical trials must have standard operating procedures (SOPs) outlined for appropriate documentation. Items should be documented in a consistent fashion throughout the clinical trial. In addition, all staff must receive instruction on the appropriate method used to correct errors and to document items. Compliance with simple documentation rules is essential. Corrections to source documentation should never obscure the initial entry (ie, scribbled out or covered with correction fluid). A single line should be drawn through an incorrect entry and the correct entry should be written next to it. The person making the correction should initial and date next to the correction (see example in **Box 10-1**). This method provides an audit trail for anyone, including study monitors, sponsor representatives, internal review boards, and possibly the Food and Drug Administration (FDA), reviewing source documentation.

> ## BOX 10-1
> ### Correction to Source Documentation
>
> tam 6-29-11
>
> Example: Patient complains today of pain rated as a 5 6 on a 0–10 scale.

STANDARD OPERATING PROCEDURES

Any institution participating in investigational protocols *must* have written SOPs to outline how protocol requirements will be met. Each department that is involved in the clinical trial process should have department-specific SOPs that outline their roles and responsibilities for clinical trial participation. Every department must document appropriate training for each staff member involved in the conduct of the clinical trial. These training records must be available for review by sponsors, clinical research organizations, and auditors, including the FDA.

The process that is followed at the institution should be governed by existing SOPs, which outline the role of each healthcare professional in ensuring patients are appropriate candidates for the investigational trial and are eligible for treatment. At the authors' institution, the individuals involved in the cycle 1, day 1 process include, but are not limited to, a principal or subinvestigator, research nurse or study coordinator, pharmacist, pharmacokinetic (PK) technician, and treatment nurse. Every piece of data must be documented and double checked by at least one other individual. Remember, if the information in the chart is not documented appropriately, the event did not happen. This is especially the case for clinical trials, where source documentation information has to be available for everything that is stated to have been completed. Checklists (**Box 10-2**) may be developed for staff to use to ensure each item is verified by monitors, auditors, and agencies such as the investigational review board (IRB) and FDA.

BOX 10-2
Course 1, Day 1 Investigational Drug Service Checklist

Eligibility Checklist:

☐ Labs meet criteria   ☐ Patient meets criteria
☐ Allergies/adverse reactions checked

Registration Received?

☐ Study number provided   ☐ Dose level provided

Consent:

☐ Patient signed   ☐ Patient dated
☐ All check boxes answered   ☐ Patient answered yes to all
                                       questions

☐ Physician signed   ☐ Physician dated

Orders (verify each item was performed *and* is within the protocol-specified time frame):

☐ Labs   ☐ Physical exam
☐ Neurological exam   ☐ Neurological form completed,
                                       if applicable

☐ ECG   ☐ ECHO/MUGA
☐ CT/MRI/PET scans   ☐ Patient questionnaire(s)
                                       completed, if applicable

☐ Ophthalmologic exam   ☐ Ophthalmologic form
                                       completed, if applicable

☐ Dose level correct on orders   IBW = ____   Actual BW = ____
☐ Research nurse contacted about dose based on patient's weight
☐ Does dose need rounding on orders?
☐ Dose needs to be changed on the orders?   ☐ Done

Pending items:

The following items must be verified before the patient is treated on

cycle 1, day 1: _____

CASE STUDY 10-1
Case Presentation Part A

A case study of a patient entering a phase I clinical trial
KL is a 51-year-old male with hormone refractory metastatic
prostate cancer who has been consented to enroll in a phase I
clinical trial at your institution with an oral taxane agent, WD1234.
You are processing his cycle 1, day 1 packet for treatment initiation
tomorrow. The patient's height is 69.5 inches, his weight is 419.7
pounds, and his BSA is 2.85 m². His ECOG performance status is 1.
His laboratory values are reported in the table that follows.

Laboratory Value (Normal Range)

ANC: 3800/mm³ (1500–8500/mm³)	Plt: 185,000/mm³ (130,000–400,000/mm³)
Hb: 11.6 g/dL (14–18 g/dL)	INR: 1.02 (0.9–1.1)
PTT: 27.6 seconds (24–33 seconds)	PSA: 27.2 ng/mL (0.0–0.4 ng/mL)
Glucose: 140 mg/dL (70–110 mg/dL)	K+: 4.3 mmol/L (3.5–5.1 mmol/L)
Mg: 2.2 mg/dL (1.8–2.4 mg/dL)	Phos: 3.3 mg/dL (2.5–4.9 mg/dL)
SCr: 1.2 mg/dL (0.6–1.3 mg/dL)	Estimated CrCl: 74 mL/min
Amylase: 56 U/L (25–115 U/L)	Lipase: 131 U/L (73–393 U/L)

Baseline toxicity assessment: grade 1 peripheral neuropathy and
urinary retention.

Patient's concomitant medications include:
Metformin hydrochloride 1000 mg twice daily
Glimepiride 2 mg PO daily
Olmesartan 20 mg PO daily
Tamsulosin 0.4 mg PO daily
Simvastatin 20 mg PO daily
Hydrocodone 10 mg/acetaminophen 325 mg 1–2 tabs Q 4–6 hours
PRN pain
Loperamide 2 mg PRN diarrhea

Pertinent inclusion criteria per protocol:

1. ECOG performance status ≤ 2
2. Adequate bone marrow, hepatic, and renal function defined as:
   a. Absolute neutrophil count (ANC) $\geq 1500/mm^3$
   b. Platelet count $\geq 100,000/mm^3$
   c. Hemoglobin ≥ 9 g/dL
   d. Aspartate aminotransferase (AST) and alanine aminotransferase (ALT) ≤ 2.5 times the upper limit of normal ($\times$ ULN) or, in the presence of liver metastasis, $\leq 5 \times$ ULN
   e. Serum creatinine $\leq 1.5 \times$ ULN or calculated CrCl ≥ 60 mL/minute
3. Patient has recovered from the effects of prior surgery or other therapy, including immunotherapy, radiation therapy, cytokine, biologic, or vaccine therapy with an approved or investigational agent, and it has been at least 4 weeks since dosing
4. Expected survival ≥ 3 months
5. For subjects enrolled in the 30 mg/m^2 dose, BSA between 1.6 m^2 and 2.1 m^2

Pertinent exclusion criteria per protocol:

How would you process this cycle 1, day 1 packet?

1. Recurrent diarrhea, defined as more than 3 episodes in any 24-hour period within 15 days prior to enrollment in this study.
2. Neuropathy $\geq$ grade 2
3. Difficulty swallowing
4. Malabsorptive disorders
5. The patient needs to continue any medication that is a potent inhibitor or inducer of the cytochrome P450 3A (CPY3A) pathway or that has P-glycoprotein activity

Explain how you would process this cycle 1, day 1 packet, including what steps you would take to verify enrollment into the research protocol and correctly dispense the drug

Examples of items to verify upon enrollment into research protocol include:

1. Patient has signed current IRB-approved consent for the clinical trial and has completed all areas appropriately. Consent has been signed by an investigator listed on the FDA 1572 form (**Box 10-3**).[4]

2. Laboratory values meet the inclusion criteria

3. Patient meets all other inclusion criteria

4. Patient has had all protocol-specific evaluations performed within the study-specified time frame, including items such as:
   - Computed tomography (CT)/magnetic resonance imaging (MRI) scans
   - Multigated acquisition (MUGA) scan/echocardiogram (ECHO)
   - Eye exam
   - Neurological exam
   - Pulmonary function tests
   - Electrocardiogram(s) (ECG)
   - Quality of life questionnaires

5. Study-specific number and dose level is correct based on the study-specific enrollment form. If this information is not provided by the sponsor on the enrollment form, then a different method must be agreed upon at study initiation to allow verification of these items.

6. Double check of all calculations has been performed, including calculation of dose. For clinical trials, it is important to answer the question, does the dose need to be rounded? If the dose is to be rounded, an SOP on how this is to occur must be in place.
   - Oral formulations need to be rounded to the nearest capsule or tablet strength
   - Intravenous (IV) formulations need to be rounded to a number that allows accurate measurement using a 1-mL syringe (ie, to the nearest single decimal point, milligram, or another value)

7. The patient does not meet any exclusion criteria

BOX 10-3

The Statement of Investigator or Form FDA 1572

The Statement of Investigator or form FDA 1572 is the agreement signed by all investigators to assure they will comply with all FDA regulations related to the appropriate conduct of a clinical trial of an investigational medication. The individuals who are listed on the study form FDA 1572 are considered qualified to order investigational medication.

ISSUES AFFECTING THE PATIENT'S ENROLLMENT IN THE CLINICAL TRIAL

When there are situations in which it is unclear how to proceed with patient enrollment because the protocol does not address the specific issues encountered in practice, the study sponsor should be contacted and apprised of the scenario so that he or she can determine how he or she would like the site to proceed. Factors that may influence the sponsor's decision include the phase of the study (ie, phase I versus phase III) and the toxicities seen to date in patients. Patients participating in phase I trials may have received previous chemotherapy and/or radiation therapy, which may limit their bone marrow reserves. Phase III trials tend to limit the number of prior regimens a patient may have received and may include first-line patients who may have better performance status, have less damage to their bone marrow, have experienced less toxicity, or have a more rapid recovery from the toxicities of therapy.

CASE STUDY 10-1
Case Presentation Part B

Do any issues affecting the patient's enrollment in the clinical trial exist? What steps should be taken to address these issues?

1. The patient is morbidly obese
2. The patient reports as-needed loperamide dosing and recurrent diarrhea
3. The patient's concomitant drugs have drug–drug interactions

DuBois Equation for BSA (m^2)

$0.007184 \times$ **Ht (cm)$^{0.725} \times$ Wt (kg)$^{0.425}$**

Ideal Body Weight Equations:

Female: $45.5 + (2.3 \times$ each inch > 60 inches)

Male: $50 + (2.3 \times$ each inch > 60 inches)

Adjusted Weight

IBW + [40% $\times$ (actual body weight – ideal body weight)]

1. The only information about overweight patients is inclusion criterion No. #5. For illustration, we will say the patient is enrolled

in the dose level of 20 mg/m^2 PO once every 21 days, which then makes inclusion criterion No. #5 not applicable as the patient's dose level is not 30 mg/m^2.

The possible doses the patient could receive based on his height of 69.5 inches (69.5 inches × 2.54 [conversion factor to change inches to centimeters] = 176.5 cm) and a weight of 419.7 pounds (419.7 lb/2.2 [conversion factor to change pounds to kilograms] = 190.8 kg) are:

Actual weight dose:

o Actual BSA = 0.007184 × 176.5 (cm)$^{0.725}$ × 190.8 (kg)$^{0.425}$ = 2.85 m^2
o Calculated patient dose: 20 mg/m^2 × 2.85 m^2 = 57 mg
o Round dose to 60 mg based on capsule size (5 mg and 25 mg available)

Ideal weight dose:

o Ideal body weight = 50 kg + (2.3 × 9.5 inches) = 71.8 kg.
o Ideal BSA = 0.007184 × 176.5 (cm)$^{0.725}$ × 71.8 (kg)$^{0.425}$ = 1.88 m^2.
o Calculated patient dose: 20 mg/m^2 × 1.88 m^2 = 37.6 mg.
o Round dose to 40 mg based on capsule size (5 mg and 25 mg available).

Adjusted weight dose:

o Adjusted body weight = 71.8 kg + [40% × (190.8 kg – 71.8 kg)] = 119.4 kg.
o Adjusted BSA = 0.007184 × 176.5 (cm)$^{0.725}$ × 119.4 (kg)$^{0.425}$ = 2.33 m^2.
o Calculated patient dose: 20 mg/m^2 × 2.33 m^2 = 46.6 mg.
o Round dose to 50 mg based on capsule size (5 mg and 25 mg available).

Because the protocol has no recommendations at this dose level, the study sponsor should be contacted and notified of the patient's high BSA and determine how he or she would like the site to proceed, since this is a phase I study and determining maximally tolerated dose is the goal. The American Society of Clinical Oncology recently published a guideline recommendation on chemotherapy dosing for obese patients.[5] This guideline does not specifically address dosing in obese patients undergoing an investigational trial, however it is an excellent resource to reference when speaking to sponsors.

2. Patient reports as-needed loperamide dosing, and recurrent diarrhea is an exclusion criterion. Therefore, the patient must be questioned about normal bowel patterns, and frequency and duration of diarrhea must be documented prior to treatment to ensure patient is eligible for study participation.

The patient's concomitant medications must be reviewed to verify that none are potent inhibitors or inducers of the cytochrome P450 3A (CYP3A) pathway or that have P-glycoprotein activity. Finasteride, simvastatin, and tamsulosin are major substrates of CYP3A and may compete with the investigational agent for metabolism via CYP3A. Therefore, close monitoring is recommended based on protocol requirements.

It is important to verify with the study sponsor what resource(s) should be used to screen for drug interactions in the study. Protocols may specify using the cytochrome P450 drug interaction table maintained by David A. Flockhart, MD, PHD, in the division of Clinical Pharmacology at Indiana University of School of Medicine as the reference for drug interactions screening, which is available at http://medicine.iupui.edu/clinpharm/ddis/. Other protocols will include medication listings with the text but also state these tables are not all inclusive, which assumes the site will use additional references, such as Lexi-Comp's drug information guide or Medispan's drug database, to perform interaction screening. A method for screening of non-FDA approved medications (ie, herbal products or supplements), which are usually not included in these databases, must also be defined. Further clarification is usually necessary when screening concomitant medications for study enrollment. The site should use consistent screening based on protocol requirements for each trial when performing medication screening for eligibility. Therefore, one individual or one group of individuals who are trained and are familiar with these concomitant medication screening tools should be assigned the task of screening for concomitant medications. In addition, some protocols exclude medications that cause QTc prolongation. Once again, the site should agree on the resource to be used in conjunction with the sponsor. One very common resource is the Arizona Center for Education and Research on Therapeutics (CERT) Criteria, which is available at http://www.azcert.org/medical-pros/drug-lists/drug-lists.cfm.

Any new medication the patient is prescribed while in a study must be evaluated. At the authors' site, pharmacists perform the initial screening process for all medications. The pharmacists are contacted by physicians, nurses, and patients when a new medication is prescribed or being considered to be prescribed. All patients on clinical trials are counseled to contact the research nurse or study coordinator any time a new medication is prescribed prior to filling the prescription(s).

COMMON TERMINOLOGY CRITERIA FOR ADVERSE EVENTS

The common terminology criteria for adverse events (CTCAE) is used to grade toxicities patients experience while in a study.[6] Having a standard grading scale allows toxicities from different investigational protocols to be compared or pooled to determine the overall toxicity profile of a medication or combination of medications. To date there have been 4 versions of the CTCAE published. Investigational protocols will specify which version of the CTCAE should be used to grade patient toxicities while being studied. The latest version of the CTCAE is v4.03, which was published on June 14, 2010. Significant changes were made to the criteria, which now allow the CTCAE terms to be grouped by MedDRA (*Medical Dictionary for Regulatory Activities*) primary System Organ Class (SOC). The MedDRA classification system has been used to classify non-oncology study toxicities for some time. This change allows more standardization across investigational trials. Version 4 also defines 2 types of activities of daily living (ADLs): instrumental (eg, cooking, shopping, managing money) and self-care (eg, bathing, dressing or undressing, using the toilet).

CASE STUDY 10-1
Case Presentation Part C

Dose-Limiting Toxicities and Retreatment Criteria

KL returns for cycle 4, day 1 of investigational treatment. He states he is having increased numbness, burning, and tingling in his hands and feet. He is having difficulty using a razor to shave his face every morning. His laboratory values are reported in the table that follows.

Laboratory Value (Normal Range)

ANC: 1300/mm^3 (1500–8500/mm^3)   Plt: 135,000/mm^3
(130,000–400,000/m^3)

Hb: 10.2 g/dL (14–18 g/dL)   INR: 1.0 (0.9–1.1)

PTT: 25.4 seconds (24–33 seconds)   PSA: 20.3 ng/mL (0.0–0.4 ng/mL)

Glucose: 135 mg/dL (70–110 mg/dL)   K+: 3.9 mmol/L (3.5–5.1 mmol/L)

Mg: 2.1 mg/dL (1.8–2.4 mg/dL)   Phos: 3.1 mg/dL (2.5–4.9 mg/dL)

SCr: 1.1 mg/dL (0.6–1.3 mg/dL)   Estimated CrCl: 80.7 mL/min

Amylase 130 U/L (25–115 U/L)   Lipase 402 U/L (73–393 U/L)

The protocol-specific retreatment criteria are listed in the following section.

Hematologic Toxicity

The dose of WD1234 will be permanently reduced by 1 dose level if any one of the following criteria is met:

- Febrile neutropenia (ANC<1000/mm^3 and temperature ≥ 38.5°C) of any duration
- ANC < 500/mm^3 lasting > 5 days
- Platelet count < 25,000/mm^3
- ANC < 1500/mm^3 on day 22 or later (up to day 36)
- Platelet count < 100,000/mm^3 on day 22 or later (up to day 36)

The dose of WD1234 will be delayed if any one of the following criteria is met:

- ANC < 1500/mm^3 on day 22
- Platelet count < 100,000/mm^3 on day 22

If recovery has not occurred by day 22, the subsequent cycle of drug may be delayed through day 36. If recovery from a treatment-related event has not occurred by day 36, protocol therapy will be discontinued.

Nonhematologic Toxicity

The dose of WD1234 administered to a specific subject will be permanently reduced by 1 dose level for ≥ grade 3 treatment-related adverse events (excluding alopecia, nausea, and vomiting) based on the CTCAE v4 criteria.

Recovery From Treatment-Related Adverse Events

A subject will be considered to have recovered from a treatment-related adverse event when:

- ANC is $\geq 1500/mm^3$
- Platelet count is $\geq 100,000/mm^3$
- Any nonhematologic treatment-related toxicities (excluding alopecia) are $\leq$ grade 1 or not worse than the baseline grade

Based on the protocol requirements, the patient's treatment would be held for several reasons, including the following:

1. ANC today is $< 1500/mm^3$ so based on the protocol requirements his treatment must be held until this recovers to $\geq 1500/mm^3$
2. Patient is reporting increased numbness, burning, and tingling in his hands and feet and he is having difficult performing his ADLs. Shaving would be considered a self-care ADL, which makes this a grade 3 toxicity (severe symptoms; limiting self-care ADL) versus a grade 2 toxicity (moderate symptoms; limiting instrumental ADL).

Dose-Limiting Toxicities and/or Retreatment Criteria

The patient had a dose-limiting toxicity, which would then require dose modification based on protocol requirements. When the patient's ANC has recovered to $\geq 1500/mm^3$, his dose of WD1234 should be reduced by one level. If his ANC does not recover to $\geq 1500/m^3$ by day 36 then he must be taken out of the study.

An adverse event (AE) is defined as "any unfavorable and unintended sign (including an abnormal laboratory finding), symptom, or disease temporally associated with the use of a medical treatment or procedure that may or may not be considered related to the medical treatment or procedure."[6] A numerical system of 1 through 5 is used to grade the majority of toxicities; however, not all grades are appropriate for all AEs. The grading assigned is based on the severity of the AE with grade 1 usually being a mild toxicity and grade 5 being a death related to the AE. The CTCAE versions 3 and 4 can be downloaded from http://ctep.cancer.gov/protocolDevelopment/electronic_applications/ctc.htm.

Toxicities may be assessed by nurses, research staff, a principal investigator, or subinvestigator. Discrepancies can occur if more than one individual is involved in assigning toxicities to a patient. Therefore, a physician investigator should review all toxicities entered and resolve any discrepancies. As the investigators are ultimately responsible for the trial's conduct, they should be the people who assign the attribution of each toxicity to the investigational agent or agents.

Study sponsors and principal investigators determine dose-escalation decisions based on the toxicities patients experience on each dose level administered. The particular dose-escalation schema each study will follow will be outlined in the investigational protocol. Some examples of dose-escalation schema include:[7]

- Traditional 3 + 3 design (modified Fibonacci), which enrolls 3 patients per dose level unless a predefined toxicity occurs, and then 6 patients are enrolled
- Accelerated titration schedule, which enrolls 1 patient per dose level until a predefined toxicity occurs, at which time 3 to 6 patients are enrolled per dose level
- Continual reassessment method that uses statistical modeling to predict the maximum tolerated dose (MTD)

Protocols will specify what is considered a dose-limiting toxicity and the exact period of time that these can occur in a study. An example would be a statement stating that "dose-limiting toxicities will only be evaluated in the first cycle of investigational therapy." Dose reductions to an existing patient's treatment may occur based on protocol requirements, sponsor request, or the investigator's assessment of the patient's toxicities.

Protocols may define retreatment criteria, such as those outlined in the patient case (Box 10-1, **Case Presentation Part C**). Retreatment criteria may not be identical to criteria used to treat conventional chemotherapy patients. Therefore, each investigational protocol must be consulted to ensure patients are eligible for retreatment during the study. However, some protocols do not outline retreatment criteria. In those instances, the clinic should have some standard criteria outlined in an SOP to guide clinical staff in evaluating patients for retreatment.

CLINICAL TRIAL MEDICATION ISSUES

Drug Accountability Records

Clinical sites participating in investigational trials must maintain complete records for the disposition of the investigational agent(s). Drug accountability records (DARs) come in several versions; refer to **Box 10-4** for an example of a DAR. The National Cancer Institute (NCI) has a DAR available on its website for free use (see reference 8 for the URL).[8] Sponsors may also provide study-specific DARs to use in their specific trials. Most sponsors ask clinical sites to maintain 2 versions of DAR, with one being a global record and the other being a patient-specific record. The patient-specific DAR makes the monitoring of the study easier for the sponsor and clinical research organization. However, a global DAR contains all the information necessary for the study. Maintaining 2 DARs per drug strength and lot creates a significant amount of increased work for clinical staff. Each clinical site performing investigational trials must have an SOP outlining how drug accountability will be performed and what form or forms will be used. Refer to **Box 10-5** for an example of a completed DAR.

BOX 10-4
Example of a Drug Accountability Record (DAR)[8]

Name of Institution:_____

Dispensing Area (if applicable):_____

Protocol Title:_____

Protocol Number:_____

Agent Name:_____

Dosage Form and Strength:_____

Investigator Name:_____

Line No.	Date	Patient Initials	Patient Study ID No.	Dose (mg)	Qty Dispensed or Received	Balance Forward	Lot No.	Initials
1.								
2.								
3.								
4.								
5.								
6.								
7.								
8.								

BOX 10-5
Example of a Completed Drug Accountability Record (DAR)[8]

Name of Institution: <u>Clinical Trials R US</u>
Dispensing Area (if applicable): <u>Investigational Drug Unit</u>
Protocol Title: <u>A Phase 1 Study of WD1234 in Cancer Patients with</u>
<u>Advanced Malignancies</u>
Protocol Number: <u>WD1234.US20</u>
Agent Name: <u>WD1234</u>   Dosage Form and Strength: <u>5 mg Capsule</u>
Investigator Name: <u>Dr. Feelgood</u>

Line No.	Date	Patient Initials	Patient Study ID No.	Dose (mg)	Qty Dispensed or Received	Balance Forward	Lot No.	Initials
1.	6/1/2011	DRUG	RECEIVED		300	300	ABC123	TAM
2.	6/21/2011	KL	000001	5 mg	−7	293	ABC123	DC
3.	6/28/2011	KL	000001	5 mg	1	294	ABC123	LA
4.	6/28/2011	Pt Rtn	Destroyed	5 mg	−1	293	ABC123	LA
5.	6/28/2011	KL	000001	5 mg	−7	286	ABC123	TAM
6.	7/5/2011	KL	000001	5 mg	−7	279	ABC123	TAM
7.	7/5/2011	Pill	Dropped	5 mg	1	280	ABC123	DC
8.	7/5/2011	Pill	Destroyed	5 mg	−1	279	ABC123	DC
9.	7/5/2011	KL	000001	5 mg	1	278	ABC123	TAM

DARs should be maintained for each medication strength received by the clinical site. For example, WD1234 comes as a 5-mg and 10-mg capsule formulation. Therefore, 2 DARs should be maintained based on strength; one for 5-mg capsules and one for 10-mg capsules. If 2 different vial sizes and/or drug concentrations are received during the conduct of the clinical trial, then different DARs should be maintained. When these records are maintained by hand, it is usually easier to maintain a separate DAR based on the lot numbers of the medication in addition to the strength.

The essential information recorded on a DAR should be listed as individual entries (ie, one line per entry). The principal investigator is ultimately responsible to the sponsor and must be able to state where each and every vial, tablet, or capsule went in the conduct of the clinical trial at the investigational site. Essential information includes:

- Receipt of investigational medication, including the date and quantity received
- Date of dispensing, quantity dispensed, and unique study identification number. Subject initials may also be requested by the sponsor and/or clinical research organization
- Patient returns of empty containers and/or missed doses of medication (oral studies)
- On-site destruction of any medication, including tablets/capsules dropped on the floor, returned missed doses, and/or IV doses that were not administered to the patient
- Final disposition of remaining study inventory at study close-out

At the end of the study, the final balance on each DAR should be zero. Finally, drug accountability records should provide a snapshot of the site's perpetual inventory and aid in medication resupply requests.

Drug Preparation and Administration Issues

IV investigational medications may be provided as powder or as a solution in a vial. The protocol or pharmacy manual will usually contain specific preparation guidelines for these products. These guidelines usually contain the type of container (polyvinyl chloride [PVC] versus non-PVC) that the medication must be prepared in, the diluent to make the drug (eg, sterile water, normal saline, dextrose) and/or to infuse the drug with, the type of infusion line to administer the medication through (eg, PVC, non-PVC, filtered with 0.22 micron in-line filter), and the rate at which the drug should be infused.

Many investigational IV medications have concentration-dependent issues (ie, a minimum and/or maximum volume in which the medication can be prepared and administered). Each protocol should be carefully reviewed to identify any issues with preparation and/or infusion of the medication. Each institution should have minimum and maximum infusion rates defined for its site. Another challenge when working with IV investigational medications is short stability times, which prevent the pharmacy from preparing the medication ahead of time.

There may also be special timing needs to document the start and end of the infusion to ensure appropriate pharmacokinetic or pharmacodynamic samples are obtained per protocol. Each site must evaluate how investigational chemotherapy is administered and how the nurse will flush the IV tubing without altering the infusion process to ensure the patient receives the complete dose.

In addition to the federal regulations referenced throughout this chapter, sites should review US Pharmacopeia Chapter <797> (USP 797)—Pharmaceutical Compounding Sterile Preparation, state pharmacy regulations, and The Joint Commission guidelines as applicable to the practice site.

Dispensing Oral Agents

The dispensing of oral investigational medication requires several additional considerations and steps. Some protocols define the number of doses to be dispensed to a patient at each clinic visit or the dates of dispensing on each cycle. However, in studies where patients have daily dosing and PK samples are collected over sequential days, there is potential for the patient to self-dose prior to returning to clinic. That is, if the patient has a supply of medication, it is difficult to ensure that he or she does not take this medication prior to their PK samples being drawn. The patient may not understand directions to hold dosing until they return to the clinic to have predose PK samples drawn.

Patients need to be appropriately counseled on how to administer the oral medication outside of the clinic environment. They need to be shown how to complete the medication diary for the study, which will document their dosing times and help the site assess compliance. Finally, they need to be told to bring their diaries and medication container(s) to each clinic visit.

Most oral studies will require an assessment of patient compliance with dosing. The assessment of compliance varies from study to study and may include an equation to calculate percentage of patient compliance, the use of pill counts, or a review of patients' medication diaries. A pharmacist or research staff member must document compliance assessment for all oral investigational agents. Patient education is very important for oral dosing, and if possible, it is optimal for the patient to dose the medication at the same time every day.

Bioequivalence and Bioavailability Studies

Bioavailability studies may be conducted to compare a test drug (new formulation) to a reference standard (previous formulation). The FDA requires that random reserve samples be maintained by each site conducting the study to allow the agency to perform all release tests 5 separate times. These samples must be retained at the clinical site for a period of at least 5 years following the date on which the application or supplemental application is approved, or if not approved, at least 5 years following the date of completion of the study. The reader is referred to the FDA guidance on bioavailability and bioequivalence studies for more information.[9,10]

Hazardous Versus Biohazardous Drugs

Each clinical site performing clinical trials with investigational medication must identify whether the medications they are testing are biohazardous or hazardous. The identification of each agent will affect how the medical waste is processed. A discussion on the identification of biohazardous or hazardous substance is outside the scope of this chapter, and the reader is referred to the Environmental Protection Agency (EPA) at http://www.epa.gov/epawaste/inforesources/online/index.htm for more information.

It is important to note that while these investigational agents are being evaluated, the effects of these drugs on those handling them may not be known. All precautions should be used to assure the health and safety of the healthcare team. Maintaining empty or partially empty IV vials once the vial septum has been punctured can result in unnecessary exposure to both pharmacy and study staff. In addition, for oral investigational agents, maintaining empty stock bottles, empty bottles returned by patients, and bottles returned by patients containing missed doses of medication can also result in unnecessary exposure to both pharmacy and study staff. At the authors' institution, any medication used in the treatment of cancer is considered to be chemotherapy and therefore, potentially hazardous.

Any container that previously contained chemotherapy or has residual chemotherapy (ie, empty or partially empty IV vials, empty stock bottles or patient return bottles, bottles returned by patients containing missing doses of medication) should be disposed of immediately as biohazardous chemotherapy waste. Empty or partially empty patient return bottles should be noted in the medical record and in the study's DAR to document patient compliance with dosing. This documentation should be verified by a second member of the pharmacy staff in the DAR (eg, second set of initials).

It is essential that any location performing investigational chemotherapy trials have standard operating procedures outlining the management of biohazardous and hazardous medications and the method used for accountability. These SOPs are discussed with each study sponsor, and copies are provided at each site initiation visit.

CODE OF FEDERAL REGULATIONS TITLE 21(1) AND THE INTERNATIONAL CONFERENCE ON HARMONIZATION GUIDELINE FOR GOOD CLINICAL PRACTICE

The intent of this chapter is to provide the reader with a basic overview of important issues when conducting oncology clinical trials. Any healthcare provider participating in clinical trials should be very familiar with the Code of Federal Regulations 21(refer to **Box 10-6**) and the International Conference on Harmonization Guideline for Good Clinical Practice.[2] These guidelines are available on the Web, and the URLs are included in the references at the end of this chapter.

Sites that use electronic medical records or other software programs should closely review 21 Part 11: Electronic Records; Electronic Signatures.[2] This guidance outlines the minimum requirements the software must meet in order to be used in the conduct of clinical trials. It is important to note that even if a piece of software has a document certifying it as 21 Part 11 compliant, the FDA requires each site to conduct an independent evaluation of the software for compliance.

The National Cancer Institute (NCI) website has many useful tools for individuals participating in clinical trials. The reader is referred to that website, http://www.cancer.gov/clinicaltrials, for further information. In addition, the Cancer Therapy Evaluation Program site contains many downloadable forms that may assist with clinical trial participation. These forms can be viewed at http://ctep.cancer.gov/forms/.

BOX 10-6

Code of Federal Regulations Title 21 and Sections Pertaining to Investigational Drug Services

Part 11: Electronic Records; Electronic Signatures
Part 50: Protection of Human Subjects
Part 56: Institutional Review Boards
Part 312: Investigational New Drug Application
Part 314: Adequate and Well-Controlled Trials

SUMMARY

Oncology clinical trials grant healthcare providers the ability to provide cutting-edge medications and technology to oncology patients. Participation in clinical trials requires a commitment from all members of an organization to ensure that the protocol is followed correctly and all data is appropriately documented. Individuals who decide to participate in clinical trials need to be familiar with the federal regulations that govern the conduct of these trials.

This chapter provides an initial overview of some of the issues to be considered when conducting clinical trials. Every site participating in clinical research must develop its own standard operating procedures and document training of staff on these procedures. These SOPs must be reviewed and updated as federal guidelines change. When SOPs are not followed, the site should perform an internal investigation into the reason why this occurred and adjust the SOP as appropriate.

REFERENCES

1. US Food and Drug Administration. Code of Federal Regulations Title 21. http://www.accessdata.fda.gov/scripts/cdrh/cfdocs/cfcfr/cfrsearch.cfm. Accessed May 24, 2013.
2. US Food and Drug Administration. ICH guidance documents. http://www.fda.gov/ScienceResearch/SpecialTopics/RunningClinicalTrials/GuidancesInformationSheetsand Notices/ucm219488.htm. Accessed May 24, 2013.
3. Clinical Trials.gov. US National Institutes of Health. Understanding Clinical Trials. http://clinicaltrials.gov/ct2/info/understand. Accessed May 24, 2013.
4. US Department of Health and Human Services, Food and Drug Administration, Office of Good Clinical Practice, Center for Drug Evaluation and Research (CDER), Center for Biologics Evaluation and Research (CBER). *Information Sheet Guidance for Sponsors, Clinical Investigators and IRBs. Frequently Asked Questions—Statement of Investigators (Form FDA 1572).* http://www.fda.gov/downloads/RegulatoryInformation/Guidances/UCM214282.pdf. Accessed May 24, 2013.
5. Griggs JJ, Mangu PB, Anderson H, et al. *Appropriate Chemotherapy Dosing for Obese Adult Patients with Cancer: American Society of Clinical Oncology Clinical Practice Guideline.* http://www.asco.org/sites/default/files/dosing_guideline_u9436.pdf. Accessed May 24, 2013.
6. National Cancer Institute. US National Institutes of Health. Common Terminology Criteria for Adverse Events (CTCAE). http://ctep.cancer.gov/protocolDevelopment/electronic_applications/ctc.htm. Accessed May 24, 2013.
7. Le Tourneau C, Lee J, Siu LL. Dose escalation methods in phase I cancer clinical trials. *J Natl Cancer Inst.* 2009;101:708–720.
8. US National Institutes of Health. National Cancer Institute. Cancer Therapy Evaluation Program (CTEP). CTEP forms, templates, and documents. Investigational Drug

Accountability Record. http://ctep.cancer.gov/forms/default.htm. Accessed May 24, 2013.

9. US Department of Health and Human Services, Food and Drug Administration, Center for Drug Evaluation and Research (CDER). *Guidance for Industry: Bioavailability and Bioequivalence Studies for Orally Administered Drug Products–General Considerations.* May 2003–Revision 1. http://www.fda.gov/downloads/Drugs/GuidanceComplianceRegulatoryInformation/Guidances/UCM070124.pdf. Accessed May 24, 2013.

10. US Department of Health and Human Services, Food and Drug Administration, Center for Drug Evaluation and Research (CDER). *Guidance for Industry: Handling and Retention of BA and BE Testing Samples.* May 2004. http://www.fda.gov/downloads/RegulatoryInformation/Guidances/UCM126836.pdf. Accessed May 24, 2013.

CHAPTER 11

Pharmacogenetics and Pharmacogenomics in Cancer Therapy

Trinh Pham
Man Yee Merl
Jia Li

LEARNING OBJECTIVES

Upon completion of the chapter, the reader will be able to:

1. Understand the terms *pharmacogenomics, pharmacogenetics, somatic mutation, germ-line mutations, predictive biomarkers, prognostic biomarkers,* and *molecular diagnostics*
2. Recognize drugs that have increased risk of toxicities in the presence of polymorphism of specific metabolizing enzymes (mercaptopurine, azathioprine, thioguanine, fluorouracil, capecitabine, irinotecan)
3. Identify biomarkers that have prognostic and predictive significance and their role in the process of selecting therapy

INTRODUCTION

Understanding the cause of variable drug response has significant implications in the field of oncology because of the fatal consequences when patients do not respond to anticancer therapy. Conversely, the tumor may be sensitive to an anti-cancer drug but the effectiveness of the medication may be limited if patients experience severe, life-threatening toxicities and are not able to continue taking their medication. The factors that influence an individual's response to a drug, either toxicity or responsiveness, are varied and include intrinsic factors such as gender, age, body size, and organ and bone marrow function, along with extrinsic factors such as drug–food or drug–drug interactions and patient adherence. With advances in human genome analysis and increased knowledge of tumor biology, there is now a better understanding of genetic variations that have a role in influencing an individual's response to anticancer drug therapy. The elucidation of the genetic basis for these interindividual differences to drug response allows clinicians to select specific drugs that are more efficacious with a better safety and toxicity profile for an individual patient. In oncology, genetic testing is being applied effectively to perform risk assessment, determine prognosis, and select treatment for patients. Furthermore, the rapidly expanding genetic information has led to the development of new drugs with novel mechanisms of action that target genetically specific forms of cancer. This chapter summarizes the most recent information on genetic mutations or polymorphisms that are predictors of response, survival, and toxicity to anticancer drug therapy for cancer diagnosis. The information is not meant to be all inclusive; the intent is to present predictive and prognostic biomarkers that are commonly evaluated in clinical practice that influences anticancer drug therapy selection.

TERMINOLOGY

Pharmacogenomics refers to the study of how genetic variants influence drug efficacy (eg, tumor response, progression-free survival, overall survival) and toxicity.[1] Pharmacogenetics is considered to be a subset of pharmacogenomics and refers to the study of germ-line genetic variants and their relevance to drug response.[2] Somatic (acquired) mutations usually refer to variations found within the tumor, which can define a patient's disease and possibly the treatment choice.[1] Germ-line (inherited) mutations refer to variations present in the patient's normal tissues that can affect the pharmacokinetics and pharmacodynamics of drugs independent of the disease type.[1] In general, the germ-line genome determines how a patient's body handles and reacts to a given treatment, and the somatic genome determines the tumor's aggressiveness and responsiveness to therapy.[3] Prognostic factors/biomarkers refer to a clinical or biologic characteristic that is objectively measureable and provides information on the likely outcome of the cancer in untreated individuals.[4] Predictive factors/biomarkers refer to a clinical or biologic characteristic that provides information on the effect of treatment on the cancer (ie, identify patients who are most likely to benefit from therapy).[4] Molecular diagnostics refers to the testing of genes, gene expression, proteins, metabolites, and new treatments that target molecular mechanisms.[4] Molecular diagnostics can classify tumors based on molecular subtypes (eg, tumors with anaplastic lymphoma kinase [ALK] or epidermal growth factor receptor [EGFR] mutations, discussed later in the chapter) and guide clinicians in individualizing treatment with targeted therapy based on these specific mutations.[4]

BIOMARKERS THAT PREDICT TREATMENT TOXICITY

Adverse effects of cancer therapy represent a major challenge for cancer patients and clinicians treating these patients. An anticancer treatment regimen that is well tolerated without major toxicities contributes to a better quality of life for patients. Toxicities to some anticancer agents may be predicted based on genetic polymorphisms of metabolic enzymes involved in the biotransformation of the anticancer agents. Genotyping for polymorphisms of metabolizing enzymes to identify patients who are at risk for poor tolerance and may require dose adjustment can be applied to the following anticancer agents: mercaptopurine, azathioprine and thioguanine; fluorouracil and capecitabine; and irinotecan. It should be noted that routine testing for genetic polymorphisms of these metabolizing enzymes prior to prescribing is not the standard of practice for all of these drugs. The following enzymes will be discussed in the next section: thiopurine s-methyltransferase, dihydropyrimidine dehydrogenase, and uridine diphosphoglucuronosyltransferase 1A1 (UGT1A1). Refer to **Table 11-1** for a summary of biomarkers that predict toxicity.

Thiopurine S-Methyltransferase

Thiopurine S-methyltransferase (TPMT) is an enzyme that catalyzes the S-methylation of the thiopurines (azathioprine, mercaptopurine, and thioguanine) resulting in inactivation of these drugs.[5] The TPMT gene exhibits genetic polymorphisms where individuals may exhibit high, intermediate, or no enzymatic activity.[5] The four common variant alleles of the gene that account for more than 95% of reduced TPMT activity are *TPMT*2*, *TPMT*3A*, *TPMT*3B*, and *TPMT*3C*.[5] Individuals with two variant alleles (homozygous) have low or no TPMT activity, while those with one variant allele (heterozygous) have intermediate TPMT activity. Wild-type *TPMT*1* homozygotes (no variant alleles), on the other hand, have normal enzyme activity.[6] Patients with low

Table 11-1 Biomarkers that Predict Toxicity

Biomarker	Drug	Comments
TPMT[a,5]	Azathioprine, mercaptopurine, thioguanine	Patients with low or no TPMT enzyme activity are particularly more susceptible to drug-related hematologic toxicities, and dose reductions of the drugs metabolized by this enzyme may be necessary.
DPD[b,7,8]	Capecitabine, fluorouracil	Patients who partially or completely lack DPD activity cannot metabolize fluoropyrimidines and are at increased risk of experiencing toxicities. Patients with known DPD deficiency are not challenged with the fluorouracil or capecitabine. Testing for the gene mutation and DPD deficiency status is not a standard of practice to guide fluoropyrimidine dosing. Dose reduce or discontinue therapy if patients experience severe toxicities and symptoms due to DPD enzyme deficiency.
UGT1A1*28[c,9–12]	Irinotecan	A 2-base pair insertion in the promoter region of UGT1A1 leads to the formation of the variant allele, UGT1A1*28. Commercial genotype testing for the UGT1A1*28 variant is available from 3 companies—ARUP Laboratories, LabCorp, and EntroGen. Routine testing for the presence of UGT1A1 mutation is unclear because of variable irinotecan toxicity depending on the irinotecan dose and other concurrent chemotherapy administration.

[a] TPMT (thiopurine S-methyltransferase): an enzyme that catalyzes the S-methylation of the thiopurines (azathioprine, 6-mercaptopurine, and thioguanine) resulting in inactivation of these drugs.
[b] DPD (dihydropyrimidine dehydrogenase): the first of 3 enzymes involved in fluoropyrimidine metabolism.
[c] UGT1A1(uridine diphosphoglucuronosyltransferase 1A1): enzyme that glucuronidates SN-38, an active metabolite of irinotecan, to its inactive form.

or no TPMT enzyme activity are particularly more susceptible to drug-related hematologic toxicities. Patients with high TPMT expression may be resistant to therapy with thiopurines. Genetic testing for TPMT polymorphism is not required but recommended by the Food and Drug Administration (FDA) for patients who receive thiopurines and experience significant toxicity after dosing.

A polymerase chain reaction (PCR)-based DNA polymorphism genotyping assay can determine the allelic pattern of a patient.

Dihydropyrimidine Dehydrogenase

Fluorouracil and capecitabine (oral prodrug of fluorouracil) are fluoropyrimidines commonly used in combination chemotherapy regimens to treat patients with breast, colorectal, and other cancers. Fluorouracil requires activation to the active compound 5-fluoro-2-deoxyuridine monophosphate (5-FdUMP). Dihydropyrimidine dehydrogenase (DPD) is the first of 3 enzymes involved in fluoropyrimidine metabolism. The enzymatic activity of DPD varies due to polymorphism in its coding gene, dihydropyrimidine dehydrogenase (DPYD). Alleles that are associated with a marked decrease in DPD activity include *DPYD *2A, DYPD *9B*, and *DPYD *13*, and patients with genetic polymorphisms in the DPYD gene are at increased risk of experiencing toxicities after receiving fluoropyrimidines.[7] Patients who partially or completely lack DPD activity cannot sufficiently degrade fluoropyrimidines, resulting in prolonged exposure to 5-FdUMP and subsequent increased risk of severe or fatal toxicities that include diarrhea, mucositis, pancytopenia, and neurological toxicity (cerebellar ataxia, cognitive dysfunction, altered level of consciousness).[8] Complete loss of DPD activity is rare, but decreased level of enzymatic activity is common. Molecular analysis of patients with DPD deficiency has identified over 40 mutations and polymorphisms in the DPYD gene. Mutations or inactivation of the DPYD gene have been characterized as autosomal recessive disease in the Caucasian and African American population and affects approximately 5% of the overall population. Generally, patients with known DPD deficiency are not challenged with fluorouracil or capecitabine. Testing every patient for DPD deficiency prior to receiving fluoropyrimidine remains controversial. Currently, testing for DPYD mutation and DPD status is not a standard of practice to guide fluorouracil dosing because the correlation between genotype and phenotype is not ideal. The readers are referred to the package insert information for capecitabine dose adjustment guidelines in patients who experience severe toxicities with this agent.

Uridine Diphosphoglucuronosyltransferase 1A1

Irinotecan is a topoisomerase inhibitor that has an important role in the treatment of metastatic colorectal cancer. It commonly causes the side effects of diarrhea and neutropenia. The active metabolite of irinotecan, SN38, is further metabolized in the liver by the enzyme uridine diphosphoglucuronosyltransferase 1A1 (UGT1A1) to an inactive compound, SN38G.[9] A 2-base pair insertion in the promoter region of UGT1A1 (*UGT1A1*28*) leads to decreased expression of UGT1A1 and results in increased risk of adverse effects.[10] *UGT1A1*28* is present in 32%-39% of Caucasians and 16%-33% of Asians. The role of routine testing for the presence of UGT1A1 mutation is unclear. The reason is because in patients who are homozygous for the *UGT1A1*28* variant, toxicity is observed in patients who received high-dose irinotecan (greater than 250 mg/m^2) but not in patients who received lower doses of irinotecan (100-125 mg/m^2).[11] Furthermore, in patients with the *UGT1A1*28* variant, toxicity was observed when irinotecan was administered with oxaliplatin but not with 5-fluorouracil.[12] Thus, genotyping may be considered and is reasonable for patients who are scheduled to receive high-dose irinotecan or irinotecan plus oxaliplatin and in patients who experience severe toxicity after irinotecan dosing or in patients who are suspected of having UGT1A1 mutation. The package insert for irinotecan recommends that a reduction in the starting dose by at least one level should be considered for patients known to be homozygous for the *UGT1A1*28* allele, and subsequent dose modification may be considered on an individual basis depending on tolerance and development of specific toxicities.[13]

BIOMARKERS THAT PREDICT TREATMENT RESPONSE AND/OR PROGNOSIS

Estrogen Receptor/Progesterone Receptor

Estrogen and progesterone receptors (ER/PgR) are important biomarkers for the management of breast cancer because there is substantial benefit of endocrine therapy for ER/PgR-positive tumors. The evaluation of ER/PgR status is mandatory for all patients diagnosed with breast cancer in order to determine endocrine therapy in these patients. The American Society of Clinical Oncology (ASCO) and the College of American Pathologists have published *Guideline Recommendations for Immunohistochemical Testing of Estrogen and Progesterone Receptors in Breast Cancer* in order to provide recommendations for optimal immunohistochemical (IHC) ER/PgR testing performance and interpretation of test results.[14] Endocrine therapy for ER/PgR-positive breast cancers includes selective estrogen receptor modulators (SERMs) and aromatase inhibitors (AIs). It is beyond the scope of this chapter to provide a review of the endocrine treatment options for hormone receptor–positive breast cancer; the readers are referred to *Suggested Reading* for an in-depth discussion on this topic.[15-17] See **Table 11-2** for a summary of common predictive and prognostic markers.

Table 11-2 Predictive and Prognostic Biomarkers

Biomarker	Cancer Diagnosis	Therapy	Comment
Estrogen α and progesterone receptor (ER-α/PgR)[14 17]	Breast	*Endocrine therapy:* Tamoxifen, letrozole, anastrozole, exemestane	Tumors that express both ER-α and PgR have more favorable prognosis and respond to endocrine therapy. Expression of ER-α is the principle qualifier for endocrine therapy. ER-α -/PgR + is uncommon, but endocrine therapy is still an option. ER-α-/ PgR- tumors do not benefit from endocrine therapy.
HER2/neu[15,17-20]	Breast, gastric, esophageal	*Breast cancer:* Trastuzumab, ado-trastuzumab, lapatinib, pertuzumab *Gastric and esophageal cancer:* Trastuzumab	Overexpression/ amplification indicates poor prognosis.
Epidermal growth factor receptor (EGFR)[21-23]	Colorectal	*Anti-EGFR monoclonal antibody:* Cetuximab, panitumumab	Anti-EGFR monoclonal antibody therapy benefits patients who overexpress EGFR but are *KRAS* mutation negative. Testing for *KRAS* mutation status is necessary for colorectal cancer patients.
	Non small cell lung cancer (NSCLC); specifically, nonsquamous cell NSCLC	*Small molecule tyrosine kinase inhibitors (TKIs):* Erlotinib (United States), gefitinib (Japan, Europe)	Patients with EGFR mutations; specifically deletions in exon 19 (LREA deletion) or mutation in exon 21 (L858R) respond to TKIs. Patients with EGFR T790M mutations are resistant to TKIs.

(continues)

Table 11-2 Predictive and Prognostic Biomarkers (*continued*)

Biomarker	Cancer Diagnosis	Therapy	Comment
			Cetuximab may also be used for all patients with NSCLC including nonsquamous histology; testing for *KRAS* mutation is not necessary for this patient population.
KRAS[24-36]	Colorectal	*Anti-EGFR monoclonal antibody:* Cetuximab, panitumumab	Patients with wild-type *KRAS* (mutation negative) responds to anti-EGFR monoclonal antibody.
EML4/ALK[37-42] (echinoderm microtubule associated protein-like 4/anaplastic lymphoma kinase)	NSCLC; specifically nonsquamous cell NSCLC	Crizotinib with FDA-approved companion diagnostic test, Vysis ALK Break Apart FISH Probe Kit	The *NCCN Guidelines* for NSCLC recommends evaluation of *ALK* gene rearrangement status for all patients with nonsquamous cell NSCLC.
BRAF[43-49]	Malignant melanoma	Vemurafenib with FDA-approved companion diagnostic test, cobas 4800 BRAF V600 mutation test	Most common in melanoma, colorectal cancer, and papillary thyroid cancer. Targeted therapy with vemurafenib only has FDA-approved indication for melanoma with BRAF mutations, not for patients with wild-type BRAF.
BCR/ABL[50-52] (breakpoint cluster region/ Abelson murine leukemia) (Philadelphia chromosome)	Chronic myeloid leukemia (CML) and Acute lymphocytic leukemia (ALL)	*Small molecule TKIs:* Imatinib, dasatinib, nilotinib, bosutinib, ponatinib	Only 20%-30% of patients with ALL have the Philadelphia chromosome; it indicates a poorer prognosis. In CML, the Philadelphia chromosome is central to its diagnosis.

| PML/RARα[53-57] (Promyelocytic leukemia/ retinoic acid receptor-alpha) | Acute promyelocytic leukemia (APL) | All-trans retinoic acid; arsenic trioxide | The PML/RAR-α gene translocation is present in a unique subtype of acute myelogenous leukemia, known as APL. It is associated with a very good prognosis and cure rate. |
| Chromosome 5q deletion[58,59] | Myelodysplatic syndrome | Lenalidomide | Very responsive to lenalidomide therapy |

Human Epidermal Growth Factor Receptor 2

Human epidermal growth factor receptor 2 (HER2), also known as Neu or ErbB-2, is a member of the epidermal growth factor receptor (EGFR/ErbB) family. HER2 is encoded by ERBB2, a known protooncogene located at the long arm of human chromosome 17 (17q12). Overexpression of this gene has been shown to play an important role in the pathogenesis of some types of cancers, and HER2/Neu has become an important biomarker and target for tumors such as breast and gastric cancer. Approximately 30% of breast cancers overexpress HER2/Neu that is detectable by fluorescent in situ hybridization (FISH) or IHC staining. The presence of HER2/Neu is associated with a poor prognosis. Overexpression of HER2/Neu is predictive for response to trastuzumab, a monoclonal antibody that targets HER2/Neu. In HER2-positive breast cancer patients, the addition of trastuzumab to chemotherapy was associated with higher response rate, longer progression-free survival and overall survival when compared with patients receiving chemotherapy alone.[18] Clinical benefit of trastuzumab requires HER2 3+ expression measured by standardized IHC methods or HER2 gene amplification demonstrated by FISH.[19]

The benefit of trastuzumab was investigated in HER2/Neu positive gastric and esophageal tumors in the ToGA trial (Trastuzumab in Combination with Chemotherapy versus Chemotherapy Alone for Treatment of HER2-positive Advanced Gastric or Gastro-esophageal Junction Cancer). The results showed that patients receiving cisplatin and fluorouracil (or capecitabine) in combination with trastuzumab achieved statistically longer progression-free survival and overall survival when compared with chemotherapy without trastuzumab.[20]

Trastuzumab has FDA-approved indications for gastric cancer along with advanced and metastatic breast cancer that overexpress HER2.[60] Other agents that target HER2 include lapatinib, pertuzumab, and ado-trastuzumab. Lapatinib is a dual HER2/EGFR tyrosine kinase inhibitor (TKI) that has synergistic effect with trastuzumab without cross-resistance.[19] It has FDA-approved indication in combination with capecitabine for patients with metastatic breast cancer who have failed anthracycline, taxane, and trastuzumab or as concurrent therapy with letrozole for postmenopausal breast cancer patients positive for HER2 overexpression.[61] Pertuzumab is a monoclonal antibody that sterically blocks dimerization of HER2 with HER1, 3 and 4; thus inhibiting signaling from HER2/HER1 and HER2/HER3 heterodimers.[19] Pertuzumab and trastuzumab bind to different epitopes in the extracellular domain of HER2. Pertuzumab is indicated for use in combination with trastuzumab and docetaxel for the treatment of patients with HER2-positive metastatic breast cancer who have not received prior anti-HER2 therapy or chemotherapy for metastatic disease.[62] Ado-trastuzumab is trastuzumab covalently linked to the fungal toxin maytansine DM1, a microtubule inhibitory drug.[19] It has FDA-approved indication as a single agent for the treatment of patients with HER2-positive, metastatic breast cancer who previously received trastuzumab and a taxane and developed disease recurrence during or within 6 months of completing adjuvant therapy.[63] Refer to the National Comprehensive Cancer Network (NCCN) *Clinical Practice Guidelines in Oncology* (also known as the *NCCN Guidelines*) for breast cancer for a more comprehensive discussion on the use of anti-HER2 drug therapy in breast cancer patients.[15]

Epidermal Growth Factor Receptor

The EGFR is the prototypical member of the ErbB family of receptor tyrosine kinases that includes ErbB2, ErbB3, and ErbB4. ErbB proteins are important regulators of proliferation, survival, and differentiation. EGFR has been found to be mutationally activated and/or overexpressed in a variety of human cancers including lung, head and neck, colon, pancreas, breast, ovary, bladder, and kidney, and in gliomas.[21,22] In general, patients with tumors that show high expression of EGFR tend to have a poorer prognosis.[22] Mutations in EGFR may occur either in the extracellular domain or the tyrosine kinase domain. About 90% of the EGFR mutations are either small deletions encompassing 5 amino acids from codons 746–750 (ELREA) or missense mutations resulting in a substitution of leucine with arginine at codon 858 (L858R).[22] EGFR mutations are mainly present in the first 4 exons—18 (G719x), 19, 20, and 21 (L858R)—of the gene encoding the tyrosine kinase domain.[22] Mutations of exons 18, 19 (45%), and 21 (40%) are associated with sensitivity to EGFR inhibitors, and mutation of exon 20 is associated with resistance to EGFR inhibitors.[23] The following section reviews treatment options for patients with EGFR mutations in lung and colorectal cancer.

In non–small cell lung cancer (NSCLC), mutational activation of EGFR through small in-frame deletions in exon 19 or missense mutations in exon 21 (both within the kinase domain) occurs in approximately 10% of American and European and 25%-50% of Asian patients.[21] Higher EGFR mutation frequency is also observed in nonsmokers, women, and nonmucinous cancers.[22,24] These mutations are the most reliable predictors of response to TKIs.[21]

In colorectal cancer, EGFR overexpression is found in 19% of patients. The BOND study (Cetuximab Monotherapy and Cetuximab plus Irinotecan in Irinotecan-Refractory Metastatic Colorectal Cancer) showed that the intensity of IHC staining of EGFR in colorectal tumor cells did not correlate with the response rate to anti-EGFR monoclonal antibody therapy (eg, cetuximab, panitumumab).[25] Therefore, the *NCCN Guidelines* for colorectal cancer recommends that patients should not be excluded from cetuximab or panitumumab therapy on the basis of EGFR test results.[26]

There are 2 types of EGFR targeting agents available—monoclonal antibodies (eg, cetuximab, panitumumab) and small molecule ATP-competitive TKIs (eg, erlotinib, gefitinib). Cetuximab and panitumumab are FDA approved as single-agent therapies for the treatment of EGFR expressing, metastatic colorectal cancer with disease progression on or following fluoropyrimidine-, oxaliplatin-, and irinotecan-containing chemotherapy regimens. Patients who are prescribed cetuximab or panitumumab for colorectal cancer should have wild-type *KRAS* (*KRAS* mutation negative).[64,65] Cetuximab also has FDA-approved indication for head and neck cancer.[65] Erlotinib is the TKI prescribed in the United States as first-line treatment of patients with metastatic NSCLC whose tumors have EGFR exon 19 deletions or exon 21 (L858R) substitution mutations as detected by an FDA-approved test.[66] Gefitinib is more commonly used in Japan and Europe.

K-RAS

The *KRAS* protein, also called p21, is located on human chromosome 12 and is a member of the *Ras* superfamily of proteins.[27] It is a small GTPase (GTP cleaving) enzyme that is involved in intracellular signal transduction and is an essential component of the EGFR signaling cascade.[27] *KRAS* mutations occur in 20%-30% of adenocarcinomas; it is most prevalent in pancreatic, thyroid, colorectal, and lung cancers.[27,28] *KRAS* mutations are distinct for specific cancer types, and these different *KRAS* mutations may confer differences in prognosis, metastasis, and survival.[28] *KRAS* mutation is found in 35%-45% of colorectal cancers, and 95% of the mutations are on codon 12 and 13.[27] In lung cancer, *KRAS* mutation is not observed in small cell lung cancer but is detected in 20%-30% of NSCLC, usually in adenocarcinomas and rarely in squamous cell carcinomas.[24,28] Wild-type *KRAS* refers to negative detection of common mutations in this protein.

The clinical utility of determining *KRAS* mutation is to predict the benefit of therapy such as chemotherapy, EGFR TKIs, and anti-EGFR monoclonal antibodies. *KRAS* mutation is a candidate molecular biomarker for anti-EGFR therapy because it is the most frequent mutated factor downstream of EGFR signaling pathway.[27] The clinical significance of *KRAS* mutation status and its role in defining treatment options is different for colorectal cancer (CRC) compared with lung cancer. In CRC, it has been demonstrated that patients with wild-type *KRAS* have better response rates, progression-free survival, or overall survival when treated with cetuximab or panitumumab (either as monotherapy or in combination with chemotherapy) compared to patients with *KRAS* mutations.[29-35] Based on this data, the *NCCN Guidelines* for colorectal cancer, ASCO, and FDA labeling of cetuximab and panitumumab recommend testing for *KRAS* gene mutation in codons 12 and 13 in patients with advanced CRC, and if *KRAS* mutation is detected, cetuximab or panitumumab should not be prescribed.[26,36,64,65] See **Case 11-1**.

In lung cancer, *KRAS* mutation is associated with a poorer prognosis; however, there is little clinical utility in testing for *KRAS* mutation in this patient population because it has not been found to be a predictive factor for the benefit of chemotherapy or EGFR monoclonal antibodies.[28] Cetuximab is an option for the treatment of advanced NSCLC in patients without EGFR mutations or *ALK* rearrangements and, unlike CRC treatment, testing for *KRAS* mutation status is not required prior to initiating cetuximab.[28,37] Intrinsic resistance to TKIs is associated with *KRAS* mutations, but routine testing of *KRAS* mutation is not necessary to prescribe EGFR TKIs because EGFR and *KRAS* mutations are mutually exclusive and determination of EGFR mutation is a strong predictor of response to EGFR TKIs.[24,28]

CASE 11-1

JP is a 45-year-old male diagnosed with metastatic colorectal cancer. After receiving his first cycle of FOLFIRI (folinic acid [leucovorin], fluorouracil, irinotecan) with an irinotecan starting dose of 180 mg/m², the patient experienced grade 3 diarrhea and grade 2 neutropenia and recovered with supportive care. Genotyping was performed for this patient due to his experiencing severe side effects, and the results showed *UGT1A1*28* [UGT1A1 6/7 (heterozygous)]; *KRAS* mutation-negative (wild type); and EGFR-expressing tumor.

1. How should his treatment be modified based on these genotyping results?

EML4-ALK Fusion Gene

Activating mutations or translocations of the anaplastic lymphoma kinase (*ALK*) gene occur in cancers such as anaplastic large cell lymphoma and neuroblastoma.[38] In NSCLC, the fusion of the *ALK* gene with the echinoderm microtubule associated protein-like 4 (*EML4*) results in an aberrant fusion gene, *EML4-ALK*, which encodes a cytoplasmic chimeric protein with constitutive kinase activity.[38] *ALK* and *EML4* are both located in the short arm of chromosome 2.[39] The *EML4-ALK* fusion gene is a predictive biomarker that has been identified in 2%-7% of all NSCLC and is commonly observed in patients with adenocarcinoma histology who have never smoked or have a light smoking history.[38,40] Unlike patients with EGFR mutations, these patients are likely to be men and are younger.[40] *ALK* gene arrangements are largely mutually exclusive with EGFR or *KRAS* mutations.[41] In advanced-stage NSCLC, the presence of EML4-ALK translocation strongly predicts for sensitivity to the *ALK* tyrosine kinase inhibitor, crizotinib. A molecular diagnostic test for detection of the *ALK* fusion gene using FISH has been approved by the FDA and is required prior to initiating treatment with crizotinib.[42] The *NCCN Guidelines* for NSCLC recommends evaluation of *ALK* gene rearrangement status for all patients with nonsquamous NSCLC.[37] In an early phase trial, with mean treatment duration of 6.4 months with crizotinib in patients with advanced NSCLC positive for the *EML4-ALK* fusion gene, the overall response rate was 57% with a 72% estimated probability of 6-month progression-free survival.[38]

BRAF

The *BRAF* molecule is a serine/threonine kinase that is 1 of 3 members (*ARAF, BRAF, CRAF/RAF-1*) of the *Raf* kinase family and a key player of the MAPK (mitogen-activated protein kinase) [*RAS/RAF/MEK/ERK*] pathway.[43] The *RAF* protein kinases activate the MAPK pathway and mediate the transduction of proliferative and differentiative signals from cell surface receptors to the nucleus, catalyzing the phosphorylation of hydroxyl groups on specific serine and threonine residues.[43] Persistent and/or inappropriate activation of *RAF* results in abnormal differentiation, proliferation, apoptosis, and cancer development.[43] *BRAF* point mutations occur in approximately 8% of human tumors with the most common frequency in melanoma, papillary thyroid, and colorectal carcinomas.[43-45]

Mutations in the gene encoding *BRAF* (specifically, *BRAF V600*) occur in approximately 40%-60% of advanced melanomas, and in 80%-90% of these cases, it is due to substitution of glutamic acid for valine at amino acid 600 (V600E mutation) in exon 15.[45,46] Advanced melanomas with mutations in *BRAF* are associated with a more aggressive clinical course. Vemurafenib is a potent kinase inhibitor with specificity for the *BRAF V600E* mutation and has been shown to improve progression-free survival and overall survival in patients with either previously untreated or treated metastatic melanoma.[46,47] Roche has developed an FDA-approved companion biomarker real time PCR (RT-PCR), cobas 4800 *BRAF V600* mutation test, for the detection of the *BRAF V600E* mutation prior to prescribing vemurafenib.

BRAF mutation occurs in 9%-18% of patients with colorectal cancer, and it is mutually exclusive of *KRAS* mutations.[44,48] Mutations in *BRAF* are a strong prognostic marker, and patients with BRAF-mutated colorectal cancers have significantly shorter median progression-free and median overall survival than patients with wild-type-*BRAF* CRC.[48] The role of *BRAF* mutation as a predictive marker is less clear. According to the *NCCN Guidelines* for colorectal cancer, there are insufficient data to guide the use of anti-EGFR therapy in the first-line setting with active chemotherapy based on *BRAF V600E* mutation status.[26] BRAF genotyping may be considered in patients with wild-type *KRAS* gene; however, it is considered optional and is not a necessary test in the process of deciding to initiate anti-EGFR therapy.[26]

In papillary thyroid carcinoma (PTC) *BRAF V600E* mutation is the most common genetic alteration and the reported frequency is 39%-45%.[45,49] *BRAF* mutation is associated with a poor prognosis and aggressive behavior including extrathyroidal extension, multicentricity, local recurrence, lymph node metastasis, and distant metastases.[49] Ongoing studies are evaluating the role of *BRAF*-targeted therapy in the treatment of PTCs.

BCR/ABL Chromosomal Translocation (Philadelphia Chromosome)

The fusion of the Abelson murine leukemia (ABL) gene on chromosome 9q34 with the breakpoint cluster region (BCR) gene on chromosome 22q11.2 (t [9;22] [q34;q11.2]) results in the generation of a BCR-ABL fusion gene, which translates into a BCR-ABL oncoprotein.[50] This rearrangement is also known as the Philadelphia chromosome. BCR-ABL is a constitutively active tyrosine kinase that promotes growth and replication through downstream pathways such as RAS, RAF, JUN kinase, MYC and STAT and results in increased proliferation, altered differentiation, and inhibition of apoptosis.[50,51] The presence of the Philadelphia chromosome (Ph) is central to the diagnosis of chronic myeloid leukemia (CML), and it is seen in about 20%-30% of adults diagnosed with acute lymphoblastic leukemia (ALL).[50,52] In ALL, the presence of the Philadelphia chromosome is associated with a poorer prognosis where patients have an increased risk for central nervous system involvement and an aggressive clinical disease course, compared with Ph-negative ALL.[52] Treatment of patients with Ph-positive leukemia involves the use of tyrosine kinase inhibitors such as imatinib, dasatinib, nilotinib, bosutinib, and ponatinib.[50,51] Please refer to *Suggested Reading* for more in-depth discussion on the treatment of CML and ALL.[50,51]

Promyelocytic Leukemia/Retinoic Acid Receptor-Alpha

Acute promyelocytic leukemia (APL) is a unique subtype of acute myeloid leukemia that is characterized by the reciprocal translocation of the promyelocytic leukemia (PML) gene on chromosome 15 with the retinoic acid receptor-alpha (RAR-α) gene on chromosome 17 (t[15;17][q22;q21]).[53] APL is associated with distinct clinical features including leukopenia and life-threatening coagulopathy.[53] Treatment for patients with APL is different from other subtypes of acute myelogenous leukemia due to the addition of all-trans retinoic acid (ATRA or tretinoin) as a component of induction, consolidation, and maintenance therapy.

The addition of all-trans retinoic acid to anthracycline based induction chemo-therapy regimens results in complete remission rates in excess of 90% and cure rates of approximately 80%.[54-57]

Deletion of Chromosome 5q

Interstitial deletion in the long arm of chromosome 5 in the band q32-33 occurs in 16%-28% of patients with myelodysplastic syndrome (MDS).[58,59] Patients with this cytogenetic abnormality present with hypoproliferative anemia and dysplastic megakaryocytes in the bone marrow, and most patients become dependent on red-cell transfusions.[58] The use of lenalidomide in patients with 5q-MDS has been shown to reduce transfusion requirements and reverse cytologic and cytogenetic abnormalities.[58]

O^6-Methyl Guanine Methyl Transferase

The MGMT gene encodes for O^6-methyl guanine methyl transferase (MGMT), a cellular DNA repair protein that removes alkyl groups from the O^6 position of guanine, a critical site of DNA alkylation.[67] Tumor cells that have high levels of MGMT are protected from the effects of alkylating anticancer agents and are resistant to treatment with these agents.[67,68] Silencing of the MGMT gene by methylation of its promoter region is associated with decreased MGMT expression and has been observed in several tumor types.[67,68] Thus, determination of MGMT promoter methylation status may allow the selection of patients most likely to benefit from alkylating anticancer therapy. The relationship between MGMT gene silencing and response to therapy with the alkylating agent temozolomide has been tested in patients with glioblastomas.[67,68] MGMT promoter methylation was found to be an independent favorable prognostic marker, irrespective of treatment, and a predictive marker for therapy with temozolomide in patients with glioblastomas.[67] Patients with MGMT promoter methylation who are receiving temozolomide have improved median survival.[67] However, the overall survival curve for patients receiving temozolomide versus no temozolomide was similar for the first 9 months of follow-up; furthermore, not all patients with MGMT promoter methylation respond to alkylating agents.[67,68] Relapse also eventually occurs in patients who respond to initial therapy.[68] At present, there are no standard recommendations or guidelines for determination of MGMT promoter methylation status to determine responsiveness to alkylating therapy.

CASE 11-1
Answers

1. Cetuximab was added to the patient's FOLFIRI regimen based on the patient's *KRAS* wild type and EGFR-expressing cancer because it has been shown to improve response rate and progression-free survival in patients with colorectal cancer. His irinotecan dose was reduced per package insert recommendations by 1 dose level based on the toxicities he experienced and testing positive for the *UGT1A1*28* heterozygous genotype variant.

SUMMARY

Incorporation of the pharmacogenomics information is a great promise for personalized medicine in the oncology field. However, genotype-guided dosing is beneficial for only a small proportion of individuals with certain genotypes associated with extremes of drug elimination or metabolism. Furthermore, only a few polymorphisms have shown clinical relevance, and genotype alone cannot take into account the multiple environmental factors that affect drug disposition.[9] At the present time, advances in genetic analysis have enabled the use of targeted therapy for specific genetic mutations in cancers such as melanoma, colorectal cancer, and non–small cell cancer and have resulted in significant benefit to patients.

In order to help guide clinicians choose the appropriate therapy for patients based on pharmacogenomics data available to date on the efficacy and toxicity of specific drugs, the Food and Drug Administration (FDA) provides a table of pharmacogenomic biomarkers in drug labels.[69] The drug labels may contain information such as drug exposure and clinical response variability, risk for adverse effects, genotype-specific dosing, polymorphic drug target and disposition genes, and mechanisms of drug action. The biomarkers mentioned in the label may include gene variants, functional deficiencies, expression changes, and chromosomal abnormalities. When indicated, the label also includes the FDA-approved genetic test that should be used for a specific biomarker prior to prescribing of a specific drug. It is important to note that not all the labels include specific actions to be taken based on the genetic information, and sound clinical judgment should be exercised in interpreting the data.

REFERENCES

1. Wheeler HE, Maitland ML, Dolan ME, Cox NJ, Ratain MJ. Cancer pharmacogenomics: strategies and challenges. *Nature Reviews Genetics*. 2013;14:23–34.
2. O'Donnell P, Ratain M. Germline pharmacogenomics in oncology: decoding the patient for targeting therapy. *Molecular Oncology*. 2012;6:251–259.
3. Hertz D, McLeod H. Use of pharmacogenetics for predicting cancer prognosis and treatment exposure, response and toxicity. *J Hum Genet*. 2013:1–7.
4. Kalia M. Personalized oncology: recent advances and future challenges. *Metab Clin Exp*. 2013;62:S11–S14.
5. Evans W. Pharmacogenetics of thiopurine S-methyltransferase and thiopurine therapy. *Ther Drug Monit*. 2004;26:186–191.
6. Black A, McLeod H, Capell H, et al. Thiopurine methyltransferase genotype predicts therapy-limiting severe toxicity from azathioprine. *Ann Intern Med*. 1998;129:716–718.
7. Morel A, Boisdron-Celle M, Fey L, et al. Clinical relevance of different dihydropyrimidine dehydrogenase gene single nucleotide polymorphisms on 5-fluorouracil tolerance. *Mol Cancer Ther*. 2006;11:2895–2904.
8. Longley D, Harkin D, Johnson P. 5-fluorouracil: mechanisms of action and clinical strategies. *Nature Reviews Cancer*. 2003;3:330–338.
9. Gao B, Klumpen H, Gurney H. Dose calculation of anticancer drugs. *Expert Opin Drug Metab Toxicol*. 2008;4:1307–1319.
10. Innocenti F, Undevia S, Lyer L, et al. Genetic variants in the UDP-glucuronosyltransferase 1A1 gene predicts the risk of severe neutropenia of irinotecan. *J Clin Oncol*. 2004;22:1382–1388.
11. Swen J, Nijenhuis M, de Boer A, et al. Pharmacogenetics: from bench to byte-an update of guidelines. *Clin Pharmacol Ther*. 2011;89:662–673.
12. McLeod H, Sargent D, Marsh S, et al. Pharmacogenetic predictors of adverse events and response to chemotherapy in metastatic colorectal cancer: results from North American Gastrointestinal Intergroup Trial N9741. *J Clin Oncol*. 2010;28:3227–3233.
13. Camptosar (irinotecan) [package insert] Pfizer; July 2012. NY, NY.
14. Hammond M, Hayes D, Dowsett M, et al. American Society of Clinical Oncology/College of American Pathologists guideline recommendations for immunohistochemical testing of estrogen and progesterone receptors in breast cancer. *J Clin Oncol*. 2010;28:2784–2795.
15. National Comprehensive Cancer Network clinical practice guidelines in oncology. Breast cancer. Version 3.2013. Updated 2013. www.nccn.org. Accessed June 27, 2013.
16. Barrios C, Forbes J, Jonat W. The sequential use of endocrine treatment for advanced breast cancer: where are we? *Ann Oncol*. 2012;23:1378–1386.
17. Patani N, Martin L, Dowsett M. Biomarkers for the clinical management of breast cancer: international perspective. *Int J Cancer*. 2013;133:1–13.
18. Slamon D, Leyland-Jones B, Shak S, et al. Use of chemotherapy plus a monoclonal antibody against HER2 for metastatic breast cancer that overexpresses HER2. *N Engl J Med*. 2001;344:783–792.
19. Nielsen D, Kümler I, Palshof J, Andersson M. Efficacy of HER2-targeted therapy in metastatic breast cancer. Monoclonal antibodies and tyrosine kinase inhibitors. *Breast*. 2013;22:1–12.

20. Bang YJ, Van Cutsem E, Feyereislova A, et al. Trastuzumab in combination with chemotherapy versus chemotherapy alone for treatment of HER2-positive advanced gastric or gastro-oesophageal junction cancer (ToGA): A phase 3, open-label, randomised controlled trial. *Lancet.* 2010;376:687–697.

21. Vivanco I, Mellinghoff I. Epidermal growth factor receptor inhibitors in oncology. *Curr Opin Oncol.* 2010;22:573–578.

22. Mitsudomi T, Yatabe Y. The epidermal growth factor receptor in relation to tumor development: EGFR gene and cancer. *FEBS J.* 2010;277:301–308.

23. Yasuda H, Kobayashi S, Costa DB. EGFR exon 20 insertion mutations in non–small-cell lung cancer: preclinical data and clinical implications. *Lancet Oncol.* 2012;13:e23-e31.

24. Suda K, Tomizawa K, Mitsudomi T. Biological and clinical significance of KRAS mutations in lung cancer: an oncogenic driver that contrasts with EGFR mutation. *Cancer Metastasis Rev.* 2010;29:49–60.

25. Cunningham D, Humblet Y, Salvatore S, et al. Cetuximab monotherapy and cetuximab plus irinotecan in irinotecan-refractory metastatic colorectal cancer. 2004;351:337–345.

26. National Comprehensive Cancer Network. NCCN clinical practice guidelines in oncology: colon cancer. Version 3.2013. www.nccn.org. Published November 26, 2012. Updated 2012. Accessed June 20, 2013.

27. Tan C, Du X. KRAS mutation testing in metastatic colorectal cancer. *World J Gastroenterol.* 2012;18:5171–5180.

28. Roberts PJ, Stinchcombe TE. *KRAS* mutation: Should we test for it, and does it matter? *J Clin Oncol.* 2013;31:1112–1121.

29. Karapetis C, Khambata-Ford S, Jonker D, et al. K-ras mutations and benefit from cetuximab in advanced colorectal cancer. *N Engl J Med.* 2008;359:1757–1765.

30. Amado R, Wolf M, Peeters M, et al. Wild-type KRAS is required for panitumumab efficacy in patients with metastatic colorectal cancer. *J Clin Oncol.* 2008;26:1626–1634.

31. Van Cutsem E, Köhne C, Hitre E, et al. Cetuximab and chemotherapy as initial treatment for metastatic colorectal cancer. *N Engl J Med.* 2009;360:1408–1417.

32. Bokemeyer C, Bondarenko I, Makhson A, et al. Fluorouracil, leucovorin, and oxaliplatin with and without cetuximab in the first line treatment of metastatic colorectal cancer. *J Clin Oncol.* 2009;27:663–671.

33. Peeters M, Price T, Cervantes A, et al. Randomized phase III study of panitumumab with fluorouracil, leucovorin, and irinotecan (FOLFIRI) compared with FOLFIRI alone as second-line treatment in patients with metastatic colorectal cancer. *J Clin Oncol.* 2010;28:4706–4713.

34. Douillard J, Siena S, Cassidy J, et al. Randomized, phase III trial of panitumumab with infusional fluorouracil, leucovorin, and oxaliplatin (FOLFOX4) versus FOLFOX4 alone as first-line treatment in patients with previously untreated metastatic colorectal cancer: the PRIME study. *J Clin Oncol.* 2010;28:4697–4705.

35. Van Cutsem E, Köhne C, Láng I, et al. Cetuximab plus irinotecan, fluorouracil, and leucovorin as first-line treatment for metastatic colorectal cancer: updated analysis of overall survival according to tumor KRAS and BRAF mutation status. *J Clin Oncol.* 2011;29:2011–2019.

36. Allegra C, Milburn Jessup J, Somerfield M, et al. American Society of Clinical Oncology provisional clinical opinion: testing for *KRAS* gene mutations in patients with metastatic colorectal carcinoma to predict response to anti epidermal growth factor receptor monoclonal antibody therapy. *J Clin Oncol.* 2009;27:2091–2096.

37. National Comprehensive Cancer Network. NCCN clinical practice guidelines in oncology: non–small cell lung cancer. Version 2.2013. www.nccn.com. Updated 2013. Accessed June 20, 2013.

38. Kwak E, Bang Y, Camidge R, et al. Anaplastic lymphoma kinase inhibition in non–small cell lung cancer. *N Engl J Med.* 2010;363:1693–1703.

39. Koivunen J, Mermel C, Zejnullahu K, et al. EML4-ALK fusion gene and efficacy of an ALK kinase inhibitor in lung cancer. *Clin Cancer Res.* 2008;14:4275–4283.

40. Shaw A, Yeap B, Mino-Kenudson M, et al. Clinical features and outcome of patients with non–small cell lung cancer who harbor *EML4-ALK. J Clin Oncol.* 2009;27:4247–4253.

41. Takahashi T, Sonobe M, Kobayashi M, et al. Clinicopathologic features of non–small cell lung cancer with EML4-ALK fusion gene. *Ann Surg Oncol.* 2010;17:889–897.

42. Xalkori (crizotinib) [package insert] Pfizer; February 2012. NY, NY

43. Santarpia L, Lippman S, El-Naggar A. Targeting the MAPK-RAS-RAF signaling pathway in cancer therapy. *Expert Opin Ther Targets.* 2012;16:103–119.

44. Davies H, Bignell G, Cox C, et al. Mutations of the BRAF gene in cancer. *Nature.* 2002;417:949–954.

45. Vakiani E, Solit D. KRAS and BRAF: drug targets and predictive biomarkers. *J Pathol.* 2011;223:219–229.

46. Chapman P, Hauschild A, Robert C, et al. Improved survival with vemurafenib in melanoma with BRAF V600E mutation. *N Engl J Med.* 2011;364:2507–2516.

47. Sosman J, Kim K, Schuchter L, et al. Survival in BRAF V600–mutant advanced melanoma treated with vemurafenib. *N Engl J Med.* 2012;366:707–714.

48. Tol J, Nagtegaal I, Punt C. BRAF mutation in metastatic colorectal cancer. *N Engl J Med.* 2009;361:98–99.

49. Melck A, Yip L, Carty S. The utility of BRAF testing in the management of papillary thyroid cancer. *Oncologist.* 2010;15:1285–1293.

50. Jabbour E, Kantarjian H. Chronic myeloid leukemia: 2012 update on diagnosis, monitoring, and management. *Am J Hematol.* 2012;87:1039–1045.

51. National Comprehensive Cancer Network. NCCN clinical practice guidelines in oncology: chronic myelogenous leukemia. Version 4.2013. www.nccn.org. Updated 2013. Accessed June 26, 2013.

52. Liu-Dumlao T, Kantarjian H, Thomas D. Philadelphia-positive acute lymphoblastic leukemia: current treatment options. *Curr Oncol Rep.* 2012;14:387–394.

53. Tallman M, Altman J. How I treat acute promyelocytic leukemia. *Blood.* 2009;114:5126–5135.

54. Baljevic M, Park JH, Stein E, Douer D, Altman JK, Tallman MS. Curing all patients with acute promyelocytic leukemia: are we there yet? *Hematol Oncol Clin N Am.* 2011;25:1215–1233.

55. Fenaux P, Le Deley M, Castaigne S, et al. Effect of all trans retinoic acid in newly diagnosed acute promyelocytic leukemia. Results of a multicenter randomized trial. European APL 91 Group. *Blood.* 1993;82:3241–3249.

56. Tallman M, Andersen J, Schiffer C, et al. All-trans-retinoic acid in acute promyelocytic leukemia. *N Engl J Med.* 1997;337:1021–1028.
57. Sanz M, Vellenga E, Rayón C, et al. All-trans retinoic acid and anthracycline monochemotherapy for the treatment of elderly patients with acute promyelocytic leukemia. *Blood.* 2004;104:3490–3493.
58. List A, Dewald G, Bennett J. Lenalidomide in the myelodysplastic syndrome with chromosome 5q deletion. *N Engl J Med.* 2006;355:1456–1465.
59. Voutsadakis I, Cairoli A. A critical review of the molecular pathophysiology of lenalidomide sensitivity in 5q-myelodysplastic syndrome. *Leuk Lymphoma.* 2012;53:779–788.
60. Herceptin (trastuzumab). [package insert] Genentech; October 2010. San Francisco, CA.
61. Tykerb (lapatinib) [package insert]. GlaxoSmithKline; June 2013. Thousand Oaks, CA.
62. Perjeta (pertuzumab) [package insert] Genentech; April 2013. San Francisco, CA.
63. Kadcyla (ado-trastuzumab) [package insert] Genentech; May 2013. San Francisco, CA.
64. Vectibex (panitumumab) [package insert] Amgen; June 2013. Thousand Oaks, CA.
65. Erbitux (cetuximab) [package insert] Bristol Meyers Squibb; March 2013. Princeton, NJ
66. Tarceva (erlotinib) [package insert] Genentech; May 2013. San Francisco, CA
67. Hegi M, Diserens A, Gorlia T, et al. MGMT gene silencing and benefit from temozolomide in glioblastoma. 2005;352(10):997. *N Engl J Med.* 2005;10:997–1003.
68. Hegi M, Liu L, Herman J, et al. Correlation of O6-methylguanine methyltransferase (MGMT) promoter methylation with clinical outcomes in glioblastoma and clinical strategies to modulate MGMT activity. *J Clin Oncol.* 2008;26:4189–4199.
69. US Food and Drug Administration. Table of pharmacogenomic biomarkers in drug labels. http://www.fda.gov/drugs/scienceresearch/researchareas/pharmacogenetics/ucm083378.htm. Updated 2013. Accessed June 12, 2013.

SUGGESTED READING

* Allegra C, Milburn Jessup J, Somerfield M, et al. American Society of Clinical Oncology provisional clinical opinion: testing for *KRAS* gene mutations in patients with metastatic colorectal carcinoma to predict response to anti epidermal growth factor receptor monoclonal antibody therapy. *J Clin Oncol.* 2009;27:2091–2096.
* Barrios C, Forbes J, Jonat W. The sequential use of endocrine treatment for advanced breast cancer: where are we? *Ann Oncol.* 2012;23:1378–1386.
* Hammond M, Hayes D, Dowsett M, et al. American Society of Clinical Oncology/College of American Pathologists guideline recommendations for immunohistochemical testing of estrogen and progesterone receptors in breast cancer. *J Clin Oncol.* 2010;28:2784–2795.
* Hertz D, McLeod H. Use of pharmacogenetics for predicting cancer prognosis and treatment exposure, response and toxicity. *J Hum Genet.* 2013:1–7.
* Jabbour E, Kantarjian H. Chronic myeloid leukemia: 2012 update on diagnosis, monitoring, and management. *Am J Hematol.* 2012;87:1039–1045.
* Kalia M. Personalized oncology: recent advances and future challenges. *Metab Clin Exp.* 2013;62:S11–S14.

- Liu-Dumlao T, Kantarjian H, Thomas D. Philadelphia-positive acute lymphoblastic leukemia: current treatment options. *Curr Oncol Rep*. 2012;14:387–394.
- National Comprehensive Cancer Network. NCCN clinical practice guidelines in oncology: chronic myelogenous leukemia. Version 4.2013. www.nccn.org. Updated 2013. Accessed June 26, 2013.
- National Comprehensive Cancer Network. NCCN clinical practice guidelines in oncology: colon cancer. Version 3.2013. www.nccn.org. Published November 26, 2012. Updated 2012. Accessed June 20, 2013.
- National Comprehensive Cancer Network. NCCN clinical practice guidelines in oncology: non–small cell lung cancer. Version 2.2013. www.nccn.com. Updated 2013. Accessed June 20, 2013.
- Patani N, Martin L, Dowsett M. Biomarkers for the clinical management of breast cancer: international perspective. *Int J Cancer*. 2013;133:1–13.
- Roberts PJ, Stinchcombe TE. *KRAS* mutation: should we test for it, and does it matter? *J Clin Oncol*. 2013;31:1112–1121.
- Tallman M, Altman J. How I treat acute promyelocytic leukemia. *Blood*. 2009;114:5126–5135.

Index

Note: Page numbers followed by *b*, *f*, or *t* indicate material in boxes, figures, or tables, respectively.

A

Abelson murine leukemia (ABL), 339
ABIM. *See* American Board of Internal
    Medicine
abiraterone, 152
    acetate, 32
ABL. *See* Abelson murine leukemia
Abraxane (albumin-bound paclitaxel), 48
ABW. *See* actual body weight
accounting methods to manage inventory,
    204–205
accrual-based accounting system, 204–205
acellular pertussis vaccine, 256*t*
acral erythema. *See* hand-foot syndrome
acrolein, 16
active chemotherapeutic agents in treatment of
    neuroblastoma, 280*t*
actual body weight (ABW), 80
acute GVHD
    clinical grading of, 237*t*
    clinical staging of, 237*t*
    description, 236–237
    pharmacologic prophylaxis of, 238–239,
        240*t*–241*t*
    prevention of, 238
    supportive care for, 246
    treatment, 239, 244–245
acute leukemias
    ALL, 271–274, 272*t*
    AML, 274–275, 275*t*
    APL, 276
    description, 271

acute lymphoblastic leukemia (ALL), 270–274,
    339
    Down syndrome and, 274
    treatment backbone for, 272*t*
acute myeloid leukemia (AML), 270, 274–275
    cumulative chemotherapy doses and related
        outcomes, 275*t*
    Down syndrome and, 275
acute promyelocytic leukemia (APL), 22, 276,
    339
ADCs. *See* automated dispensing cabinets
administration
    chemotherapy errors, 183–185, 185*b*–186*b*
        wrong patient, 183–184
        wrong rate, 184
    for oral cancer therapy, 141–145
ado-trastuzumab emtansine (Kadcyla), 48
Adria (doxorubicin), 47
ADT. *See* androgen deprivation therapy
adverse event (AE), 315
    reporting, 195
afatinib, 28
Affordable Care Act, 212
agents
    erythropoiesis-stimulating, 196
    oral cancer therapy. *See* oral cancer therapy,
        agents
    targeted/biologic, 141
        cancer treatment with approval dates, 139,
            140*t*
        emergence of, 145
AIs. *See* aromatase inhibitors

albumin-bound paclitaxel (Abraxane), 48

ALCL. *See* anaplastic large cell lymphoma

Aldesleukin (interleukin-2), 10*t*, 281

alemtuzumab (Campath), 8*t*

Alimta (pemetrexed), 13*t*

ALK. *See* anaplastic lymphoma kinase

alkylating agents, 15

    nitrogen mustard, 15–16

    nitrosoureas, 16

    nonclassical, 16

ALL. *See* acute lymphoblastic leukemia

allogeneic HSCT, 226, 226*t*, 246

American Board of Internal Medicine (ABIM), 41

American College of Clinical Pharmacy, 41

American Society of Clinical Oncology (ASCO), 66*t*, 76, 148, 161, 234, 311, 330

American Society of Health-System Pharmacists (ASHP), 41, 125

aminohydrolase, 23

AML. *See* acute myeloid leukemia

amplifications, genetic mutations, 4*t*

anaplastic large cell lymphoma (ALCL), 277

anaplastic lymphoma kinase (ALK), 277

anastrozole, 31

ancillary medications, 62, 62*t*

androgen deprivation therapy (ADT), 152

angiogenesis inhibitors, 26

anteroom, 119

anthracene derivatives, 21–22

anthracyclines, 21, 189–190, 274

antiandrogens, 31–32, 152

anticancer agents, 8*t*–14*t*

    computerized provider-order-entry for, 45–46

    for intrathecal administration, 60–61

anticancer drugs, variations in dosing of, 53

anticancer regimens, abbreviation for, 49–51

anticancer therapy, 43–44

    nononcology indications for, 68–69

    regimen cycle, 51–52

anticancer therapy dosing

    adjustment recommendations, 89

    and administration modification in HD setting, 102–105

    hepatic function assessment, 105–106

    renal function assessment

        estimation of, 99–100

        IDMS method, 101–102

        renal impairment, classifications of, 100–101

antiestrogens, 30

antifolates, 19–20

antimetabolites, 17

    antifolates, 19–20

    cytidine analogs, 18–19

    purine, 19

    pyrimidines, 18

antimicrobial scrub brushes, 121*b*

antimotility agents, 245

antineoplastics. *See* chemotherapy, agents

antithymocyte globulin, 245

APL. *See* acute promyelocytic leukemia

APPRISE. *See* Assisting Providers and Cancer Patients with Risk Information for the Safe use of ESAs

aprepitant, 234

area under the curve (AUC), 82

Aredia (pamidronate), 47

aromatase inhibitors (AIs), 30–31, 151, 330

arsenic trioxide, 22

Arzerra (ofatumumab), 11*t*–12*t*

ASCO. *See* American Society of Clinical Oncology

ASCO/ONS Chemotherapy Administration Safety Standards, 46

ASCO/ONS Chemotherapy Administration Safety Standards Including Standards for the Safe Administration and Management of Oral Chemotherapy, 58–59

aseptic technique, 116

ASP. *See* average sales price

asparaginase, 23, 286*t*

Assisting Providers and Cancer Patients with Risk Information for the Safe use of ESAs (APPRISE), 285

AUC. *See* area under the curve

autologous HSCT, 226, 226*t*

automated dispensing cabinets (ADCs), 126–128, 127*f*

Avastin (bevacizumab), 8*t*

average sales price (ASP), 215

axitinib, 28

azacitidine, 18

azathioprine, 86

B

barrier isolators

    advantages and disadvantage, 115

    biologic safety cabinet *vs.,* 113–115

BCOP. *See* board certification in oncology
    pharmacy
BCR. *See* breakpoint cluster region
BCR-ABL fusion gene, 27, 272
bendamustine, 16
bevacizumab (Avastin), 8*t*, 26, 63
bexarotene, 24
Bexxar (tositumomab), 14*t*
bioavailability and bioequivalence studies, clinical
    trial medication issues, 320–321
biohazardous drugs, hazardous *vs.*, 321
biologic safety cabinet (BSC)
    advantages and disadvantage, 115
    decontamination, 123
    vs. isolator, 113–115
biologic therapies, 4
Blenoxane (bleomycin), 8*t*, 23, 85
bleomycin (Blenoxane), 8*t*, 23, 85
board certification in oncology pharmacy
    (BCOP), 41, 135
Board of Pharmacy Specialties, 41
body surface area (BSA), 141, 143
    adult amputees, 81–82
    body weight equations, 75, 77
    formula, 75, 77
    obese and underweight patients, 78–81
    principles, 78, 79
bone marrow support, pediatric oncology, 285
bone marrow transplantation (BMT). *See* hema-
    topoietic stem cell transplantation
bortezomib, 29
bosutinib, 27–28
BRAFV600E, 28
breakpoint cluster region (BCR), 339
breast cancer
    hormonal agents for treatment, 145, 151
    tamoxifen for, 153
"brown bagging," 210
BSA. *See* body surface area
BSC. *See* biologic safety cabinet
Burkitt's lymphoma, 2
busulfan (Busulfex, Myleran), 9*t*, 16, 230*t*
Busulfex (busulfan), 9*t*

C

cabazitaxel (Jevtana), 7, 9*t*
cabozantinib, 28
CAIs. *See* compounding aseptic isolators
calcineurin inhibitors (CNIs), 238, 258

Calvert formula, 17
Campath (alemtuzumab), 8*t*
Camptosar (irinotecan), 11*t*
camptothecin derivatives, 20–21
cancer
    agents, abbreviation for, 49
    cells, 2
    childhood mortality, 267, 268*f*
    definition of, 1
    diagnosis, 65*t*
cancer therapy prescription, 44
    anticancer therapy regimen cycle, 51–52
    CPOE for anticancer agents, 45–46
    documentation of, 44–45
    dose calculation, 52–54
    investigational anticancer regimens/
        medications, 54–55
    strategies to prevent errors in, 46–49, 49*t*–51*t*
capecitabine, 86
    dosing for, 142
    for metastatic breast cancer, 145, 166–167
carboplatin (Paraplatin), 9*t*, 17, 190*f*, 230*t*, 286*t*
    dosing
        AUC, 82
        Calvert equation, 83–85
        renal function, 82
carcinogenesis, 3
cardiovascular side effects of oral cancer therapy,
        146*t*, 148–149
carfilzomib, 29
carmustine, 16, 230*t*
cash-based accounting for inventory control, 204
CE opportunities. *See* continuing education
        opportunities
cell-cycle, 2, 5
    nonspecific drugs, 5
    specific drugs, 5
CellCept (mycophenolate mofetil), 241*t*
Center for Education and Research on Therapeu-
        tics CERT, 312
Centers for Medicare & Medicaid Services
        (CMS), 213
central nervous system (CNS) tumors, 278–280,
        279*b*
cerebrospinal fluid (CSF), 60
CERT. *See* Center for Education and Research
        on Therapeutics
certified pharmacy technicians (CPhT), 136
CETA. *See* Controlled Environment Testing
        Association

cetuximab (Erbitux), 9*t*
chain-of-custody laws, 211*f*
chemical safety glasses, 125
chemo gown, 125
chemoregimen website, 66*t*
chemotherapy, 226
    agents, 4, 5
        alkylating agents. *See* alkylating agents
        antimetabolites. *See* antimetabolites
        heavy metal compounds, 17
        microtubule-targeting drugs. *See*
            microtubule-targeting drugs
        topoisomerase inhibitors. *See* topoisomerase
            inhibitors
    CNS tumors, 279
    dispensing, 125
    dosing in infants, 290–292, 290*t*–291*t*
    for Ewing's sarcoma, 283, 283*t*
    medication errors, 172
        administering, 183–185, 185*b*–186*b*
        compounding/dispensing, 179–183
        monitoring, 186
        prescribing, 177–178
        prevention, 186–194, 198*b*–199*b*
        procurement, 174–177, 176*b*–177*b*
        transcribing/documenting, 178–179
        types of, 174–186
    in pediatric population, unique features, 286,
        286*t*–288*t*
    preparation, 113
    products with look-alike names, 182*t*–183*t*
    spill kit, 124, 125*b*, 126*f*
    standardized order forms and checking pro-
        cess, 188–194
    treatments, 303–304
chemotherapy-induced nausea and vomiting
        (CINV), 233–235, 284–285
    case study, 234–235, 257–258
    pediatric oncology, 284–285
chemotherapy-sensitive tumors, 226
childhood cancers, 267, 268*f. See also* pediatric
        oncology
    malignant CNS tumors of, 279*b*
    signs and symptoms of, 269*b*
    solid tumors. *See* solid tumors of childhood
children
    and adolescents with HL, 277
    obese, 293
    rituximab administration in, 278

Children's Oncology Group (COG), 66*t*,
        268–269
chronic GVHD
    clinical manifestations of, 248*t*–249*t*
    description, 246
    pathogenesis of, 246–247
    signs and symptoms, 260
    treatment of, 247, 251–252
chronic myelogenous leukemia (CML), 27, 270,
        339
    imatinib for, 160, 167–168
CINV. *See* chemotherapy-induced nausea and
        vomiting
cisplatin (Platinol), 9*t*, 17, 63, 190*f*, 287*t*
cladribine, 19
cleanroom
    environment control, 113–120
    processes
        chemotherapy spills, 124
        cleaning regimens, 123–124
        personal protective equipment, 120–123
        refrigeration, 128–131
        safe disposal of hazardous drug waste,
            131–133
        storage and dispensing, 124–128
clinical benefit response, 33*t*
clinical trials, 305
    issues affecting patient's enrollment in,
        310–313
    medication issues
        bioequivalence and bioavailability studies,
            320–321
        DARs, 316–319, 317*b*, 318*b*
        dispensing oral agents, 320
        drug preparation and administration issues,
            319–320
        hazardous *vs.* biohazardous drugs, 321
    phase I case study, 307–309
    phases, 304, 310
    SOPs, 305
clofarabine, 19
closed system transfer devices (CSTDs), 116,
        117, 117*b*
    advantages and disadvantages, 118*b*
    implementation, 118*b*
    opponents of, 119*b*
CML. *See* chronic myelogenous leukemia
CMS. *See* Centers for Medicare & Medicaid
        Services

CNIs. *See* calcineurin inhibitors
CNS tumors. *See* central nervous system tumors
Cockcroft-Gault (CG) equation, 101
Code of Federal Regulations Title 21, 322, 322*b*
COG. *See* Children's Oncology Group
common terminology criteria for adverse events (CTCAE), 313–316
communication plan for healthcare providers, 196
complete response (CR), 33*t*
compounding aseptic containment isolators (CACIs), 114
compounding aseptic isolators (CAIs), 114
compounding/dispensing errors, 179–183
wrong dose, 181
computerized physician order entry (CPOE), 193
for anticancer agents, 45–46
conditioning regimen, 224*t*
constipation, 150
continuing education (CE) opportunities, 43
Controlled Environment Testing Association (CETA), 116
cooperative research groups, role in pediatric oncology, 268–269
corticosteroids, 233, 239, 245, 247
counseling of oral cancer therapy, 156–158, 157*b*
CPOE. *See* computerized physician order entry
CR. *See* complete response
crizotinib, 28
CSF. *See* cerebrospinal fluid
CSTDs. *See* closed system transfer devices
CTCAE. *See* common terminology criteria for adverse events
cure response, 33*t*
cyclophosphamide, 15, 230*t*
cyclosporine (Gengraf, Neoral, Sandimmune), 238, 240*t*, 242*t*
CYP450. *See* cytochrome P450
CYP3A. *See* cytochrome P450 3A
CYP17A1 enzyme, 31
cytarabine (Cytosar), 9*t*, 18, 60, 230*t*
cytidine analogs, 18–19
cytochrome P450 (CYP450), 153
cytochrome P450 3A (CYP3A), 308, 312
cytochrome P450 3A4 pathway, 258

cytopenias, 235–236
Cytosar (cytarabine), 9*t*, 18, 60, 230*t*
cytotoxic cancer therapy, 141, 145, 165
with approval dates, 139, 140*t*
cytotoxic drugs, detectable levels of, 119
cytotoxic medications, 116
cytotoxicity, mechanism of, 18

D
dabrafenib, 28
dacarbazine, 16
dactinomycin, 287*t*
DARs. *See* drug accountability records
dasatinib, 27
data collection thermometers, 129
daunorubicin, 287*t*
decitabine, 18
defibrotid, 253, 254
degarelix, 31
deletions, genetic mutations, 4*t*
dermatologic side effects of oral cancer therapy, 146*t*
dexamethasone, 164, 287*t*
dexterity, 121
diagnosis-related group (DRG) system, 213
diarrhea, oral cancer therapy and, 146*t*, 149–150, 150*b*
digital range thermometers, 129
dihydropyrimidine dehydrogenase (DPD), 86, 329
dimethyl sulfoxide (DMSO), 232
diphtheria, 256*t*
disposable gowns, 123*b*
disposal bag, 125
District of Columbia, 42
DLT. *See* dose-limiting toxicity
DMSO. *See* dimethyl sulfoxide
DNA damage, 2, 15
docetaxel (Taxotere), 6–7, 10*t*, 176, 191*f*
dosage forms, standardized formulary of drugs and, 187
dose-escalation schema, 316
dose-limiting toxicity (DLT), 226
and retreatment criteria, 313–316
dosing
for capecitabine, 142
chemotherapy errors, 178
for oral cancer therapy, 141–145

dosing calculations
of anticancer agent, 52–54
anticancer therapy dosing
dose adjustment recommendations, 89
dose and administration modification in
HD setting, 102–105
hepatic function assessment, 105–106
renal function assessment, 88, 101–102
BSA
adult amputees, 81–82
body weight equations, 75, 77
formula, 75, 77
obese and underweight patients, 78–81
principles, 78, 79
drug preparation process, 88
flat fixed-dose dosing system, 74
genotype
DPYD gene, 86–87
polymorphic gene expression, 85–86
UGT1A1*28, 87
methods for, 74
pharmacokinetic, 82–85
Down syndrome
and ALL, 274
and AML, 275
Doxil (liposomal doxorubicin), 48
doxorubicin (Adria), 47, 287*t*
DPD. *See* dihydropyrimidine dehydrogenase
DRG system. *See* diagnosis-related group
system
drug accountability records (DARs), 316–319,
321
drug-induced adverse events, 195
drug interactions with oral cancer therapy,
152–156
drug packaging, 119
drug therapy, 4

E

Eastern Cooperative Oncology Group (ECOG)
scale, 33, 34*t*
education for cancer treatment, 43–44
EF. *See* ejection fraction
EGFR. *See* epidermal growth factor receptor
ejection fraction (EF), 77
electrolytes, 65*t*
elements to assure safe use (ETASU), 196, 206
Eloxatin (oxaliplatin), 12*t*
employ technology to medication occurrences,
193

engraftment, 224*t*
environmental controls
creation of negative pressure, 119
in production area, 113
Environmental Protection Agency (EPA), 131,
133, 321
enzalutamide, 31–32, 152
EOB. *See* explanation of benefits
EPA. *See* Environmental Protection Agency
epidermal growth factor receptor (EGFR), 27,
334–335
epothilones, 7
EPS. *See* extrapyramidal side effects
Epstein-Barr virus, 2
equipment, cleaning, 123
ER. *See* estrogen receptor
Erbitux (cetuximab), 9*t*
eribulin, 14
erlotinib, 27
errors, medication. *See* medication, errors
erythropoiesis-stimulating agents (ESAs), 196,
285
ES. *See* Ewing's sarcoma
ESAs. *See* erythropoiesis-stimulating agents
Escherichia coli, 23
ESFT. *See* Ewing's sarcoma family of tumors
estramustine, 15
estrogen receptor (ER), 330
ETASU. *See* elements to assure safe use
etoposide, 21, 230*t*, 287*t*
everolimus, 29
Ewing's sarcoma (ES), 282–283, 283*t*
Ewing's sarcoma family of tumors (ESFT),
282–283
explanation of benefits (EOB), 218
extrapyramidal side effects (EPS),
284–285

F

fatigue of oral cancer therapy, 150–151
FDA. *See* Food and Drug Administration
FDAAA. *See* Food and Drug Administration
Amendments Act
febrile neutropenia (FN), 68
fee-for-service plan, private insurance, 216
filgrastim (Neupogen), 47, 231
financial assistance for oral cancer therapy, 165,
166*t*
FISH. *See* fluorescent in situ hybridization
Flockhart, David A., 312

FLT3 ITD. *See* internal tandem duplications of *FLT3*
fluconazole, 261
fludarabine, 230*t*
fluid management, pediatric oncology, 289–290, 289*t*
fluid retention, 7
fluorescent in situ hybridization (FISH), 333
fluorouracil, 86
FOLFOX regimen, 53
Folotyn (pralatrexate), 13*t*
Food and Drug Administration (FDA), 14, 195, 328
Food and Drug Administration Amendments Act (FDAAA), 196
food interactions with oral cancer therapy, 152–156
Form FDA 1572, 309*b*
frost-free refrigerators, 128–129
full-size refrigerators, 128

G

G-CSFs. *See* granulocyte colony-stimulating factors
garbing procedure, 122*b*–123*b*
gastrointestinal side effects of oral cancer therapy, 146*t*, 149–150
GBM. *See* glioblastoma multiforme
gemcitabine, 18
genetic mutations, types of, 4*t*
Gengraf (cyclosporine), 240*t*
GFR. *See* glomerular filtration rate
glioblastoma multiforme (GBM)
  temozolomide dosing for, 143, 143*b*
glomerular filtration rate (GFR), 82
glove boxes. *See* barrier isolators
gloves, 121–122, 125
glucose moiety, 16
GM-CSF. *See* granulocyte-macrophage colony-stimulating factor
GOG. *See* Gynecologic Oncology Group
GPOs. *See* group purchasing organizations
graft-versus-host disease (GVHD), 224*t*
  acute. *See* acute GVHD
  case study, 250–251, 259–262
  chronic GVHD
    clinical manifestations of, 248*t*–249*t*
    description, 246
    pathogenesis of, 246–247
    treatment of, 247, 251–252

description, 236
  risk factor for, 259
  steroid refractory. *See* steroid refractory GVHD
  treatment, 239, 244–245
graft-versus-tumor (GVT) effect, 227, 239
granulocyte colony-stimulating factors (G-CSFs), 47, 68
granulocyte-macrophage colony-stimulating factor (GM-CSF), 281
group purchasing organizations (GPOs), 207
GVHD. *See* graft-versus-host disease
GVT effect. *See* graft-versus-tumor effect
Gynecologic Oncology Group (GOG), 67*t*

H

Haemophilus influenzae type b (Hib) vaccine, 256*t*
HAMA. *See* human antimouse antibodies
hand-foot syndrome (HFS), 146*t*, 147, 147*b*
hand-washing procedure, 121*b*
haploidentical transplantation, 239
hazardous drugs, 113
  vs. biohazardous drugs, 321
  CACI for, 115
  waste, safe disposal of, 131–133
HD. *See* hemodialysis
HDAC inhibitors. *See* histone deacetylase inhibitors
health maintenance organizations (HMOs), 217
healthcare providers, 43
  communication plan for, 196
heavy metal compounds, 17
hedgehog pathway, 29
hematologic cancers, 65*t*
hematologic malignancies, treatment of, 25
Hematology/Oncology Pharmacy Association (HOPA), 41, 67*t*
hematopoietic stem cell transplantation (HSCT)
  clinical pearls for immunosuppressive therapy in, 242*t*–243*t*
  collection of, 229, 231
  conditioning regimens for, 228*t*–229*t*
  description, 223–224
  infusion of, 231–233
  recipients
    infections in, 255*t*
    vaccination recommendations for, 256*t*
  stem cell source and type, 224, 226*t*

hematopoietic stem cell transplantation (HSCT) (*Contd.*)
    supportive care and transplant-related complications
        CINV, 233–235
        cytopenias, 235–236
        GVHD. *See* graft-versus-host disease
    terminology and definitions, 224, 224*t*–225*t*
    toxicities in, 230*t*
    types of, 226–227
hematopoietic stem cells (HSCs), 223, 224*t*
    infusion guidelines, 232*t*
hemodialysis (HD), 102
HER2. *See* human epidermal growth factor receptor 2
Herceptin (trastuzumab), 14*t*, 48
HFS. *See* hand-foot syndrome
Hib vaccine. *See Haemophilus influenzae* type b vaccine
high-efficiency particulate air (HEPA) filtration, 113–114, 119
histone deacetylase (HDAC) inhibitors, 23
HL. *See* Hodgkin's lymphoma
HLA. *See* human leukocyte antigen
HMOs. *See* health maintenance organizations
hoarseness, 6
Hodgkin's lymphoma (HL), 15, 276–277
HOPA. *See* Hematology/Oncology Pharmacy Association
hormonal agents, 30
    antiandrogens, 31–32
    antiestrogens, 30
    aromatase inhibitors, 30–31
    cancer treatment, 145
        with approval dates, 139, 140*t*
    LHRH analogs and antagonists, 31
    toxicities of, 151–152
hormonal therapies
    for breast cancer, 151
    for prostate cancer, 152
    side effects of, 151
hormone-sensitive prostate cancer cells, 15
HSCs. *See* hematopoietic stem cells
HSCT. *See* hematopoietic stem cell transplantation
human antimouse antibodies (HAMA), 25
human epidermal growth factor receptor 2 (HER2), 27, 333
human leukocyte antigen (HLA), 224*t*
hydration, 65*t*
    HSCs, 232*t*

hydrocortisone, 244
hydroxyurea, 23
hyperleukocytosis, 270
hypersensitivity, 23, 25
hypertension, 146*t*, 148
hyperuricemia, 65*t*

I

ibritumomab tiuxetan (Zevalin), 10*t*
ICP. *See* intracranial pressure
idarubicin, 287*t*
ideal staffing, 137
IDMS. *See* isotope dilution mass spectrometry
ifosfamide, 15, 287*t*
IHC. *See* immunohistochemical (IHC)
imatinib, 27, 160, 167–168
immunohistochemical (IHC), 330
immunomodulators, 26
inactivated influenza vaccine, 256*t*
infants, chemotherapy dosing in, 290–292, 290*t*–291*t*
infusion-related reactions, 63
initiation, carcinogenesis, 3
insertions, genetic mutations, 4*t*
Institute for Safe Medication Practices (ISMP), 179, 193–194
Institute for Safe Medication Practices-Canada (ISMP-Canada), 178, 179, 183, 194
Institute of Medicine (IOM) report, 172, 177
interferon-alfa (Roferon-A, Intron A), 10*t*, 30
interleukin-2 (Aldesleukin), 10*t*, 30
internal tandem duplications of *FLT3* (*FLT3* ITD), 276
International Conference on Harmonization Guideline for Good Clinical Practice, 322
intracellular activity, 5
intracranial pressure (ICP), 279
intrathecal administration, anticancer agents for, 60–61
intrathecal anticancer therapy, 60–62
intrathecal therapy, wrong-route errors associated with, 192–193
intrathecal vincristine injection, 61–62
intravenous (IV) anticancer therapies, 141
intravenous (IV) busulfan, 252–253
intravenous (IV) cancer therapies, 141, 156
    safe prescribing and dispensing practices, 160–163
intravenous (IV) formulations, 21, 309

intravenous (IV) investigational medications, 319–320
intravenous (IV) vials, 321
Intron A (interferon-alfa), 10t
inventory control
  accounting, 204–205
  definition, 204
  management, 209
  purchasing, 206–211
  340B pricing, 212
investigational agents, 303
investigational anticancer regimens/medications, 54–55
investigational drugs
  clinical trial medication issues
    bioequivalence and bioavailability studies, 320–321
    DARs, 316–319
    dispensing oral agents, 320
    drug preparation and administration issues, 319–320
    hazardous vs. biohazardous drugs, 321
  CTCAE, 313–316
  documentation, 304–305, 305b
  patient's enrollment in clinical trial, 310–313
  service, 322b
    checklist, 306b
  SOPs, 305
IOM Committee on Identifying and Preventing Medication Errors, 174
IOM report. See Institute of Medicine report
irinotecan (Camptosar), 11t, 87, 288t
ISMP. See Institute for Safe Medication Practices
ISMP-Canada. See Institute for Safe Medication Practices-Canada
ISO Class 5 device, 113
isotope dilution mass spectrometry (IDMS), 85, 101
isotretinoin, 287t
itraconazole, 187
ixabepilone (Ixempra), 7, 11t
Ixempra (ixabepilone), 7, 11t

J
Jevtana (cabazitaxel), 9t
Joint Commission standards, 46, 178, 195

K
Kadcyla (ado-trastuzumab emtansine), 48
Karnofsky score, 33

Kidney Disease Outcomes Quality Initiative's (KDO/QI), 89

L
L-asparagine, 23
lapatinib, 27
  for metastatic breast cancer, 145, 166–167
LASA medication. See look-alike, sound-alike medication
left ventricular dysfunction, 146t, 148
lenalidomide, 26
  REMS requirements for, 162b–163b
letrozole, 31
leucovorin, 18
LHRH. See luteinizing hormone-releasing hormone
liposomal doxorubicin (Doxil), 48
liposomal formulation, 18
liver enzyme, 31
lomustine, 16
look-alike, sound-alike (LASA) medication
  preventing errors, 189–192
  wrong medication associated with product, 180
lorazepam, 258
lung cancer, 336
luteinizing hormone-releasing hormone (LHRH), 31, 152
lymphomas
  Hodgkin's, 276–277
  non-Hodgkin's, 277–278

M
maintenance therapy, 5
mammalian target of rapamycin (mTOR) inhibitors, 29
MAO inhibitor. See monoamine oxidase inhibitor
MASCC. See Multinational Association of Supportive Care in Cancer
matched related donor, 225t
matched unrelated donor (MUD), 225t
materiality threshold, in accounting, 205
maximum tolerated dose (MTD), 316
MDRD. See Modification of Diet in Renal Disease
MDS. See myelodysplastic syndrome
measles, mumps, rubella (MMR) vaccine, 256t
mechlorethamine, 15

MedDRA. *See* Medical Dictionary for Regulatory
    Activities
Medicaid, 216
Medical Dictionary for Regulatory Activities
    (MedDRA), 313
Medicare, 213–216
    coverage, 217–218
    peer-reviewed journals recognized by, 219*t*
Medicare Modernization Act (MMA), 165
Medicare Part A, 213, 214*t*, 216*t*
Medicare Part B, 213, 214*t*, 216*t*
Medicare Part D, 165, 213
medication
    cancer therapy, 5
    errors, 172
        categories for, 173*t*
        causes of, 194
        chemotherapy. *See* chemotherapy, medica-
            tion errors
        NCC MERP Index for, 174*t*
        patient and medication information in,
            172*t*
        prevention, 172
            LASA, 189–192
        reporting, 194
    guide, REMS program components, 196
    information, access to, 187–188
    preparation process, 190
        cleanroom garb for IV, 121
MEDMARX, 194
MedWatch program, 195, 196
MEK inhibitor. *See* mitogen-activated protein
    kinase inhibitor
melphalan, 230*t*, 257–258
MEMS. *See* Micro Electronic Monitoring System
mercaptopurine, 19, 86, 288*t*
mesna, 16
metastatic breast cancer, 151
    capecitabine and lapatinib for, 145, 166–167
metastatic colorectal cancer, 53
methotrexate (Trexall), 11*t*, 19–20, 63, 238,
    240*t*, 243*t*, 288*t*
metoclopramide, 284–285
MGMT. *See* O⁶-methyl guanine methyl transfer-
    ase (MGMT)
Micro Electronic Monitoring System (MEMS),
    159
Micromedex, 69
microtubule-targeting drugs, 5–6
    epothilones, 7
    eribulin, 14
    estramustine, 15
    taxanes, 6–7, 8*t*–14*t*
    vinca alkaloids, 6
microtubules, 6
minimal residual disease (MRD), 271–272
minitransplant, 225*t*
mismatched related donor, 225*t*
mismatched unrelated donor, 225*t*
mitogen-activated protein kinase (MEK)
    inhibitor, 28
mitotic inhibitors, 5, 7
mitoxantrone, 21
MMA. *See* Medicare Modernization Act
MMR vaccine. *See* measles, mumps, rubella
    vaccine
MoABs. *See* monoclonal antibodies (MoABs)
mobilization regimen, 225*t*
modalities of cancer treatment, 4
Modification of Diet in Renal Disease (MDRD),
    101
monitoring, chemotherapy errors, 186
monoamine oxidase (MAO) inhibitor, 155
monoclonal antibodies (MoABs), 24–25, 25*t*
monotherapy, 31
MPJE. *See* Multistate Pharmacy Jurisprudence
    Exam
MRD. *See* minimal residual disease
MTD. *See* maximum tolerated dose
mTOR inhibitors. *See* mammalian target of
    rapamycin inhibitors
MUD. *See* matched unrelated donor
multidisciplinary team, 133–137
Multinational Association of Supportive Care in
    Cancer (MASCC), 67*t*
Multistate Pharmacy Jurisprudence Exam
    (MPJE), 41
Musculoskeletal side effects of breast cancer,
    151
mutations, 4*t*
mycophenolate mofetil (CellCept, Myfortic),
    238, 241*t*, 243*t*
myeloablative conditioning, 225*t*
myelodysplastic syndrome (MDS), 340
myelosuppression, 7, 18, 226
Myfortic (mycophenolate mofetil), 241*t*
Myleran (busulfan), 9*t*

N

NAPLEX. *See* North American Pharmacist
    Licensure Examination

National Cancer Institute (NCI), 67*t*, 128, 316, 322
National Comprehensive Cancer Network (NCCN), 67, 148, 150, 334
   Guidelines for Treatment of Cancer, 32
National Coordinating Council for Medication Error Reporting and Prevention (NCC MERP), 172
   taxonomy of medication error, 194
National Institute for Occupational Health and Safety (NIOSH), 125
National Kidney Disease Education Program (NKDEP), 101
National Wilms' Tumor Study (NWTS), 281
NCC MERP. *See* National Coordinating Council for Medication Error Reporting and Prevention
NCC MERP Index for medication errors, 174*t*, 194
NCCN. *See* National Comprehensive Cancer Network
NCI. *See* National Cancer Institute
negative pressure in cleanroom, 119
nelarabine, 19
neoadjuvant therapy, 5
Neoral (cyclosporine), 240*t*
nephrotoxicity, prevention of, 63*t*
Neu/ErbB-2, 333
Neulasta (pegfilgrastim), 47
Neupogen (filgrastim), 47
neuroblastoma, 280–281, 280*t*
neurotoxicity, 6
NHL. *See* non-Hodgkin's lymphoma
nilotinib, 27
nitrogen mustard, 15–16
nitrosoureas, 16
NKDEP. *See* National Kidney Disease Education Program
nodular lymphocyte predominant HL, 277
non-Hodgkin's lymphoma (NHL), 271, 277–278
nonclassical alkylating agents, 16
nonhazardous medications, 114
nonmyeloablative conditioning, 225*t*
nononcology indications for anticancer therapies, 68–69
non–small cell lung cancer (NSCLC), 335
North American Pharmacist Licensure Examination (NAPLEX), 41, 134
NSCLC. *See* non–small cell lung cancer (NSCLC)

nurses, 41, 42*t*, 135–136
NWTS. *See* National Wilms' Tumor Study

O

O^6-methyl guanine methyl transferase (MGMT), 340
obese children, 293
Occupational Safety and Health Administration (OSHA), 125
octreotide, 246
ofatumumab (Arzerra), 11*t*–12*t*
Ommaya reservoir, 60
ONCC. *See* Oncology Nursing Certification Corporation
oncogenes, 2
oncology, 156
   dangerous abbreviations/symbols in, 179
   education and certification information, websites for, 42*t*
   healthcare professionals, 61, 69
   training, 40–42
oncology certified nurses (OCNs), 135
oncology-focused FDA REMS programs, 197*t*
Oncology Nursing Certification Corporation (ONCC), 41
Oncology Nursing Society (ONS), 40–41, 67, 125, 161
ondansetron, 258
ONS. *See* Oncology Nursing Society
OPPS. *See* Outpatient Prospective Payment Systems
OR. *See* overall response
oral anticancer therapy, 58–59, 59*t*
oral cancer therapy, 139–168. *See also* intravenous cancer therapies
   adherence to, 158–160, 158*t*
   administration for, 141–145
   agents, 164
      administration of, 144*t*
      with approval dates, 139, 140*t*
      approved REMS for, 163*t*
      with cytochrome P450 interactions, 154*t*–155*t*
      with emetogenic potential, 149*t*
      types of, 142–143
      use of, 141, 164
   counseling and monitoring, 156–158, 157*b*
   dosing for, 141–145
   drug and food interactions with, 152–156
      examples of, 141

oral cancer therapy (*Contd.*)
  financial considerations, 165–166, 166*t*
  prescribing and dispensing recommendation
      of, 161, 161*b*–162*b*
  REMS, 141
      requirements, 162–163, 162*b*–163*b*
  safe handling of, 141, 164–165
  safety practices, 160–163
  side effects of, 145–152, 146*t*
      cardiovascular toxicity, 148–149
      fatigue, 150–151
      gastrointestinal toxicity, 149–150
      hormonal agents toxicity, 151–152
      skin toxicity, 147–148
oral chemotherapy formulations, pediatric
      oncology, 294, 296–297
oral investigational medication, 320
oral nonabsorbed steroids, 244
OS response. *See* overall survival response
osteosarcoma, 282
Outpatient Prospective Payment Systems
      (OPPS), 214–215
outpatient setting, medication errors in, 294,
      295*t*–296*t*
overall response (OR), 33*t*
overall survival (OS) response, 33*t*
oxaliplatin (Eloxatin), 12*t*, 17

P

p53 gene, 2
PA. *See* physician assistant
paclitaxel (Taxol), 6, 12*t*, 191*f*
palmar-plantar erythrodysesthesia. *See* hand-foot
      syndrome
pamidronate (Aredia), 47
panitumumab (Vectibix), 12*t*
Paraplatin (carboplatin), 9*t*
partial response (PR), 33*t*
patient assistance programs, 218–220
patient enrollment, in clinical trial, 310–313
PBSCs. *See* peripheral blood stem cells
PCP infection. *See* Pneumocystis jiroveci infection
PCR. *See* polymerase chain reaction (PCR)
pediatric oncology. *See also* childhood cancers
  acute leukemias
      ALL, 271–274, 272*t*
      AML, 274–275, 275*t*
      APL, 276
      description, 271

  bone marrow support, 285
  case study, 293, 297–298
  chemotherapy dosing in infants, 290–292,
      290*t*–291*t*
  CINV, 284–285
  CNS tumors, 278–280, 279*b*
  cooperative research groups role in, 268–269
  description, 267, 268*f*
  fluid management, 289–290, 289*t*
  initial presentation, 269
  lymphomas
      Hodgkin's, 276–277
      non-Hodgkin's, 277–278
  medication errors in outpatient setting, 294,
      295*t*–296*t*
  obese children, 293
  oncologic emergencies, 270–271
  oral chemotherapy formulations, 294,
      296–297
  outpatient, 297
  solid tumors of
      Ewing's sarcoma, 282–283, 283*t*
      neuroblastoma, 280–281, 280*t*
      osteosarcoma, 282
      retinoblastoma, 283–284
      rhabdomyosarcoma, 281–282
      Wilms' tumor, 281
  special dosing considerations, 286, 286*t*–288*t*
  supportive care, 284
  survivorship and long-term toxicities,
      285–286
pedigree laws, 211
pegfilgrastim (Neulasta), 47, 285
pemetrexed (Alimta), 13*t*, 20
pentostatin, 19
performance status scales, 33, 34*t*
peripheral blood stem cells (PBSCs), 229
personal protective equipment (PPE), 112,
      120–123
personnel cancer therapy preparation, 133–137
pertinent patient information, access to,
      186–187
PFS response. *See* progression free survival
      response
PgR. *See* progesterone receptor (PgR)
pharmaceutical waste, 132*f*, 133
pharmacists, 41, 42*t*, 134–135
pharmacokinetic, monitoring, 159
pharmacy technician, 136
phases of cell division, 2

physical agents, carcinogens, 2
physician assistant (PA), 42, 42*t*
physicians, 41, 42*t*
PK samples, 320
Platinol (cisplatin), 9*t*
plerixafor, 231
PML. *See* promyelocytic leukemia (PML)
PNET. *See* primitive neuroectodermal tumor
pneumococcal vaccine, 256*t*
Pneumocystis jiroveci (PCP) infection, 254
podophyllotoxin derivatives, 21
point mutations, 4*t*
point-of-service (POS), 217
polyethylene-coated polypropylene gowns, 121
polymerase chain reaction (PCR), 329
pomalidomide, 26
POMALYST REMS, 26
ponatinib, 27
POS. *See* point-of-service
potential causes of cancer, 3*t*
powder-free gloves, 122*b*
PPE. *See* personal protective equipment
PPOs. *See* preferred physician provider
        organizations
PR. *See* partial response
pralatrexate (Folotyn), 13*t*
prednisolone, 287*t*
prednisone, 287*t*
preferred physician provider organizations
        (PPOs), 217
premedication, HSCs, 232*t*
prescribing errors, 177–178
    types, 177
    wrong dose, 177*b*–178*b*
*Preventing Medication Errors: Quality Chasm
        Series* (IOM), 177
primitive neuroectodermal tumor (PNET),
        282–283
principles of cancer therapy preparation, 112
private insurance, 216–217
procarbazine, 155, 156
prochlorperazine, 284–285
procurement, chemotherapy errors, 174–177
    risk-reduction strategies, 176*b*–177*b*
progesterone receptor (PgR), 330
Prograf (tacrolimus), 240*t*, 242*t*
progression free survival (PFS) response, 33*t*
progression stage, neoplastic growth, 4
promotion, carcinogenesis, 3

promyelocytic leukemia (PML), 339
prostate cancers, hormonal agents for treatment,
        145, 151
proteasome, 29
proto-oncogenes, 2
protocols, 316, 320
purchasing, cancer drug therapies, 206–211
purine antimetabolites, 19
pyrimidines, 18

Q

QTc prolongation, side effects of oral cancer
        agents, 146*t*, 149

R

raloxifene, 30
Rapamune (sirolimus), 241*t*, 243*t*
RAR-α. *See* retinoic acid receptor-alpha (RAR-α)
rasburicase, 288*t*
RECIST. *See* response evaluation criteria in solid
        tumors
reduced intensity conditioning (RIC), 225*t*
reduced toxicity conditioning, 225*t*
refrigeration, 128–130
    failure, 130–131
registered nurse, 135
regorafenib, 28
reimbursement
    coverage, 217–218
    patient assistance programs, 218–220
    payers, 212
        Medicaid, 216
        Medicare, 213–216
        private insurance, 216–217
relapsed disease, 277
REMS. *See* risk evaluation and mitigation
        strategy
renal tubular necrosis, 20
response evaluation criteria in solid tumors
        (RECIST), 32
response, to cancer treatment, 32, 33*t*
retinoblastoma, 283–284
retinoic acid receptor-alpha (RAR-α), 339
retinoic acid syndrome, 24
retinoids, 23
RevAssist program, 26
REVLIMID REMS, 26
rhabdomyosarcoma, 281–282
RIC. *See* reduced intensity conditioning

risk evaluation and mitigation strategy (REMS), 141
  for oral cancer agents, 163*t*
  programs, 196–197, 206
  requirements, 162–163
  for lenalidomide, 162*b*–163*b*
Rituxan (rituximab), 13*t*
rituximab (Rituxan), 13*t*
Roferon-A (interferon-alfa), 10*t*
romidepsin, 23

S

safe disposal of hazardous drug waste, 131–133
safe handling principles, 116
safe work environment, 193–194
Sandimmune (cyclosporine), 240*t*
scrubs, 122*b*
SD. *See* stable disease
selective estrogen receptor modulators (SERMs), 30, 330
selective serotonin reuptake inhibitors (SSRIs), 153
sentinel event report, 194–195
SERMs. *See* selective estrogen receptor modulators
sinusoidal obstruction syndrome (SOS)
  description, 252
  diagnosis of, 252, 253*t*
  infection in HSCT patients, 254, 255*t*, 256–257, 256*t*
  risk factors for, 252
  treatment of, 253–254
sirolimus (Rapamune), 238, 241*t*, 243*t*
skin rashes, oral cancer therapy and, 147–148
smart pump technology, 193
solid tumors of childhood
  Ewing's sarcoma, 282–283, 283*t*
  neuroblastoma, 280–281, 280*t*
  osteosarcoma, 282
  retinoblastoma, 283–284
  rhabdomyosarcoma, 281–282
  Wilms' tumor, 281
SOPs. *See* standard operating procedures
sorafenib, 27
spill kit, chemotherapy, 124, 125*b*, 126*f*
SSRIs. *See* selective serotonin reuptake inhibitors
St. Jude Children's Research Hospital staging system, 277–278
stable disease (SD), 33*t*

standard operating procedures (SOPs), 304–305, 305*b*
standardized forms, anticancer prescription, 45–46
Statement of Investigator, 309*b*
S.T.E.P.S. program. *See* System for Thalidomide Education and Prescribing Safety program
sterile product, 116
steroid refractory GVHD
  acute GVHD, supportive care, 246
  chronic GVHD
    clinical manifestations of, 248*t*–249*t*
    description, 246
    pathogenesis of, 246–247
    treatment of, 247, 251–252
  description, 245–246
Stevens-Johnson syndrome, 147
streptozocin, 16
sunitinib, 27
superior vena cava (SVC) syndrome, 270
syngeneic transplant, 226*t*
System for Thalidomide Education and Prescribing Safety (S.T.E.P.S.) program, 26
systemic corticosteroids, 244

T

T-cell acute lymphoblastic leukemia, 19
T-cell lymphoma, 23
tacrolimus (Prograf), 238, 239, 240*t*, 242*t*, 261–262
tamoxifen, 30, 151
  for breast cancer, 153
  and SSRIs, 153
tandem transplant, 225*t*
targeted/biologic agents, 141
  cancer treatment with approval dates, 139, 140*t*
  emergence of, 145
targeted therapies, 4, 24
  angiogenesis inhibitors, 26
  immunomodulators, 26
  interferon-alfa and interleukin-2, 30
  miscellaneous agents, 29
  MoABs, 24–25, 25*t*
  TKIs, 26–29
taxanes, 6–7, 8*t*–14*t*
Taxol (paclitaxel), 12*t*
Taxotere (docetaxel), 10*t*
Taxus baccata, 7

Taxus brevifolia, 6
temozolomide, 16, 142, 143
    dosing for diagnosed GBM, 143*b*
temsirolimus (Torisel), 13*t*, 29
tenfold dosing error, 178
teniposide, 21
tetanus, 256*t*
thalidomide, 143, 150
THALOMID REMS, 26
thioguanine, 19, 288*t*
thiopurine methyltransferase (TPMT), 19, 86,
    273, 327–329
thiotepa, 16
340B program, 212
thrombosis, risk factors for, 146*t*, 148
time to progression (TTP) response, 33
"the time value of money," 207
TKIs. *See* tyrosine kinase inhibitors
TLS. *See* tumor lysis syndrome
TMD. *See* transient myeloproliferative disorder
*To Err Is Human: Building a Safer Health Care
    System,* (IOM), 172
topoisomerase II inhibitors, 21
topoisomerase inhibitors, 20
    anthracene derivatives, 21–22
    camptothecin derivatives, 20–21
    miscellaneous agents, 22–24
    podophyllotoxin derivatives, 21
toremifene, 30
Torisel (temsirolimus), 13*t*, 29
tositumomab (Bexxar), 14*t*
total body irradiation, 230*t*
toxicity treatment, biomarkers
    BCR/ABL chromosomal translocation, 339
    BRAF, 338–339
    chromosome 5q, deletion of, 340
    DPD, 329
    EGFR, 334–335
    EML4-ALK fusion gene, 337–338
    ER/PgR, 330–333
    HER2, 333–334
    K-RAS, 335–337
    O⁶-MGMT, 340
    promyelocytic leukemia/RAR-α, 339–340
    TPMT, 327–329
    UGT1A1, 329–330
TPMT. *See* thiopurine methyltransferase
trametinib, 28
transcribing/documenting errors, 178–179
transformation phase, carcinogenesis, 3

transient myeloproliferative disorder (TMD),
    275
transporter-based interactions, with oral cancer
    therapy, 156
trastuzumab (Herceptin), 14*t*, 48
treatment-based algorithms, 188
tretinoin, 23
Trexall (methotrexate), 11*t*
triamcinolone, 244
TTP response. *See* time to progression response
tumor lysis syndrome (TLS), 64, 65*t*, 270,
    297–298
tumor suppressor genes, 2
tyrosine kinase inhibitors (TKIs), 26–29, 148,
    334

U

UCB. *See* umbilical cord blood
UGT1A1. *See* uridine diphosphoglucuronosyl-
    transferase 1A1 (UGT1A1)
umbilical cord blood (UCB), 225*t*
unintentional intrathecal vincristine administra-
    tion, 61
United States Pharmacopeia (USP), 112
United States Pharmacopeia (USP) 797, 119
United States Pharmacopeial Convention, 61
universal waste approach, 132*f*, 133
uridine diphosphoglucuronosyltransferase 1A1
    (UGT1A1), 87, 329
ursodiol, 246, 253

V

VAC. *See* vincristine, actinomycin D, and
    cyclophosphamide
vascular endothelial grown factor (VEGF) recep-
    tor, 148
Vectibix (panitumumab), 12*t*
VEGF receptor. *See* vascular endothelial grown
    factor receptor
venoocclusive disease (VOD). *See* sinusoidal
    obstruction syndrome
venous thromboembolism prophylaxis, 148
verification process of cancer therapy, 55–56,
    56*t*–57*t*, 58
vinblastine, 6, 191*f*
vinca alkaloids, 6, 192
    preventing administration errors, 185*b*–186*b*
vincristine, 6, 85, 178, 185, 191*f*, 192, 288*t*
    preventing administration errors, 185*b*–186*b*

vincristine, actinomycin D, and cyclophosphamide (VAC), 281–282
vinorelbine, 6
vismodegib, 29
voriconazole, 262
vorinostat, 23

W

warfarin, 153
WBC count. *See* white blood cell count
"white bagging," 210
white blood cell (WBC) count, 270
Wilms' tumor, 281

World Health Organization, 211
wrong dose
associated with stock location, 175
compounding/dispensing errors, 181
prescribing, 177*b*–178*b*
wrong-route errors, 185
associated with intrathecal therapy,
192–193
contributing factors with, 185

Z

Zevalin (ibritumomab tiuxetan), 10*t*
ziv-aflibercept, 29